USMLE™

MASTER THE BOARDS

STEP 3

Other Kaplan USMLE Titles

USMLE Medical Ethics:
The 100 Cases You Are Most Likely to See on the Exam

USMLE Diagnostic Test Flashcards:
The 200 Diagnostic Test Questions You Need to Know for the Exam

USMLE Physical Findings Flashcards:
The 200 Questions You're Most Likely to See on the Exam

USMLE Pharmacology and Treatment Flashcards:
The 200 Questions You're Must Likely to See on the Exam

USMLE Examination Flashcards:
The 200 "Most Likely Diagnosis" Questions You Will See on the Exam

USMLE Step 1 QBook

USMLE Step 2 CK QBook

USMLE Step 2 Clinical Skills

USMLE Step 2 CS Complex Cases

USMLE Step 3 QBook

USMLE™
MASTER THE BOARDS

STEP 3

Conrad Fischer, MD
Sonia Reichert, MD

© 2009 by Conrad Fischer, MD and Sonia Reichert, MD
Edited by Sailesh C. Harwani, MD, PhD
All images courtesy of Conrad Fischer, MD

Published by Kaplan Publishing, a division of Kaplan, Inc.
1 Liberty Plaza, 24th Floor
New York, NY 10006

Printed in the United States of America

10 9 8 7 6 5

ISBN-13: 978-1-4277-9833-6

Kaplan Publishing books are available at special quantity discounts to use for sales promotions, employee premiums, or educational purposes. Please email our Special Sales Department to order or for more information at kaplanpublishing@kaplan.com, or write to Kaplan Publishing, 1 Liberty Plaza, 24th Floor, New York, NY 10006.

Dedication

To the Reader,

This book represents the consolidation of nearly 20 years in the classroom teaching Step 3. You can be fully confident that you have, in one volume EVERYTHING you need to do well on Step 3.

To Edmund Bourke, MD,

My "Fearless Leader," teacher, and protector these many years. Dr. Bourke represents the best compilation of a "Gentleman Scholar," lifelong student, and teacher. A wise counselor and loyal friend. I dedicate this book to a "man for all seasons" whose kindness spills over onto all who are in contact with him. "Oh, for a muse of fire!"

Conrad Fischer, MD

To Mum,

I dedicate this book to you, a woman who has always exemplified dedication, determination, strength, and above all, a bright spirit that has been the guiding light for many people. You taught me to have a vision, dream big, and to always reach for the farthest and brightest star. You have shown me that dreams have no limits and boundaries. I will be eternally grateful for your love and support.

Sonia Reichert, MD

TABLE OF CONTENTS

ABOUT THE AUTHORS

CONRAD FISCHER, MD, is one of the most experienced educators in medicine today. His breadth of teaching includes medical students, USMLE prep, and Specialty Board exams. In addition, Dr. Fischer is the Associate Chief of Medicine for Educational and Academic Activities at SUNY Downstate School of Medicine, and is an Attending Physician at King's County Hospital in Brooklyn, NY. Dr. Fischer has been Chairman of Medicine for Kaplan Medical since 1999, and has held Residency Program Director positions at both Maimonides Medical Center and Flushing Hospital in New York City.

SONIA E. REICHERT, MD, previously served as Director of Curriculum for Kaplan Medical and is currently an Internal Medicine Resident at SUNY Downstate at Brooklyn. Dr. Reichert is a regular participant of National Board conferences and has many years of experience in the creation and development of Kaplan Medical's online, print, DVD, and other media related-educational tools in the medical and allied health fields. She is the leading national expert in the content, scoring, and structure of medical licensing and allied health exams.

INTRODUCTION

ABOUT THE STEP 3 EXAM

The USMLE Step 3 is the last in a series of three USMLE examinations that all physicians applying for a license to practice medicine in the United States are required to pass. After successfully completing the three steps of the USMLE, a physician is eligible to practice medicine in an independent, unsupervised setting (some period of U.S. postgraduate training is also required).

This test is not merely a more advanced and detailed version of the Step 2 CK or CS exams. Understanding this concept is key to this challenging exam. Step 3 tests whether a physician not only can assimilate data and diagnose clinical conditions but also has acquired the ability to make clinical decisions about patient management in a way that ensures appropriate management in an unsupervised setting.

How can the Step 3 test all first-year interns if they are working in such varied subspecialty settings? The same concepts that medicine house-officers learn about managing a diabetic with heart failure can be equally applied to the postsurgical patient with heart failure.

HOW IS STEP 3 DIFFERENT?

Unlike the Step 2 exams, which emphasizes diagnosis of medical conditions, Step 3 evaluates your ability to evaluate the severity of a patient's condition and discern the most appropriate clinical management based on the presenting scenario. This assessment of your *clinical judgment* distinguishes Step 3 from Step 2. In Step 3, you are required to think beyond the diagnosis (which is often implicit in the question itself) and make decisions in management. The cases presented will include options that may all appear appropriate; however, for the presented situation, there is only ever one correct answer. Your interpretation of laboratory data, imaging, and elements of the presenting history and physical examination will assist you in selecting the correct management.

CLINICAL ENCOUNTER FRAMES

Multiple-choice and case-simulation questions are presented in one of three *clinical encounter frames:* initial care, continuing care, and urgent care. The encounter frame determines the amount of history, as well as clinical and laboratory test results, that are available to you. More importantly, the encounter frame influences how you'll proceed with management. For example, a longstanding patient with a history of repeated hospitalizations for asthma who presents with shortness of breath would be approached differently than if she were presenting for the first time to a clinic complaining of periodic dyspnea or if she presented to the emergency department with an acute asthma attack. The majority of test items (50 to 60 percent) in Step 3 involve the management of continuing-care patients. In the continuing-care setting, you are tested on your ability to recognize new problems in an existing condition, assess severity, establish prognosis, monitor therapy, and perform long-term management.

CLINICAL SETTINGS

There are three clinical settings in Step 3: office/health center, inpatient facility, and the emergency department. As with the encounter frame, knowing the clinical setting influences your management decisions. As will be discussed in the "Examination Structure" section, test questions will be arranged in blocks based on one of the three clinical settings.

PHYSICIAN TASKS

For any given clinical encounter frame in a clinical setting, you'll be challenged with a finite number of skills. The six physician tasks that are tested on the Step 3 exam are representative of what all physicians practicing unsupervised medical management are expected to know.

Task	Tests your ability to...
Obtaining a history and performing a physical examination	• identify key facets of the history or physical exam and relate them to the presenting problem or condition. • predict the most likely additional physical finding or examination technique that would result in the finding.
Using laboratory and diagnostic studies	• select the appropriate *routine* or *initial* lab or diagnostic test either to ensure effective therapy or to establish diagnosis. • predict the most likely lab or diagnostic test result.
Formulating the most likely diagnosis	• determine the diagnosis and use it to manage the patient.
Evaluating the severity of the patient's problems	• assess the severity of a patient's condition and identify indications for consultations or further diagnostic workup. • recognize factors in history, physical exam, or lab studies that affect prognosis or determine a change in therapy.
Managing the patient	• manage a patient in the following four areas: 1. Health maintenance (i.e., implementing preventative measures by identifying risk factors) 2. Clinical intervention (i.e., knowing appropriate postsurgical/postprocedural management and follow-up measures) 3. Clinical therapeutics (i.e., properly utilizing pharmacotherapeutic options) 4. Legal/ethical and health care system issues, including patient autonomy, physician-patient relationships, and managed-care protocols
Applying scientific concepts	• identify processes responsible for an underlying condition and interpret results of clinical or epidemiologic experiments

STEP 3 EXAMINATION STRUCTURE

The USMLE Step 3 is a two-day computerized examination. The first day and a half tests your knowledge with a total of 480 traditional multiple-choice questions, which are arranged in blocks organized by one of the three clinical settings. Within a block, you may answer the items in any order, review responses, and change answers. However, after exiting a block, you can no longer review questions or change answers within that block. A link to view standard lab values, as well as access a calculator, is available at any time within the block of questions.

Day 1 includes 336 multiple-choice items divided into seven 60-minute blocks of 48 items. A total of 60 minutes is allowed for completing each block of questions, for a maximum of seven hours of testing. A minimum of 45 minutes of break time and an optional 15-minute tutorial complete the eight-hour day. Extra break time can be gained by completing question blocks or the tutorial before the allocated time.

INITIAL HISTORY SCREEN

The initial history screen gives you a comprehensive description of the history of present illness, past medical history, family history, social history, and review of systems. Read this section carefully, as key diagnostic information is given here. After reading the history of present illness, you should be able to establish a short differential diagnostic list. Make note of any key features in the past medical, family, and social history and review of systems that support or refute your differential diagnosis. At the end of the initial history, click the **OK** button; this will mark the end of the prompted section of the case.

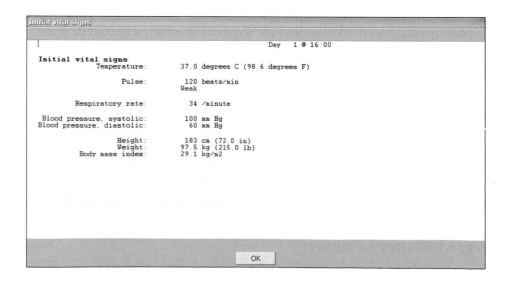

Initial history

Initial history
Reason(s) for Visit:
Chest pain; respiratory distress

History of Present Illness:
The patient, a 65-year-old accountant, is brought to the emergency department by ambulance from the trucking company where he works. About 10 minutes before the ambulance arrived, the patient developed excruciating, sharp pain in the right side of his chest and marked respiratory distress. He rates the pain as 8 on a 10-point scale. The pain increases with respiration. He is unable to answer questions. A coworker who accompanied the patient to the hospital says that this never happened before, but the patient has had emphysema and asthma for years. Oxygen was administered during transport.

All other history unobtainable.

OK

Initial vital signs

Day   1 @ 16:00

Initial vital signs
Temperature: 37.0 degrees C (98.6 degrees F)

Pulse: 120 beats/min
                          Weak

Respiratory rate: 34 /minute

Blood pressure, systolic: 100 mm Hg
Blood pressure, diastolic: 60 mm Hg

Height: 183 cm (72.0 in)
Weight: 97.5 kg (215.0 lb)
Body mass index: 29.1 kg/m2

OK

CASE MANAGEMENT

This section of the case is driven by your actions rather than prompts from the software. There are four buttons at the top of the screen, which you will use to manage the case. You will be able to access any of these buttons until the last five minutes, at which point you are automatically brought to the final stage.

The **History/Physical** button allows you to order a follow-up history, as well as either a comprehensive or system-focused physical exam.

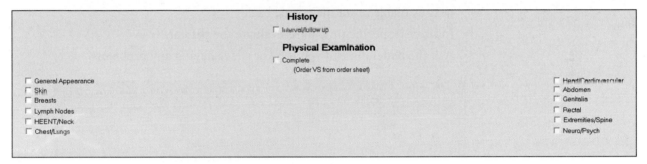

The **Write Orders/Review Chart** button brings up a number of other chart options, including an order sheet, progress notes, vital signs, lab reports, imaging studies, other tests, and a treatment record.

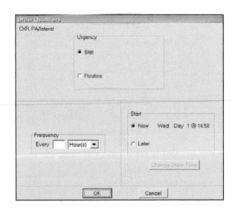

The **clock button** allows you to manipulate the **case time clock (virtual time)**. This is a completely separate from the real-time clock, found at the bottom right part of the screen throughout the case. In real test time, you have up to a maximum of 20 to 25 minutes to manage the case from beginning to end. But to get results or schedule a time to re-evaluate the patient, you'll need to move the **case time clock** ahead. You may move the clock ahead in any of the following ways:

• Move the clock ahead to a selected time so that you can get a specific result back.

• Move the clock automatically to when the first result comes back. Remember that you will still need to manage the case in the interim period before the next available result may come back.

• Indicate a specific time to re-evaluate the patient.

• Ask the patient to call you if he or she is having any problems.

At the end of the case, you must enter your diagnosis on the screen provided. When you click **OK,** the case closes, and you move onto the next case.

SCORE REPORTING

The minimum passing score for Step 3 is 187. This corresponds to answering approximately 60 to 70 percent of the items correctly. The USMLE does not report performance as percentiles. There will be a three-digit and a two-digit score on your score report. The two-digit score is derived from the three-digit score to meet the requirements of some medical licensing authorities that the passing score be reported as 75. A graphical report of performance on the reverse side of your score sheet indicates relative strengths and weaknesses. This graphical report is not seen by anyone but you and is not provided to institutions or licensing bodies.

REGISTRATION FOR STEP 3

For registration and more information, contact:

FSMB
Department of Examination Services
P.O. Box 619850
Dallas, TX 75261-9850
Website: *www.fsmb.org*
Telephone: (817) 868-4041
Fax: (817) 868-4098
Email: usmle@fsmb.org
or your state **medical licensing authority** (see the USMLE website at http://usmle.org).

SECTION 1
INTERNAL MEDICINE

INFECTIOUS DISEASES 1

INTRODUCTION TO ANTIBIOTICS

STAPHYLOCOCCUS AUREUS: BONE, HEART, SKIN, JOINT

- **Sensitive staph (MSSA):**
  - IV: Oxacillin/nafcillin, dicloxacillin, or cefazolin (first-generation cephalasporin)
  - Oral: Dicloxacillin or cephalexin (first-generation cephalosporin)
- **Resistant staph (MRSA):**
  - Severe infection: Vancomycin, linezolid, daptomycin, or tigecycline
  - Minor infection: Trimethoprim/sulfamethoxazole (TMP/SMX), clindamycin
- **Penicillin allergy:**
  - Rash: Safe to use cephalosporins
  - Anaphylaxis: Macrolides (azithromycin, clarithromycin) or clindamycin
  - Severe infection: Vancomycin, linezolid, daptomycin
  - Minor infection: Macrolides (azithromycin, clarithromycin), clindamycin, TMP/SMX

STREPTOCOCCUS

The medications above will cover streptococcus as well as staphylococcus. The following medications are *specific* for streptococcus:

- Penicillin
- Ampicillin
- Amoxicillin

GRAM-NEGATIVE BACILLI (RODS): E. COLI, ENTEROBACTER, CITROBACTER, MORGANELLA, PSEUDOMONAS, SERRATIA

All of the following medications are essentially equal in their efficacy for gram-negative bacilli.

Cephalosporins	Penicillins	Monobactam	Quinolones	Aminoglycosides	Carbapenems
Cefepime Ceftazidime	Piperacillin Ticarcillin	Aztreonam	Ciprofloxacin Levofloxacin Gatifloxacin Moxifloxacin	Gentamicin Tobramycin Amikacin	Imipenem Meropenem Ertapenem

Exceptions

- **Ertapenem** is the only carbapenem that does *not* cover pseudomonas.
- **Piperacillin** and **ticarcillin** *also* cover streptococci and anaerobes.
- **Levofloxacin, gatifloxacin,** and **moxifloxacin** are *excellent* pneumococcal drugs.
- **Aminoglycosides** work *synergistically* with other agents to treat staph and strep.
- **Carbapenems** are *excellent* anti-anaerobic medications, They cover streptococci and all sensitive staphylococcus (MSSA).
- **Tigecycline** covers MRSA and is broadly active against gram-negative bacilli.

ANAEROBES

- **Gastrointestinal anaerobes (bacteroides)**
  - **Metronidazole** is the *best* medication for abdominal anaerobes.
  - **Carbapenems, piperacillin,** and **ticarcillin** are equal in efficacy for abdominal anaerobes compared to metronidazole.
  - **Cefoxitin** and **cefotetan** (in the cephamycin class) are the *only* cephalosporins that cover anaerobes.
- **Respiratory anaerobes (anaerobic strep)**
  - **Clindamycin** is the *best* drug for anaerobic strep.
- Medications with *no* anaerobic coverage
  - **Aminoglycosides, aztreonam, fluoroquinolones, oxacillin/nafcillin,** and all the **cephalosporins** *except* cefoxitin and cefotetan

CCS Tip

CCS does *not* require you to know doses, but you *are* expected to know the route of administration.

A man is admitted for endocarditis. His blood cultures grow staph aureus, and vanco-mycin is started while awaiting sensitivity testing. He develops red skin, particularly on the neck. What should you do?

Answer: Slow the rate of the infusion. Vancomycin is associated with "red man syndrome," which is red, flushed skin from histamine release. This happens from rapid infusion of vanco-mycin. There is no specific therapy, and you do not need to switch the medication. If the rate of infusion is slowed, the reaction will not occur.

ANTIVIRAL AGENTS

- **Acyclovir, valacyclovir, famciclovir** (*Herpes simplex, Varicella zoster*): All three of these agents are equal in efficacy.
- **Ganciclovir** and **foscarnet (Cytomegalovirus [CMV]):** These are essentially equal in efficacy. They also cover *Herpes simplex* and *varicella*. They can have the following **adverse effects:**
  - Ganciclovir: Neutropenia and bone marrow suppression
  - Foscarnet: Renal toxicity
- **Oseltamivir** and **zanamivir** (neuraminidase inhibitors): Influenza A and B
- **Ribavirin:** Hepatitis C (in combination with interferon), respiratory syncy-tial virus (RSV)
- **Lamivudine, interreron, adefovir, entecavir,** and **telbivudine:** Chronic Hepatitis B

ANTIFUNGAL AGENTS

- **Fluconazole:** *Candida* (*not Candida krusei or Candida glabrata*), *Cryptococcus*, oral and vaginal candidiasis as an alternative to topical mediations
- **Itraconazole:** Largely equal to fluconazole but less easy to use; rarely the best initial therapy for anything
- **Voriconazole:** Covers *all Candida*; *best* agent against *Aspergillus*. Adverse effect:
  - Some visual disturbance
- **Echinocandins** (caspofungin, micafungin, anidulafungin):
  - *Excellent* for neutropenic fever patients.
  - Does *not* cover *Cryptococcus*.
  - Better than amphotericin for neutropenia and fever (less mortality).
  - Adverse effect—Echinocandins have *no* significant human toxicity because they affect/inhibit the 1,4 glucan synthesis step, which does not exist in humans.
- **Amphotericin:** Effective against *all Candida, Cryptococcus,* and *Aspergillus*:
  - *Aspergillus:* Voriconazole superior to amphotericin
  - **Neutropenic fever**: Caspofungin superior to amphotericin
  - *Candida:* Fluconazole is equal to amphotericin for efficacy but has *much fewer* adverse effects (see box).

> ## Adverse effects of amphotericin:
> - Renal toxicity (increased creatinine)
> - Hypokalemia
> - Metabolic acidosis
> - Fever, shakes, chills

OSTEOMYELITIS

Is the infection in the soft tissue (skin) only? Or has it spread into the bone?

Osteomyelitis in adults almost always presents as a patient with **diabetes, peripheral vascular disease, or both with an ulcer or soft tissue infection.** You can also think about osteomyelitis in patients with direct trauma and a history of orthopedic surgery, but the case with diabetes and peripheral vascular disease is more likely to show up on the exam. The "Next best step?" question fundamentally asks if you know what to do to distinguish the difference between a soft tissue infection and a contiguous spread into the bone.

Diagnostic Testing
- Best **initial test:** Plain **X-ray**
- Best **second-line test** (if there is high clinical suspicion and X-ray is negative): **MRI**

You must lose more than 50 percent of the calcium content of the bone before the X-ray becomes abnormal. Although it may take up to two weeks for osteomyelitis to become severe enough to make the X-ray abnormal, the X-ray is *still* the first test. (You would not skip an EKG and go straight to a stress test; you would not skip a chest X-ray and go straight to a chest CT scan.)

Which of the following is the earliest finding of osteomyelitis on an X-ray?

a. Periosteal elevation

b. Involucrum

c. Sequestrum

d. Punched-out lesions

e. Fracture

*Answer: **A.** The earliest finding of osteomyelitis on an X-ray is elevation of the periosteum. Involucrum and sequestrum are terms applied to the formation of abnormal new bone in the periosteum and chunks of bone chipped off from the infection. Punched-out lesions are seen in myeloma, not osteomyelitis. Osteomyelitis does not have an association with fracture.*

On Step 3, you can get the X-ray result in two ways as part of a question:

1. Single best answer: The stem of the question simply states, "X-ray of the bone is normal."
2. CCS: You move the clock forward, and the X-ray result will pop up as you pass the time when it says "report available."

A 67-year-old man with diabetes and peripheral arterial disease comes in having had pain in his leg for two weeks. There is an ulcer with a draining sinus tract. The X-ray is normal. What is the next best step in determining a diagnosis?

a. Bone scan

b. CT scan

c. MRI

d. ESR

e. Biopsy

Answer: The MRI (C) is the next best test to do to determine the diagnosis of osteomyelitis if the X-ray is normal. A bone scan does not have the specificity of an MRI.

Diagnostic Testing

The *most accurate* diagnostic test is a bone biopsy and culture.

X-ray is *always* the best initial test. If the X-ray is normal, an MRI is *far* superior to a bone scan with a nuclear isotope. The bone scan is very poor at being able to distinguish between infection in the bone and infection of the soft tissue above it. The sedimentation rate is the best method of following a response to therapy. Remember that osteomyelitis is *most* commonly caused by **direct contiguous spread from overlying tissue,** but hematogenous (blood) infection can also be present as a cause or result of osteomyelitis, so a blood culture (especially if the patient looks septic) is not a bad idea. However, perform the MRI first.

Which test has greater sensitivity, the MRI or the bone scan? Answer: They are **equal** in sensitivity. The MRI and bone scan both have an equal ability to exclude osteomyelitis if they are normal. The MRI, however, is *far* more specific. A swab of the ulcer for culture is extremely inaccurate. We cannot tell what is growing inside the bone for sure by growing something from the superficial ulcer. Would you allow yourself to be treated by weeks to months of intravenous antibiotics with only a 50/50 chance that you are treating the right organism?

How do we know how long to treat if 90 percent of patients have no fever and a normal white cell count? By following the sedimentation rate. If the sedimentation rate (ESR) is still markedly elevated after 4–6 weeks of therapy, further treatment and possible surgical debridement is necessary.

Never culture the draining sinus tract or swab an ulcer.

Treatment

Staphylococcus: This is still the *most* common cause of osteomyelitis. If the organism is sensitive, **oxacillin** or **nafcillin** intravenously for 4–6 weeks is the treatment. MRSA is treated with **vancomycin, linezolid,** or **daptomycin.** You *cannot* use oral therapy for staphylococcal osteomyelitis.

> You *must* do a bone biopsy/culture to treat osteomyelitis appropriately.

- **Gram-negative bacilli** (**salmonella** and **pseudomonas** are the ones to consider): This is the *only* form of osteomyelitis that can be successfully and reliably treated with oral antibiotics.
  - You *must* confirm it is a gram-negative with a bone biopsy.
  - The organism *must* be sensitive to antibiotics.
  - There is no urgency to treating chronic osteomyelitis. You can obtain the biopsy, move the clock forward, and treat what you find on the culture.

HEAD AND NECK INFECTIONS

OTITIS EXTERNA

Presents with **itching** and **drainage** from the external auditory canal. This is a form of cellulitis of the skin of the external auditory canal. It is often difficult to visualize the tympanic membrane because of the swelling of the canal. It is also painful, especially when the tragus of the ear is manipulated.

It is associated with **swimming,** because swimming washes out the acidic environment normally found in the external auditory canal. Other causes include **foreign objects** in the ears (e.g., repeated use of cotton swabs, hearing aids, etc.).

Diagnostic Testing

No specific tests are necessary; diagnosis is based on exam. Do *not* perform a routine culture of the ear canal.

Treatment

Topical antibiotics, such as *ofloxacin* or *polymyxin/neomycin.* Add **topical hydrocortisone** to decrease swelling and itching. Adding **acetic acid and water solution** to reacidify the ear can help eliminate the infection.

MALIGNANT OTITIS EXTERNA

This is an *extremely* different disease from simple otitis externa. Malignant otitis externa is really **osteomyelitis of the skull** from pseudomonas in a patient with diabetes. It is an extremely serious disease, because it can lead to a brain abscess and destruction of the skull. Treat it like osteomyelitis: X-ray, MRI, bone biopsy/culture.

Diagnostic Testing

- Best **initial** test: **Skull X-ray** or **MRI**
- Most **accurate** test: **Biopsy**

Treatment

Treat with **surgical debridement** and **antibiotics active against pseudomonas,** such as piperacillin, cefepime, a carbapenem, or aztreonam.

OTITIS MEDIA

There is *no* radiologic test to confirm the diagnosis, which is based entirely on physical examination. Patients may complain of decreased or muffled hearing.

Key features include the following:

- Redness
- Bulging
- Decreased hearing
- Loss of light reflex
- Immobility of the tympanic membrane

Although all of the findings above can be present, the *most* sensitive is the presence of **immobility of the tympanic membrane.** If the tympanic membrane is freely mobile on insufflations of the ear, then otitis media is not present. The physical exam may also describe the absence of the light reflex.

Treatment

- Best initial therapy: **Amoxicillin.** Usual course is 7–10 days; longer for younger patients and shorter for older patients.
- Next step: Perform the most accurate test, **tympanocentesis and aspirate of the tympanic membrane for culture.** This is rarely necessary and is only done for recurrent or persistent cases that fail therapy.

CCS Tip

On CCS, advance the clock forward 3 days. If the infection is not improving, switch the amoxicillin to one of the following:

- Amoxicillin-clavulanate
- Cefdinir
- Ceftibuten
- Cefuroxime
- Cefprozil

SINUSITIS

Look for a patient with nasal discharge, headache, facial tenderness, teeth pain, bad taste in the mouth, and decreased transillumination of the sinuses. Most cases are viral, but bacterial causes include the same group that cause otitis media: *S. pnuemoniae, H. influenzae,* and *M. catarrhalis.*

Treatment

- Same as for otitis media
- Use **amoxicillin** if there is
  - fever and pain;
  - persistent symptoms despite 7 days of decongestants; and
  - purulent nasal discharge.

Diagnostic Testing

- Best initial test: **X-ray**
- Most accurate diagnostic test: **Sinus aspirate for culture.** This is *more* accurate than a CT or MRI; you cannot stain or culture a radiologic test.

PHARYNGITIS

The diagnosis of streptococcal pharyngitis is certain if the following are present:

- **Pain/sore throat**
- **Exudate**
- **Adenopathy**
- *No* cough/hoarseness

Diagnostic Testing

- Best initial diagnostic test: **"Rapid strep test."** A positive rapid strep test is just as specific as a positive throat culture. The rapid strep test is able to be performed instantly and can tell if the organism is of the type (group A strep) that might lead to rheumatic fever or glomerulonephritis. In adults, the sensitivity of the rapid strep test is enough. If the rapid strep test is negative in an adult, no further testing or treatment with antibiotics is necessary.
- Most accurate diagnostic test: **Culture**

Treatment

- **Penicillin** or **amoxicillin**
- **Penicillin allergy:** Use azithromycin or clarithromycin.

INFLUENZA

Look for a patient with **arthralgia, myalgia, cough, headache, fever, sore throat,** and **feeling of tiredness.**

Diagnostic Testing

- **Viral antigen detection** testing of a nasopharyngeal swab (next best step)

Treatment

Oseltamivir or **zanamivir** if the patient presents within the first 48 hours after the onset of symptoms. These are neuraminidase inhibitors that work against *both* influenza A and B. Amantadine and rimantadine will be *wrong* answers; they are only effective against influenza A.

Vaccination Against Influenza

- COPD, CHF, dialysis patients, steroid use, health care workers, everyone >50

SKIN INFECTIONS

IMPETIGO

This is the *most superficial* of the bacterial skin infections. It is from *Strep. pyogenes* or *Staph. aureus* infecting the epidermal layer of the skin. Because it is so superficial, there is **weeping, crusting,** and **oozing** of the skin. A specific microbiologic diagnosis is rarely made or necessary. Look for "weeping, oozing, honey-colored lesions."

Treatment

- **Topical mupirocin or bacitracin** (mupirocin has greater activity against MRSA)
- Severe disease: **Oral dicloxacillin or cephalexin**
- Community-acquired MRSA (CA-MRSA): **TMP/SMZ;** clindamycin is sometimes useful
- **Penicillin allergy:**
  - Rash: Cephalosporins are safe.
  - Anaphylaxis: Macrolides (azithromycin, clarithromycin) or clindamycin
  - Severe infection with anaphylaxis: Vancomycin, linezolid, daptomycin

ERYSIPELAS

This is a **group A (pyogenes) streptococcal infection** of the skin. The skin is **very bright red** and **hot** because of dilation of the capillaries of the dermis due to locally released inflammatory mediators. As with most bacterial skin infections, a specific microbiologic diagnosis is rarely made.

> The face is often the site of erysipelas.

Diagnostic Testing

Blood cultures may be positive in erysipelas. Order blood cultures in CCS, but go straight to treatment on the single best multiple-choice answer.

Treatment

- Best initial treatment: **Oral dicloxacillin or cephalexin.** Topical antiobiotics are useless.
- If the organism is *confirmed* as group A beta hemolytic streptococci, you may treat with **penicillin VK.**

CELLULITIS

Look for a **warm, red, swollen, tender skin.** Likely to present in the arm or leg but can present in any skin. If presented with a case of cellulitis in a leg, make sure you order a **lower extremity Doppler** to exclude a blood clot. *Both* clotting and cellulitis can cause a fever.

Staphylococcus aureus and *Streptococcus pyogenes* are nearly equal in the cause of cellulitis.

Treatment

- Minor disease: **Dicloxacillin or cephalexin orally**
- Severe disease: **Oxacillin, nafcillin, or cefazolin IV**
- **Penicillin allergy:**
  - Rash: Use cephalosporins such as cefazolin.
  - Anaphylaxis: Use vancomycin, linezolid, or daptomycin. For minor infections, macrolides or clindamycin can be useful.

> *Can erysipelas lead to rheumatic fever?* No. Only pharyngeal infection can lead to rheumatic fever. Skin infections can lead to glomerulonephritis, however. Remember: Skin (erysipelas) goes to kidneys (glomerulonephritis) only. Throat (pharyngitis) goes to kidneys (glomerulonephritis) *and* heart (rheumatic fever).

What skin infection does Staphylococcus epidermidis *cause?* None. *Staph epi* is a normal commensal inhabitant of the skin. It lives there and does *not* cause skin infection.

FOLLICULITIS < FURUNCLES < CARBUNCLES < BOILS

These are **Staph. aureus-related skin infections** beginning at the hair follicle. The only difference between them is *size*. Folliculitis is the smallest and most minor. Furuncles are larger, carbuncles larger than that, and boils even larger. An "abscess" would be considered the largest.

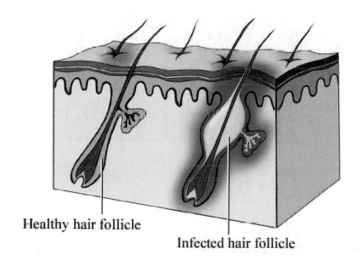

Healthy hair follicle

Infected hair follicle

Folliculitis

Treatment

Antibiotic therapy is **identical to that described for cellulitis.** Larger infections, such as boils, respond to **drainage.** As with all other skin infections, the patient can develop post-streptococcal glomerulonephritis but not rheumatic fever.

FUNGAL INFECTIONS OF SKIN AND NAILS

Common symptoms in skin infections are severe itching of the scalp, dandruff, and bald patches where the fungus has rooted itself in the skin. In onuchomycosis, nails may be thickened, yellow, cloudy, and appear fragile and broken.

Best Initial Diagnostic Test

• KOH preparation

1. Scrape the skin or nail.
2. Place the scraping on a slide with KOH and acid and heat it.
3. The epithelial cells will dissolve and leave the fungal forms behind, visible on the slide.

KOH Prep

Treatment

- **Topical antifungal medication** (if no hair or nail involvement): **Clotrimazole, miconazole, ketoconazole, econazole, terconazole, nystatin,** or **ciclopirox**
- **Oral antifungal medication** for scalp (tinea capitis) or nail (onychomycosis)

  - **Terbinafine:** Causes increased liver function tests
  - **Itraconazole**
  - **Griseofulvan** (for tinea capitis): Has less efficacy than either terbinafine or itraconazole

SEXUALLY TRANSMITTED DISEASES

URETHRITIS

Look for a **urethral discharge.** There can also be symptoms of dysuria, such as frequency, urgency, and burning. Discharge *without* dysuria is still considered urethritis. With dysuric symptoms but not discharge, the patient does not necessarily have urethritis; the patient could just have cystitis (i.e., a urinary tract infection).

Best Initial Diagnostic Test

- **Urethral swab** for gram stain, culture, and DNA probe
- **Nucleic acid amplification** tests are highly effective as well

Treatment

Urethritis gets treated with *two* medications. Use one drug active against **gonorrhea** and one drug active against **Chlamydia,** because these are very often present in coinfection.

Gonorrhea medications	*Chlamydia* medications
• Ceftriaxone IM • Cefixime oral • Cefpodoxime oral • Ciprofloxacin oral (2nd line)	• Azithromycin (single dose) • Doxycycline (for a week)
Pregnant patients • Ceftriaxone IM	Pregnant patients • Azithromycin

A patient develops recurrent episodes of gonorrhea. What should he be tested for?

a. Presence of a spleen

b. HIV

c. Terminal complement deficiency

d. Steroid use

e. Malabsorption

*Answer: Terminal complement deficiency **(C)** predisposes a patient to recurrent episodes of Neisseria infection. This includes any form of Neisseria infection, including genital and CNS infection.*

CERVICITIS

This presents with **cervical discharge** that should be swabbed for stain, culture, and DNA testing in the same way as for urethritis.

Treatment

Treat in exactly the same way as **urethritis** above.

PELVIC INFLAMMATORY DISEASE (PID)

Patients present with **lower abdominal pain, tenderness, fever,** and **cervical motion tenderness.** They may also have dysuria and/or vaginal discharge.

Diagnostic Testing

- There are *no* specific blood tests. **Leukocytosis** is a measure of severity.
- **Best initial diagnostic test: Pregnancy test,** then **cervical culture** and **DNA probe** for *Chlamydia* and gonorrhea.
- **Most accurate test: Laparoscopy.** This is rarely needed. Only done for recurrent or persistent infection despite therapy or for cases in which the diagnosis is not clear.

A 30-year-old woman comes to the emergency department with lower abdominal pain and tenderness, fever, leukocytosis and cervical motion tenderness. What is the next best step in the management of this patient?

a. Cervical culture

b. Pelvic sonogram

c. Urine pregnancy test

d. Laparoscopy

e. Ceftriaxone and doxycycline

*Answer: The most important thing to do in a woman with lower abdominal pain or tenderness is to **exclude an ectopic pregnancy.** Perform a urine pregnancy test first and then get a cervical culture and start therapy.*

Treatment

- Outpatient: **Ceftriaxone (IM)** and **doxycycline (oral)**
- Inpatient: **Cefoxitin (IV)** and **doxycycline** and maybe metronidazole. Cefotetan can be used instead of cefoxitin.

Antibiotics that are safe in pregnancy are the following:

- Penicillins
- Cephalosporins
- Aztreonam
- Erythromycin
- Azithromycin

EPIDYDIMO-ORCHITIS

Presents with an extremely **painful and tender testicle** with a **normal position** in the scrotum. Testicular torsion is different, because it presents with an elevated testicle in an abnormal transverse position.

Treatment

- < 35 years of age: **Ceftriaxone** and **doxycycline**
- > 35 years of age: **Fluoroquinolone**

ULCERATIVE GENITAL DISEASES

All forms of ulcerative genital disease can be associated with enlarged lymph nodes. Sexual history is not as important as the presence of ulcers.

CHANCROID

The ulcer will be **painful** (*Hemophilus ducreyi*).

Diagnostic Testing

The best initial diagnostic test is a **swab for gram stain** (gram-negative coccobacilli) and culture (will require specialized medium: Nairobi medium or Mueller-Hinton agar).

Treatment

Single **IM shot of ceftriaxone** or single oral dose of azithromycin.

LYMPHOGRANULOMA VENEREUM (LGV)

Large tender nodes are present in addition to the ulcer. The enlarged nodes, sometimes called "buboes" may develop a suppurating, draining sinus tract. Diagnose with serology for *Chlamydia trachomatis*. Aspirate the bubo. Treat with doxycycline.

HERPES SIMPLEX VIRUS TYPE 2 (HSV2) (I.E., GENITAL HERPES)

A 34-year-old man comes to the clinic with multiple vesicles on his penis. There is enlarged adenopathy in the inguinal area. What is the next step in management?

a. Tzanck prep
b. Viral culture
c. Valacyclovir
d. Ganciclovir

Answer: When there are clear vesicular lesions present, there is no need to do a specific diagnostic test for herpes. If the question describes multiple vesicles, then treatment with **acyclovir, valacyclovir,** *or* **famciclovir for 7–10 days** *is the next best step in management. Daily suppressive therapy can be prescribed for recurrent genital herpes. If the roofs come off the vesicles and the lesion becomes an ulcer of unclear etiology, then the best initial diagnostic test is a tzanck prep. The most accurate test for herpes is a viral culture. If there are clear vesicles, this is not necessary; go straight to treatment. Ganciclovir is therapy for cytomegalovirus (CMV).*

SYPHILLIS

The responsible pathogen is *Treponema pallidum*.

A man comes to the clinic having had a **painless, firm genital lesion** *for the last several days. The inguinal adenopathy is painless.*

What is the most accurate diagnostic test?

a. VDRL

b. RPR

c. FTA

d. Darkfield microscopic exam

*Answer: The VDRL and RPR are only 75 percent sensitive in primary syphilis. There is a false negative rate of 25 percent. The most accurate test in primary syphilis is darkfield microscopy, answer **D**. Darkfield microscopy is far more sensitive than a VDRL or RPR in primary syphilis.*

Primary Syphilis:

- Symptoms: **Chancre, adenopathy**
- Treatment: **Single IM shot of penicillin**. Use doxycycline for the penicillin-allergic.

Secondary Syphilis:

- Symptoms: **Rash, mucous patch, alopecia areata, condylomata lata**
- Initial diagnostic test: **RPR** and **FTA**
- Treatment: **Single IM shot of penicillin.** Use Doxycycline for the penicillin-allergic.

Tertiary Syphilis:

- Neurological involvement: **Tabes dorsalis, Argyll-Robertson pupil, general paresis,** rarely a gumma or aortitis
- **Initial diagnostic test: RPR** and **FTA, lumbar puncture** for neurosyphilis (test CSF with VDRL and FTA)
- Treatment: **IV penicillin.** Desensitize if penicillin-allergic.

A man comes with a painless ulcer and adenopathy. The edges of the ulcer are firm. The VDRL is negative. What is the next best step in management?

a. Repeat the VDRL

b. RPR

c. FTA

d. Darkfield microscopic exam

e. Order antiphospholipid antibody

Answer: Perform a darkfield examination. The VDRL and RPR can be negative in 25 percent of cases of primary syphilis.

If the patient is allergic to penicillin, desensitization is the answer for

- Neurosyphilis
- Pregnant women

Syphilis by Stage			
Stage	**Primary**	**Secondary**	**Tertiary**
Presentation	Chancre	• Rash • Alopecia • Condylomata lata • Mucous patch	• Neurosyphilis: Tabes doralis, general paresis, Argyll-Robertson pupil • Gummas • Aortitis
Test	• Darkfield (most sensitive) • RPR or VDRL • FTA	• RPR or VDRL • FTA	• RPR or VDRL • FTA • Lumbar puncture
Treatment	1. Single IM penicillin 2. Doxcycline if allergic	1. Single IM penicillin 2. Doxcycline if allergic	1. IV penicillin 2. Desensitization if allergic

GRANULOMA INGUINALE

This is indicated by a **rare, beefy red genital lesion that ulcerates.**

Initial Diagnostic Test

• **Biopsy** or **"touch prep"**

Treatment

• **Doxycycline** or **TMP/SMX**

Pediculosis and Scabies	
Pediculosis	**Scabies**
• Larger • In hair-bearing areas, such as the pubic area or axilla • Visible on the surface	• Small • Burrows in web spaces • Scrape and magnify
Treat with permethrin or lindane.	Treat with permethrin or lindane.

WARTS

All warts (condylomata accuminata, verrucous wart, Molluscum contagiousum) are diagnosed by **how they look.** They are treated with **mechanical removal:**

• Perform surgical removal if large.

• Imiquimod is an immunostimulant that leads to sloughing off of the wart.

• Cryotherapy, laser removal, and melting with podophylin are other options.

URINARY TRACT INFECTION

CYSTITIS

This often presents with **urinary frequency, urgency, burning,** and **dysuria.**
Young, otherwise healthy women are the most common case presented.

Diagnostic Testing

- Best initial test: **Urinalysis**
- Most accurate diagnostic test: **Urine culture**

Treatment

- **Uncomplicated cystitis** is treated with **TMP/SMX orally for three days,** if
  E. coli resistance in that area is low. If resistance is > 20 percent, then use
  ciprofloxacin or **levofloxacin.**
- **"Complicated" cystitis** is treated with **7 days of TMP/SMX** or **ciprofloxacin.** *Complicated* means an anatomic abnormality is present, such as a stone,
  stricture, tumor, or obstruction.

*A 25-year-old, generally healthy woman comes to the office with burning on urination.
There are 50 white cells on the urinalysis. What is the next best step in management?*

a. Wait for results of urine culture.
b. Obtain urine culture.
c. Treat with TMP/SMX for three days.
d. Treat with ciprofloxacin for seven days.
e. Perform a renal ultrasound.

*Answer: When there are clear symptoms of cystitis and white cells in the urine, it is not
necessary to obtain a urine culture or to wait for results of either the culture or a sonogram.
For uncomplicated cystitis, go straight to treatment for three days, answer **C.** Ultrasound is
important in male patients, as it is unusual for a male patient to have a urinary tract infection in the absence of an anatomic abnormality.*

> **Asymptomatic bacteriuria:**
> Only pregnant women
> should be treated. Do
> *not* treat asymptomatic
> bacteriuria, unless the
> patient is pregnant.

PYELONEPHRITIS

Patient presents with urinary frequency, urgency, burning, and dysuria in the
same way as cystitis, *and* there is **flank pain** and **tenderness.** Pyelonephritis
is also a more severe disease, so there is a higher fever and the patient is much
more ill.

Best Initial Diagnostic Test

- Urinalysis and urine culture the same as for cystitis

Treatment

Any of the medications for gram-negative bacilli are effective. The recommendation is for **ciprofloxacin** for outpatient treatment and **ampicillin/gentamicin** for inpatient therapy.

Radiologic testing and urinary tract infections:

Neither cystitis nor pyelonephritis is diagnosed by a radiologic study (sonogram or CT). Sonography and CT scanning are used to determine the etiology of the urinary tract infection.

If there is pyelonephritis...Is there a stone? Stricture? Tumor? Obstruction? Is there an anatomic defect that has led to the infection that must be corrected so that the infection will not recur?

- Dysuria + White cells in urine + Suprapubic tenderness = **Cystitis**
- Dysuria + White cells in urine + Flank pain + fever = **Pyelonephritis**

Urinalysis: For infections, we are concerned mainly with the presence of **white cells (WBC)**. Numerous squamous epithelial cells suggest an improperly collected specimen, and unless symptomatic, you would not treat. **Leukocyte esterase** is derived from granulocytic white blood cells and serves as indirect evidence of the presence of bacteriuria. Nitrites are indicative of gram-negative bacteria. Protein is very nonspecific in a urinalysis. Protein can be from both infection and glomerular disorders. Red cells are nonspecific as well.

PERINEPHRIC ABSCESS

This is a rare complication of pyelonephritis. Look for a patient with pyelonephritis who **does not respond to treatment after 5–7 days.** The patient remains febrile and still shows white cells on urinalysis. Perform a sonogram or CT of the kidneys to find the collection.

Most Accurate Diagnostic Test:
- **Biopsy:** This is the only way to determine a precise microbiologic diagnosis to guide therapy.

Treatment
- Treat with a **quinolone** and **ADD staphylococcal coverage,** such as oxacillin or nafcillin, because treatment with antibiotics for gram-negative organisms preferentially selects out for staphylococci.

PROSTATITIS

This is indicated by **frequency, urgency,** and **dysuria** and **perineal or sacral pain.** There is tenderness of the prostate, and it may be described as "boggy" on examination.

Treat with **ciprofloxacin** for an extended period of time. Prostatitis is like an abscess. Use the same drugs as for cystitis and pyelonephritis but extend the length of therapy.

INFECTIVE ENDOCARDITIS

Clinically, endocarditis is diagnosed by meeting **Duke's criteria** (2 major and 5 minor criteria). The diagnosis of endocarditis is made by the presence of 2 major, 1 major *and* 3 minor, or 5 minor criteria.

Duke's Criteria for Endocarditis	
Major	**Minor**
2 positive blood cultures with • Staphylococcus aureus • Viridans streptococci, ***Strep. bovis/epidermis,*** enterococci, gram-negative rods, ***Candida*** HACEK organisms are generally culture-negative. • *Haemophilus aphrophilus/parainfluenzae* • *Actinobacillus actinomycetemcomitans* • *Cardiobacterium hominis* • *Eikenella corrodens* • *Kingella kingae*	Fever (> 38.0°C)

Abnormal echocardiogram:
• Intracardiac mass or valvular vegetation
    OR
• Abscess
    OR
• New partial dehiscence of prosthetic valve
	Presence of risk factors:
	• IV drug use (IDU)
	• Presence of structural heart disease
	• Prosthetic heart valve
	• Dental procedures involving bleeding
	• History of endocarditis

	Vascular findings: • Janeway lesions • Septic pulmonary infarcts • Arterial emboli • Mycotic aneurysm • Conjunctival hemorrhage
	Immunological findings: • Roth spots • Osler's nodes • Glomerulonephritis
	Microbiologic findings • Positive blood culture but does not meet major criteria

Look for a patient with a risk such as the following:

- Prosthetic heart valve
- Injection drug use
- Dental procedures that cause bleeding
- Previous endocarditis
- Unrepaired or recently repaired cyanotic heart disease

- **Fever + Murmur = Possible endocarditis**
- **Fever + Murmur = Do blood cultures**

When there is **fever** and a **new murmur or change in a murmur,** the "next best step" in management is to **perform blood cultures first.** If the blood cultures are positive, then perform an **echocardiogram** to look for vegetations.

Other Physical Findings

These are rarely seen but are useful in establishing the diagnosis of endocarditis if the blood cultures are negative:

- Roth spots (retina)
- Janeway lesions (flat, painless in hands and feet)
- Osler's nodes (raised, painful, and pea shaped)
- Splinter hemorrhages (under fingernails)

Diagnosis

	Transthoracic Echocardiogram (TTE)	Transesophageal Echocardiogram (TEE)
Sensitivity	60%	90–95%
Specificity	90–95%	90–95%
	If TTE is negative, then proceed to TEE.	

- **2 positive blood cultures + Positive echo = Endocarditis**

Treatment

- The *best* empiric therapy is **vancomycin and gentamicin in combination.** This will cover the most common organisms, which are *Staph. aureus,* MRSA, and viridans group streptococci. You do *not* need to cover empirically for fungi or resistant gram-negative rods, since these are less common. Treatment is for 4–6 weeks.

- *Strep. bovis:* Perform **colonoscopy.** *Strep. bovis* is associated with colonic pathology.
- **Surgery (valve replacement):** The strongest indications for surgery are **anatomic defects,** which are hard or impossible to correct with antibiotics alone, including:
  - Valve rupture
  - Abscess
  - Prosthetic valves
  - Fungal endocarditis
  - Embolic events when already started on antibiotics

Endocarditis Prophylaxis

The *only* **cardiac defects** that need prophylaxis are the following:

- Prosthetic valves
- Unrepaired cyanotic heart disease
- Previous endocarditis
- Transplant recipients who develop valve disease

The *only* **procedures** that need prophylaxis are the following:

- Dental procedures that cause bleeding: The prophylactic antibiotic to use for dental procedures is **amoxicillin.** For penicillin-allergic patients, clindamycin is the drug of choice.
- Respiratory tract surgery
- Surgery of infected skin

The following **procedures** do *not* need prophylaxis:

- Dental fillings
- All flexible scopes
- All OB/GYN procedures
- All urinary procedures, including cystoscopy

The following **cardiac defects** do *not* need prophylaxis:

- Aortic stenosis or regurgitation
- Mitral stenosis or regurgitation
- Atrial or ventricular septal defects
- Pacemakers and implantable defibrillators
- Mitral valve prolapse, even if there is a murmur
- HOCM (IHSS)

HIV/AIDS

Following are the "must know" facts about HIV:

- Adverse effects of medications
- Needle-stick injury management
- Pregnancy/perinatal HIV management

When to start therapy?

- CD4 count < 350
- Symptomative patients with any CD4 count or viral load
- Pregnant women (see below)
- Needle-stick scenario, where patient is known to be HIV-positive

Start **triple Highly Active Antiretroviral Therapy (HAART),** which is one of the following:

- Tenofovir *and* emtricitabine *and* efavirenz (single combination pill with all of these)
- Zidovudine *and* lamivudine *and* efavirenz
- Zidovudine *and* lamivudine *and* ritonavir/lopinavir

The precise combination is not as important as knowing the adverse effects of the medications.

Class	Nucleoside Reverse Transcriptase Inhibitors	Protease Inhibitors	Nonnucleoside Reverse Transcriptase Inhibitors
Adverse effects of the class	Lactic acidosis	Hyperglycemia Hyperlipidemia	
Individual medications	Zidovudine: Anemia Didanosine: Pancreatitis and peripheral neuropathy Stavudine: Pancreatitis and neuropathy Lamivudine: None Abacavir: Rash Emtricitabine	Indinavir: Kidney stones Ritonavir Lopinavir Nelfinavir Saquinavir Darunavir Tipranavir Amprenavir Atazanavir	Efavirenz Nevirapine

NEEDLE-STICK INJURY (POSTEXPOSURE PROPHYLAXIS)

With any significant exposure to HIV-positive blood via a needle, scalpel, or penetrating injury, the answer is the same: **HAART for a month.**

This would also be true for the **exposure of mucosal surfaces** to HIV-positive blood or after **unprotected sexual contact** with a person known to be HIV-positive.

PREGNANCY/PERINATAL

- If the patient is already on antiretroviral therapy for her own health, then simply continue the same therapy.
- If the patient finds she is HIV-positive as part of prenatal care but is not already on therapy, there are two choices:
  1. **CD4 < 350:** Start HAART now.
  2. **CD4 > 350 and viral load is low:** Use HAART during the second and third trimesters only to prevent perinatal transmission.

PROPHYLAXIS

Pneumocystis Jiroveci **Pneumonia (PCP) (< 200 CD4 cells)**

- **TMP/SMX** is the *best* prophylaxis for PCP by far.
- If TMP/SMX causes a rash, switch to **atovoquone** or **dapsone.** (Dapsone *cannot* be used if there is G6PD deficiency.)
- Aerosolized pentamidine has the *poorest* efficacy and is rarely used. There is the most amount of breakthrough.

Mycobacterium Avium Intracellulare **(MAI) (< 50 CD4 cells)**

- Use **azithromycin** once a week orally.

OPPORTUNISTIC INFECTIONS

Pneumocystis Jiroveci **Pneumonia (PCP)**

This presents with **shortness of breath, dry cough, hypoxia,** and **increased LDH.**

Diagnostic Testing

- Best initial test: A **chest X-ray** will show increased interstitial markings bilaterally.
- Most accurate test: **Bronchoalveolar lavage**

Treatment

- **IV TMP/SMX**
- If there is a rash, use **IV pentamidine.**
- **Atovoquone** can be used for *mild* pneumocystis.
- **Dapsone** is not intravenous and is used for prophylaxis, *not* treatment.
- If PCP is severe (pO2 < 70 or A-a gradient > 35), then give **steroids.**

Toxoplasmosis

Look for headache, nausea, vomiting, and focal neurologic findings. Best initial test is a **head CT with contrast** showing "ring" or contrast-enhancing lesions.

Treat with **pyrimethamine and sulfadiazine for 2 weeks** and repeat the CT scan. If the lesions are smaller, then this is confirmative of toxoplasmosis. If the lesions are unchanged in size, then perform a brain biopsy, since this is most likely lymphoma.

Cytomegalovirus (CMV)

HIV with < **50 CD4 cells** and **blurry vision.** Perform a dilated ophthalmologic examination. CMV is diagnosed by the appearance of the lesions on examination.

Treat with **ganciclovir** or **foscarnet.**

Maintenance therapy is with **oral valganciclovir lifelong,** unless the CD4 goes up with HAART. If the CD4 rises, you can stop the CMV medications.

Cryptococcus

HIV and < **50 CD4 cells** with **fever and headache.** Neck stiffness and photophobia are not always present. Perform a **lumbar puncture,** finding an increase in the level of lymphocytes in the CSF. The best initial test is an **India ink stain,** which has about a 60 percent sensitivity. The most accurate test is a **cryptococcal antigen test,** which is over 95 percent sensitive and specific.

Treat initially with **amphotericin,** followed by **fluconazole.** The fluconazole is continued lifelong unless the CD4 count rises. If the CD4 count rises, all opportunistic infection treatment and prophylaxis can be stopped. The only treatment that cannot be stopped is the antiretrovirals.

Progressive Multifocal Leukoencephalopathy (PML)

HIV and < **50 CD4 cells** with **focal neurologic abnormalities.** The best initial test is a **head CT** or **MRI.** The lesions do *not* show ring enhancement and there is no mass effect.

Treatment: There is *no* specific therapy available for PML. Treat with HAART. When the CD4 count rises, PML will resolve.

Mycobacterium Avium Intracellulare (MAI)

HIV and < **50 CD4 cells.** There is wasting with **weight loss, fever,** and **fatigue. Anemia** is frequent from invasion of the bone marrow. Increased alkaline phosphatase and GGTP with a normal bilirubin is characteristic of hepatic involvement.

Diagnostic testing: **Bone marrow** is more sensitive. **Liver biopsy** is the most sensitive. Blood culture is the least sensitive.

Treat with **clarithromycin and ethambutal.**

ANIMAL-BORNE DISEASES

LEPTOSPIROSIS

This is a spirochete.

> • Animal exposure + Jaundice + Renal = Leptospirosis

There is some form of **exposure to animals** in the history. The patient has eaten food contaminated by the urine of infected animals. There is **fever, abdominal pain,** and **muscle aches** as well. Severe disease leads to altered mental status. Diagnose with serology and treat with **ceftriaxone** or **penicillin.**

TULAREMIA

Involves contact with **rabbits** in the summer. Look for a hunter or someone who has touched a small, furry animal. There is an **ulcer at the site of contact** and **enlarged lymph nodes. Conjunctivitis** is another clue. Diagnose with **serology.** Note that taking a culture is dangerous, as spores can cause severe pneumonia in lab personnel.

CYSTICERCOSIS

The CT scan of the head will show **thin-walled cysts,** which are most often **calcified.** Treat with **albendazole.** This disease is often transmitted by **infected pork** that is ingested. Infection is most likely in those who have eaten pork in endemic areas such as Mexico, South America, Eastern Europe, or India.

Below this box is the 90th percentile area. This is lower-yield material. If you *only* need to pass the exam, you do not need to read this. If you do not have a residency yet, and your Step 3 grade will be seen to make an admission decision, you should read and learn the material below to try to get a 95 or higher.

TICK-BORNE DISEASE

LYME

For USMLE, **camping and hiking** is a marker for the presence of **ticks.** Only 20 percent of those with Lyme disease remember the tick bite, because it is so small. The **rash** is shaped like **a target with a pale center and a red ring on the outside.** The cause is a spirochete named *Borrelia burgdorferi,* which is carried by the *Ixodes* genus (deer) tick. The question may say something about vacationing in the Northeast or Midwest. States in this region are Connecticut, Delaware, Maine, Maryland, Massachusetts, Minnesota, New Hampshire, New York, New Jersey, Pennsylvania, and Wisconsin.

The proper term is **"erythema migrans,"** but this is not a term that has a precise meaning.

> • Camping/hiking + Target-shaped rash = Lyme disease

A 43-year-old man presents with a target-shaped rash that has developed over the last several days. He was on a camping trip in the woods last week in Maine. What is the next best step in management?

a. Serology for IgM

b. ELISA

c. Western blot

d. Doxycycline

e. Ceftriaxone

*Answer: A rash suggestive of Lyme is enough to indicate treatment. A 5-cm-wide target-shaped rash, particularly with a history of camping/hiking, is enough to indicate the need for antibiotic treatment with doxycycline, answer **D**. A characteristic rash is more specific than serology. Ceftriaxone is used for CNS or cardiac Lyme.*

Long-term manifestations/complications of Lyme are as follows:

• Joint
• Cardiac
• Neurologic

Diagnosis

Each of these is diagnosed with serology, such as IgM, IgG ELISA, Western blot, or PCR.

• The most common **late** manifestation of Lyme: **Joint involvement**
• The most common **cardiac** manifestation: **AV conduction block/defect**
• The most common **neurologic** manifestation: **7th cranial nerve palsy (Bell's palsy)**

Treatment
- Rash, joint, Bell's palsy: **Oral doxycycline** or **amoxicillin**
- CNS or cardiac involvement: **IV ceftriaxone**

BABESIOSIS

Babesiosis is transmitted by the same *Ixodes* (deer) tick that transmits Lyme. As a result, it is also common in the Northeast. It manifests with **hemolytic anemia** and is severe in asplenic individuals.

Diagnose with a **peripheral blood smear** looking for tetrads of intraerythrocytic ring forms or do a **PCR.**

Treat with **clindamycin** and **quinine.**

EHRLICHIA

This, too, is transmitted by the *Ixodes* tick. There is **no rash.** Instead, there is elevated liver function tests (ALT and AST), **thrombocytopenia** (decreased platlets), and **leukopenia** (decreased white blood cells).

Diagnose with a **peripheral blood smear** looking for "morulae," which are inclusion bodies in the white cells or do **PCR.**

Treat with **doxycycline.**

MALARIA

This disease is rarely domestic. Look for a traveler recently returning from an endemic area with **hemolysis. GI complaints** are always present. Diagnosed by **blood smear.**

Treatment
- **Acute disease** is treated with **quinine** and **doxycycline.**
- **Prophylaxis** is with **mefloquine** (weekly) or **atovoquone/proguanil** (Malarone, administered daily). Daily doxycycline has been used for prophylaxis but would not be the best answer. Note that those being given mefloquine should be advised of neuropsychiatric side effects, sinus bradycardia, and QT prolongation.

RESPIRATORY DISEASES

NOCARDIA

This involves **immunocompromised people** (leukemia, lymphoma, steroid use, HIV). Respiratory/pulmonary disease may disseminate to any organ, with skin and brain being the most common.

Nocardia gives branching, gram-positive filaments that are weakly acid fast.

Diagnostic Testing
- Best initial test: **Chest X-ray**
- Most accurate test: **Culture**

Treatment
- **TMP/SMX**

ACTINOMYCES

Host has a **normal immune system.** There is a history of **facial or dental trauma,** which inoculated these organisms into the cervicofacial area. *Actinomyces* is a part of normal mouth flora. Trauma, such as a tooth extraction, can put it into the facial area, thorax, and abdomen.

Diagnose with **gram stain** and confirm with **anaerobic culture.** Like *Nocardia*, *Actinomyces* is a **branching, filamentous bacteria.**

Treat with **penicillin.**

HISTOPLASMOSIS

Look for **wet areas,** such as the Ohio and Mississippi River valleys. This lung disease that can present as a viral syndrome is also associated with **bat droppings from caves.** A physical exam will show **palate and oral ulcers** and **splenomegaly.**

The disseminated disease enters the bone marrow and causes **pancytopenia.** Anything tuberculosis can do, histoplasmosis can do.

Treatment
- Acute pulmonary disease is transient and requires *no* therapy.
- The disseminated disease is treated with **amphotericin.**

COCCIDIOIDOMYCOSIS

This is an acute respiratory illness that occurs in **very dry areas** like Arizona. It causes **joint pain** and **erythema nodosum.**

Treatment
- **Itraconazole**

BLASTOMYCOSIS

This is an acute pulmonary disease in the **rural Southeast.** Look for **broad budding yeast.**

Bone lesions are common.

- Broad budding yeast = Blastomycosis

Treatment

- Antifungal agents, such as **amphotericin** or **itraconazole**

ALLERGY AND IMMUNOLOGY

2

ANAPHYLAXIS

Anaphylaxis is a hypersensitivity/allergic reaction that is potentially life threatening. The most common causes are foods (e.g., peanuts, shellfish, etc.). Other causes include the following:

- **Insect stings/bites**
- **Medications** (e.g., penicillin, allopurinol, sulfa-containing drugs)

Anaphylaxis presents as **hemodynamic instability** with **hypotension and tachycardia** as well as **difficulty breathing.**

TREATMENT

Anaphylaxis treatment has been unchanged for decades. The best initial therapy is to administer all of the following:

- **Subcutaneous epinephrine in a 1:1000 concentration**
- **Corticosteroids**
- H1-inhibiting antihistamines, such as **diphenhydramine** or **hydroxyzine**

Remember that CCS does *not* require you to know doses, but you must know the route of administration and the type of the medication. Hence, you must know to give the epinephrine **subcutaneously.**

ANGIOEDEMA

Angioedema is a **sudden swelling of the face, palate, tongue, and airway** in association with **minor trauma to the face or hands** or the **ingestion of ACE inhibitors.** The question may describe a **person hit in the face with a pillow** or **wood chips hitting the arm.** The hereditary form occurs from **deficiency of C1 esterase inhibitor.** Other symptoms include the following:

- Stridor
- Abdominal pain
- A lack of response to steroids

> Consider placing people with angioedema in the ICU.

Angioedema Face

DIAGNOSTIC TESTING

The diagnosis of angioedema is based on finding **low levels of C2 and C4 in the complement pathway.** They are chronically depleted because of the deficiency of the C1 esterase inhibitor. An elevated white cell count is *not* specific.

TREATMENT

- Acute episodes: These are managed with the **infusion of fresh frozen plasma.**
- Chronic therapy: **Androgens** are used for chronic therapy. Androgens, for unknown reasons, raise the levels of C1 esterase inhibitor. The most frequently used androgens are **danazol** and **stanazol.**

A patient comes to the emergency department with shortness of breath, facial swelling, and lip swelling 30 minutes after a bee sting. There was no response to epi-pen injection in the field. Six hours after a bolus of steroid and diphenhydramine, the patient is still short of breath and still has lip swelling.

Where should the patient be placed?

Answer: This patient should be placed in the intensive care unit. If the patient comes with anaphylaxis from any cause, the placement of the patient for CCS is based entirely on the response to therapy that occurs after treatment. In this case, the source of the allergic reaction, an insect sting, is irrelevant. What matters is that after moving the clock forward, the symptoms do not resolve. Any persistent lip, facial or hemodynamic involvement after initial therapy should place the patient in the ICU.

A man comes in with neurosyphilis. He has a history of life-threatening anaphylaxis to penicillin. He has a history of essential tremor and is on propranolol. He has asthma and is on an inhaled beta agonist and inhaled steroids.

Which of the following is most appropriate?

a. Use ceftriaxone instead of penicillin
b. Stop propranolol prior to desensitizing him
c. Bolus with oral steroids prior to penicillin use
d. Add long acting beta agonists to treatment

Answer: Neurosyphilis is only effectively treated with penicillin. The patient must be desensitized. Prior for desensitization it is important to stop propranolol and all beta blockers. This is because epinephrine may have to be used in the event of anaphylaxis when you desensitize the patient. Bolusing with steroids in inappropriate, because anaphylaxis is treated first with epinephrine.

ALLERGIC RHINITIS

PRESENTATION

Allergic rhinitis presents with **recurrent episodes of nasal itching, stuffiness, rhinorrhea, and paroxysms of sneezing.** There is also often **eye itching** and **dermatitis.** Allergic rhinitis may be associated with the development of asthma. Many patients present with wheezing as well.

TREATMENT

Avoidance

The mainstay of all therapy for those with extrinsic allergies is the **avoidance of the allergen.** It is important to close windows and stay in air-conditioned rooms to avoid pollen. In addition, an allergy to animal dander may mean avoiding a pet. Mattresses and pillows must be covered with mite and dust-proof casings.

Drug Therapy

- **Antihistamines** such as loratadine, fexofenadine, and cetirizine
- **Topical corticosteroids**
- **Nasal saline spray and wash**
- **Cromolyn**
- **Ipratropium bromide**
- **Leukotriene inhibitors** (e.g., monteleukast)

Immunotherapy

For extrinsic allergens that cannot be avoided, **desensitization** therapy may work.

PRIMARY IMMUNODEFICIENCY SYNDROMES

COMMON VARIABLE IMMUNODEFICIENCY (CVID)

Presentation

CVID presents in *both* men and women and may only present when the patient is an adult. Both CVID and X-linked agammaglobulinemia present with **recurrent episodes of sinopulmonary infections,** such as bronchitis, sinusitis, pneumonia, and pharyngitis. In addition, CVID causes a **spruelike abdominal disorder.** There is malabsorption, steatorrhea, and diarrhea. Lymph nodes, adenoids, and the spleen are present and may be enlarged.

Diagnositic Testing

The machinery to make immunoglobulins is intact. The nodes and both B and T cells are present, but they do not make enough antibody. Hence **total IgG levels are low.**

Treatment

CVID is treated with **infusions of intravenous immunoglobulins.**

X-LINKED AGAMMAGLOBULINEMIA (BRUTON'S)

This presents in **male children with recurrent sinopulmonary infections.**

Diagnostic Testing

Lymph nodes, adenoids, and the spleen are diminished in size or absent. **B cells** are missing, as are the **immunoglobulins.**

Treatment

Like CVID, X-linked agammaglobulinemia is treated with **infusions of intravenous immunoglobulins.**

IGA DEFICIENCY

This is the most common primary immunodeficiency. Many people are asymptomatic. Some have **recurrent sinopulmonary infections.** There is also a **sprue-like malabsorption syndrome** as well as an increased incidence of **atopic conditions.** Some people present with **anaphylaxis** when receiving blood from donors who are not IgA deficient.

Treatment

Treat the infections as they arise. Intravenous immunoglobulins will not work since it has little IgA in it.

HYPER IGE SYNDROME

Hyper IgE syndrome presents with **recurrent skin infections from Staphylococcus.**

Treatment

Treat the infections as they arise.

A three-year-old male child comes with recurrent sinopulmonary infections. There are no nodes palpated in the cervical area and no tonsils seen on oral exam. The child has been treated for an infection nearly every 1-2 months since birth. There are no skin Infections.

What is the most likely diagnosis?

a. Hyper IgE syndrome
b. IgA deficiency
c. X-Linked agammaglobulinemia
d. Common variable Immunodeficiency

Answer: X-linked agammaglobulinemia is exclusively in male children whereas common variable immunodeficiency presents in adults. The absence of skin infection in this case goes strongly against hyper IgE syndrome. These patients are best managed with intravenous immunoglobulin infusions on a regular basis and with antibiotics for infections as episodes arise.

CARDIOLOGY

3

ISCHEMIC HEART DISEASE

Coronary artery disease (CAD) is the most common cause of death, by far, in the United States, killing ten times more women than breast cancer.

Risk factors are useful for two things:

1. They can help answer diagnostic questions in equivocal cases.
2. Modifying them can lower mortality.

> **Remember: For family history to be significant, the family member must be young (female relatives < 65, male relatives < 55).**

Emotional stress is *not* a clear risk factor. It is not possible to measure precisely.

Risk factors include the following:

- Diabetes mellitus
- Hypertension
- Tobacco use
- Hyperlipidemia
- Peripheral arterial disease (PAD)
- Obesity
- Inactivity
- Family history

PRESENTATION

Coronary artery disease (CAD) presents with chest pain that does *not* change with body position or respiration. CAD is *not* associated with chest wall tenderness. When any one of these three features is present, the patient does *not* have CAD.

Pleuritic Pain (changes with respiration)	Positional (changes with bodily position)	Tender (pain on palpation)
Pulmonary embolism Pneumonia Pleuritis Pericarditis Pneumothorax	Pericarditis	Costochondritis

The most common cause of chest pain that is *not* cardiac in etiology is a gastrointestinal (acid reflux) problem.

a) *A patient comes to the emergency department with chest pain. The pain also occurs in the epigastric area and is associated with a sore throat, a bad metallic taste in the mouth, and a cough. What do you recommend?*

b) *An alcoholic patient comes to the emergency department with chest pain. There is nausea and vomiting and epigastric tenderness. What do you recommend?*

c) *A patient comes to the emergency department with chest pain. There is right-upper quadrant tenderness and mild fever. What do you recommend?*

Answers:

a) *Give a proton pump inhibitor.*

b) *Check amylase and lipase levels.*

c) *Order an abdominal sonogram for gallstones.*

Besides chest pain, other clues to ischemic disease as the cause of chest pain are as follows:

- Dull pain
- Lasting 15–30 minutes
- Occurring on exertion
- In a substernal location
- Radiating to the jaw or left arm

PHYSICAL FINDINGS

There is nothing unique or pathognomonic about the physical findings of ischemic heart disease. Physical findings such as tenderness only tell you the patient does *not* have ischemic disease. There is no buzzword for physical examination of CAD that indicates, "Aha! This is coronary disease." However, for CCS, it is critical to know what could be abnormal so you know which pieces of the physical to choose:

Piece of Physical Exam	Findings That *Could* Be Abnormal
CV (cardiovascular)	S3 gallop: Dilated left ventricle S4 gallop: Left ventricular hypertrophy Jugulovenous distention Holosystolic murmur of mitral regurgitation
Chest	Rales suggestive of congestive heart failure
General exam	Distressed patient, short of breath, clutching chest
Extremities	Edema

Holosystolic Murmur

Systole   Diastole

S_1 S_2 S_1

Mitral Regurgitation

Heart Sounds

S4   S1   S2   S3

Jugular veins on Step 3 CCS are in the CV exam, *not* the HEENT exam.

DIAGNOSTIC TESTING

The vast majority of chest pain cases on Step 3 will hand you a clear case in terms of the diagnosis and ask you what to do next in the management. An EKG is *always* the best initial diagnostic test for ischemic-type pain. If the case presented to you is **very clearly a case of ischemic pain** and the examiners ask you to **choose** between an EKG and aspirin, nitrates, oxygen, and morphine, then choose **treatment first.**

ST Elevation

ST Depression

TWave Inversion

The wrong best initial tests or steps are troponin, CK-MB, stress testing, echo-cardiogram, or angiography. These tests do *not* eliminate the need to **give aspirin first.** In a computerized clinical case scenario (CCS), however, answer *all* of these at the same time.

When the question asks what the *most accurate* test is, answer CK-MB or troponin.

CK-MB and troponin levels both rise at 3–6 hours after the start of chest pain. They have nearly the same specificity. The **main difference between CK-MB and troponin** is that CK-MB only stays elevated 1–2 days while troponin stays elevated for 1–2 weeks. Therefore, CK-MB testing is the best test to detect a reinfarction a few days after the initial infarction.

Always the wrong answer: LDH level or LDH isoenzymes.

Myoglobin elevates as early as 1–4 hours after the start of chest pain. Myoglobin is the answer to the question "Which of the following will rise first?" when the choices are all cardiac enzymes.

Stress testing is the answer when the case is *not* acute and the initial EKG and/or enzyme tests do *not* establish the diagnosis.

> Do not answer "consultation" for single best answer questions. However, "consultation" is okay to answer as a part of CCS management. In single best answer questions, you should not need a consultant to tell you to do an EKG, check enzymes, and give aspirin to a patient with acute coronary syndrome.

A 56-year-old man comes to the office a few days after an episode of chest pain. This was his first episode of pain, and he has no risk factors. In the emergency department, he had a normal EKG and normal CK-MB and was released the next day. Which of the following is most appropriate in his further management?

a. Repeat CK-MB

b. Statin

c. LDL level

d. Stress (exercise tolerance) testing

e. Angiography

*Answer: The correct answer is **D**. Stress test when the case is equivocal or uncertain for the presence of CAD. Do not do an angiography unless the stress test is abnormal. Exercise toler-ance, or "stress," testing detects coronary artery disease when the heart rate is raised and ST segment depression is detected. This case is asking you to know that **a stress test is a way of increasing the sensitivity of detection of CAD beyond an EKG and enzymes.***

Step 3 loves the phrase "further management."

When do I answer dipyridamole or adenosine thallium stress test or dobutamine echo?	When do I answer exercise thallium testing or stress echocardiography?
Patients who cannot exercise to a target heart rate of > 85% of maximum: • COPD • Amputation • Deconditioning • Weakness/previous stroke • Lower-extremity ulcer • Dementia • Obesity	EKG is unreadable for ischemia: • Left bundle branch block • Digoxin use • Pacemaker in place • Left ventricular hypertrophy • Any baseline abnormality of the ST segment of the EKG

Sestamibi nuclear stress testing is used in obese patients and those with large breasts because of the greater ability of this radioisotope to penetrate tissue.

A 63-year-old woman is in your office for evaluation of an abnormal stress test that shows an area or reversible ischemia. She has no risk factors for CAD. What is the most accurate diagnostic test, or what is the best next step in further management?

a. Troponin level

b. Angiography

c. Coronary bypass

d. Echocardiogram

e. Nuclear ventriculogram (MUGA scan)

Answer: The correct answer is **B.** Angiography is the next diagnostic test to evaluate an abnormal stress test that shows "reversible" ischemia. **Reversible ischemia** is the most dangerous thing that a stress test can show. If the stress test shows "fixed" defects—that is, a defect unchanged between exercise and rest—this is a scar from a previous infarction. Fixed defects do not need angiography. **Coronary bypass** is the answer only if the angiogram has already been done. **Echocardiography** is the best initial test to evaluate valve function or ventricular wall motion. **Nuclear ventriculogram** is the most accurate method to evaluate ejection fraction.

A patient admitted 5 days ago for a myocardial infarction has a new episode of chest pain. Which of the following is the most specific method of establishing the diagnosis of a new infarction?

a. CK-MB

b. Troponin

c. Echocardiogram

d. Stress testing

e. Angiography

Answer: The correct answer is **A.** The CK-MB level should return to normal 2–3 days after a myocardial infarction. If a reinfarction has occurred, the level 5 days later will go back up again, while the troponin level will still be up from the original infarction. Angiography can detect obstructive, stenotic lesions but cannot detect myocardial necrosis. Stress testing should **never** be performed if the patient is having current chest pain; chest pain is a reason to stop a stress test.

The definition of **acute coronary syndrome (ACS)** is as follows:

- Causes acute chest pain
- Can be with exercise or at rest
- Can have ST segment elevation, depression, or even a normal EKG
- Is not based on enzyme levels, angiography, or stress test results
- Is based on a history of chest pain with features suggestive of ischemic disease

TREATMENT

Aspirin

The best initial therapy for all cases of ACS is **aspirin.** Aspirin can be administered orally or chewed and absorbed under the tongue. It has an **instant effect on inhibiting platelets.** Aspirin alone reduces mortality by 25 percent for acute myocardial infarction and by 50 percent for "unstable angina," which may become a non-ST segment elevation myocardial infarction (NSTEMI). **Oxygen, nitrates, and morphine** should also be administered in acute coronary syndromes, but they do *not* lower mortality.

Thrombolytics and Primary Angioplasty

Step 3 is very big on knowing which treatments will *lower mortality.* Thrombolytics and primary angioplasty both **lower mortality** in ST segment elevation myocardial infarction (STEMI) and are **dependent on time;** in other words, their benefit markedly diminishes with time.

Primary angioplasty means angioplasty during an acute episode of chest pain, and **infarction** is the single best evidence for mortality benefit with angioplasty. Angioplasty is one type of "percutaneous coronary intervention" (PCI). PCI *must* be performed within 90 minutes of arrival at the emergency department for an ST segment elevation MI. Angioplasty has *not* been shown to decrease mortality in stable angina more than medical therapy (aspirin, beta blockers, and statins) alone.

> CCS requires you to know the **route of administration of medications.**

If **PCI cannot be performed within 90 minutes** of arrival in the emergency department, the patient should receive **thrombolytics.** The question will clearly state that "the patient is at a small rural hospital" or "the nearest catheterization facility is over an hour away." The question must be clear on this point. Thrombolytics are indicated when the patient has **chest pain for < 12 hours**

When is the answer "urgent angioplasty" or PCI?

- The question asks "what has the single greatest efficacy" in lowering mortality in ST elevation MI.
- The question includes a contraindication to the use of thrombolytics.

and has **ST segment elevation in 2 or more leads. A new left bundle branch block (LBBB)** is also an indication for thrombolytic therapy. Thrombolytics should be given **within 30 minutes** of a patient's arrival in the emergency department with pain.

Beta Blockers, ACE Inhibitors, and Angiotensin Receptor Blockers

Beta blockers lower mortality, but the timing of their administration is *not* critical. Beta blockers, such as metoprolol, should be given, but they are not as urgent to give as aspirin, thrombolytics, or primary angioplasty. **ACE inhibitors** or **angiotensin receptor blockers (ARBs)** should be given to all patients with an acute coronary syndrome, but they only lower mortality if there is **left ventricular dysfunction or systolic dysfunction.** Make sure there is a lipid profile and start the patient on HMG CoA reductase inhibitors, if indicated (i.e., if LDL is not at goal).

CCS and Step 3 do *not* require you to know doses.

A 72-year-old man comes to the emergency department having had chest pain for the last hour. His initial EKG shows ST segment elevation in leads V2–V4. Aspirin has been given. Which of the following will most likely benefit this patient?

a. CK-MB

b. Stress test

c. Angioplasty

d. Metoprolol

e. Diltiazem

f. Atorvostatin

g. Digoxin

h. Amiodarone

i. Oxygen, morphine, and nitrates

j. Thrombolytics

*Answer: The correct answer is **C**. Angioplasty will lower the risk of mortality most for this patient. If it can be obtained within 90 minutes, angioplasty is the best therapy. Metoprolol lowers mortality but is not dependent on how soon you give it, as long as the patient receives it before going home.*

Statins

Statin medications, such as atorvostatin, should be given to *all* patients with an **acute coronary syndrome,** regardless of what the EKG shows or troponin or CK-MB levels

Therapy Used In Acute Coronary Syndromes

Always Lower Mortality	Lower Mortality in Certain Conditions	Do Not Lower Mortality
• Aspirin • Thrombolytics • Primary angioplasty • Metoprolol • Statins • Clopidogrel	• ACE inhibitors if ejection fraction is low • ARBs if ejection fraction is low	• Oxygen • Morphine • Nitrates • Calcium channel blockers • Lidocaine • Amiodarone

- When is **clopidogrel** the answer?
  - The patient has acute coronary syndrome and is **allergic to aspirin.**
  - Clopidogrel is a platelet antagonist but is *not* to be used routinely in ACS *unless* there is **aspirin allergy** or the patient is to **undergo angioplasty.**

- When are **calcium channel blockers** (verapamil, diltiazem) the answer?
  - The patient has an **intolerance** to beta blockers, such as severe reactive airway disease (asthma).
  - There is cocaine-induced chest pain.
  - There is coronary vasospasm/Prinzmetal's angina.

- When is a **pacemaker** the answer for acute MI?
  - Third-degree AV block
  - Mobitz II, second-degree AV block
  - Bifascicular block
  - New left bundle branch block
  - Symptomatic bradycardia

- When is **lidocaine or amiodarone** the answer for acute MI?
  - *Only* when there is ventricular **tachycardia** or ventricular **fibrillation.**
  - Do *not* give anti-arrhythmic medications to prevent ventricular arrhythmias.

COMPLICATIONS OF MYOCARDIAL INFARCTION (MI)

All the complications of myocardial infarction result in **hypotension.** Step 3 rarely asks what the diagnosis is; instead, it most often hands it to you and asks what to do in further management.

Diagnosis	Diagnostic Test	Treatment
Cardiogenic shock	Echo, Swan-Ganz (right heart) catheter	ACE inhibitors, urgent revascularization
Valve rupture	Echo	ACE, nitroprusside, intra-aortic balloon pump as a bridge to surgery
Septal rupture	Echo, right heart catheter showing a step up in saturation from the right atrium to right ventricle	ACE, nitroprusside, and urgent surgery
Myocardial wall rupture	Echo	Pericardiocentesis, urgent cardiac repair
Sinus bradycardia	EKG	Atropine, followed by pacemaker if there are still symptoms
Third-degree (complete) heart block	EKG, canon "a" waves	Atropine and a pacemaker even if symptoms resolve
Right ventricular infarction	Right ventricular leads on an EKG	Fluid loading

Post-MI Discharge Instructions

All patients post-MI should go home on aspirin, a beta blocker, a statin, and an ACE inhibitor.

A patient's wife comes to take her husband home after an MI and asks how long they should wait before they have sex. What do you tell her?

a. No waiting necessary

b. Two weeks

c. Six weeks

d. They should wait for a normal angiography.

*Answer: The correct answer is **A**. No waiting is necessary to have sex after an infarction. Sex does not significantly increase the risk of infarction, because neither the duration nor the intensity of exertion is sufficient to provoke ischemia in most cases.*

Non-ST Segment Elevation Myocardial Infarction

The predominant differences in the management of non-ST segment elevation MI (NSTEMI) are as follows:

- No thrombolytic use.
- Heparin is used routinely.
- Glycoprotein IIb/IIIa inhibitors lower mortality, particularly in those undergoing angioplasty.

A 54-year-old man with a history of diabetes and hypertension comes to the emergency department with crushing, substernal chest pain that radiates to his left arm. The pain has been on and off for several hours, with this last episode being 30 minutes in duration. He has had chest pain on exertion before, but this is the first time it has developed at rest. The EKG is normal. Aspirin, oxygen, and nitrates have been given. Troponin levels are elevated. Which of the following is most likely to benefit this patient?

a. Low molecular weight heparin

b. Thrombolytics

c. Diltiazem

d. Morphine

e. CK-MB levels

*Answer: The correct answer is **A**. Heparin is the only one of these choices that has been shown to produce lower mortality. Thrombolytics do not lower mortality, unless there is ST elevation or a new LBBB. Positive cardiac enzymes are not an indication for thrombolytics. Other answers that could be right if they were choices are **GPIIb/IIIa inhibitors**, such as eptifibatide, tirofiban, or abciximab, or the use of **angioplasty/PCI**.*

> The single greatest benefits from **GPIIb/IIIa inhibitors** with ACS come in combination with angioplasty and stent placement. Abciximab does *not* benefit ST segment elevation MI.

> **Thrombolytics** are *only* used if there is ST segment elevation or a new LBBB within 12 hours of the onset of chest pain.

> ARBs are used interchangeably with ACE inhibitors, especially if the patient has a cough with ACE inhibitors. Both ACE and ARBs cause hyperkalemia.

STABLE ANGINA

Office-based cases of further management will emphasize the same issues of mortality benefit.

Treatment

Aspirin and **metoprolol** are the two main routinely indicated medications because of their benefit on mortality. Nitrates should be used for those with angina pain but they do *not* lower mortality.

ACE inhibitors and ARBs should only be used in further management for stable cases if the question describes any of the following:

- Congestive failure
- Systolic dysfunction
- Low ejection fraction

Coronary Angiography for Further Management

Angiography is predominantly used to determine who is **a candidate for coronary artery bypass grafting (CABG).** You do not need to do angiography to diagnose CAD. Stress testing can show "reversible ischemia." However, you *must* do angiography to see who needs CABG.

You do *not* need to do angiography to initiate the following:

- Aspirin + metoprolol (mortality benefit)
- Nitrates (pain)
- ACE/ARB (low ejection fraction)

- Clopidogrel (can't tolerate aspirin)
- Statins (LDL > 70–100)

Which of the following is the main difference between saphenous vein grafts and internal mammary artery grafts?

a. There is less need for aspirin and metoprolol with internal mammary artery grafts.
b. Warfarin is necessary with saphenous vein grafts.
c. Internal mammary artery grafts remain open for 10 years.
d. Heparin is necessary for vein grafts.

*Answer: The correct answer is **C**. The main difference between saphenous vein grafts and internal mammary artery grafts is that vein grafts start to become occluded after 5 years but internal mammary artery grafts are often patient at 10 years. There is no difference in the need for medications.*

Following are the indications for CABG:

- Three coronary vessels with > 70 percent stenosis
- Left main coronary artery stenosis > 70 percent

Following are coronary artery disease equivalents:

- Diabetes mellitus
- Peripheral arterial disease
- Aortic disease
- Carotid disease

LIPID MANAGEMENT

The single strongest indication for lipid-lowering therapy is for **a statin in a patient with an acute coronary syndrome and an LDL > 130.** The goal of therapy in those with CAD is an LDL < 100. Although the evidence is strongest for an LDL > 130, you will answer "statin therapy" for *any* case of CAD *or an equivalent* with an LDL > 100.

Risk Factors

If a question asks for the LDL goal in a patient with **diabetes,** the answer is **LDL goal < 70.**

There are also other risk factors to consider. Make sure you also know how to calculate risk factors to help determine LDL goals.

Risk factors in lipid management include the following:

- Tobacco use (cigarette smoking)

- High blood pressure (≥ 140/90 mm Hg or on blood pressure medication)

- Low HDL cholesterol (< 40)

- Family history of early coronary heart disease (female relatives < 65, male relatives < 55)

- Age (males ≥ 45, females ≥ 55)

Many medications, such as statins, cholestryramine, gemfibrazol, ezetimibe, and niacin, lower LDL, lower triglycerides and total cholesterol, and raise HDL. Which of the following is the most important reason for using statins?

a. Fewer adverse effects
b. Lower cost
c. Greater patient acceptance
d. Greatest mortality benefit
e. Greatest effect on lowering LDL

*Answer: The correct answer is **D**. The statins have a greater effect on lowering mortality compared with the other medications.*

When is the goal of therapy an LDL < 70?

a. CHF
b. Diabetes
c. Coronary disease and carotid disease
d. Coronary disease and diabetes
e. Diabetes and hypertension

*Answer: The correct answer is **D**. The goal of LDL can be < 70 for patients at the very highest risk of infarction. This includes those with acute coronary syndromes or the combination of coronary disease and a very severe risk factor, such as diabetes.*

> Remember: Give statins with CAD and an LDL > 100.

Side Effects

The most common adverse effect of statin medications is **liver toxicity.** As many as 1 percent of patients will stop a statin because of its effect on raising transaminases. Liver function tests should be routinely checked. Rhabdomyolysis is *not* the most common adverse effect. There is no routine indication to check CPK levels.

SEX AND THE HEART

A man develops erectile dysfunction after an infarction. What is the most common cause?

a. Metoprolol

b. Nitrates

c. ACE inhibitors

d. Aspirin

e. Anxiety

Answer: The correct answer is **E.** *Anxiety is the most common cause of erectile dysfunction postinfarction. Although beta blockers may be the most common medication associated with erectile dysfunction, anxiety is still a more common cause of erectile dysfunction than beta blockers.*

A man develops erectile dysfunction postinfarction. You are planning to start sildenafil. Which of the following medications must you stop?

a. Metoprolol

b. Nitrates

c. ACE inhibitors

d. Aspirin

Answer: The correct answer is **B.** *Nitrates are contraindicated when medications such as sildenafil are to be used. When used at the same time, they can cause a dangerous level of hypotension.*

CONGESTIVE HEART FAILURE (CHF)

Step 3 as an examination of testing and treatment will spend little time asking for mechanism of disease. The only part of mechanism that matters for congestive failure has to do with the difference in treatment between **systolic dysfunction with a low ejection fraction and diastolic dysfunction** and a **normal ejection fraction.** There is *no* clear way to distinguish systolic from diastolic dysfunction from symptoms alone. Clues in the history are **hypertension, valvular heart disease,** and **myocardial infarction.**

PRESENTATION OF CHF

CHF presents with shortness of breath, particularly on exertion, in a person with any of the following:

- Edema
- Rales on lung examination
- Ascites
- Jugular venous distention
- S3 gallop
- Orthopnea
- Paroxysmal nocturnal dyspnea
- Fatigue

A 63-year-old woman comes to the emergency department with acute, severe shortness of breath; rales on lung exam; S3 gallop; and orthopnea. Which of the following is the most important step?

a. Chest X-ray
b. Oxygen, furosemide, nitrates, and morphine
c. Echocardiogram
d. Digoxin
e. ACE inhibitors
f. Carvedilol

*Answer: The correct answer is B. Oxygen, furosemide, nitrates, and morphine are the mainstay of therapy for **acute pulmonary edema**. Although they are not associated with a concrete mortality benefit, they are the standard of care for pulmonary edema, which is the worst manifestation of CHF. Removing volume from the vascular system and, therefore, the lungs is more important than any form of diagnostic testing. Pulmonary edema is a **clinical diagnosis**. Shortness of breath, rales, S3, and orthopnea are more important in establishing the diagnosis than any single test.*

On CCS, move the clock forward *no more than 15–30 minutes* at a time for acutely unstable ICU or emergency department patients.

DIAGNOSTIC TESTING

All of the following should be ordered on the first screen on the CCS portion of the exam. They should be ordered with the initial therapy (i.e., with the oxygen, furosemide, nitrates, and morphine).

Initial Tests to Be Ordered	What the Tests Show
Chest X-ray	• Pulmonary vascular congestion • Cephalization of flow • Effusion • Cardiomegaly
EKG	• Sinus tachycardia • Atrial and ventricular arrhythmia
Oximeter (consider ordering arterial blood gases, ABG)	• Hypoxia • Respiratory alkalosis
Echocardiogram	• Distinguishes systolic from diastolic dysfunction

> Cases of pulmonary edema and myocardial infarction should be placed in the intensive care unit.

On CCS, the order in which the tests and treatments are written on the screen does not matter, as long as they are written at the same time. *Pulmonary edema* is the perfect example of a CCS in which all the tests should be ordered at the same time as the treatment

> Digoxin is *never* the right answer as an acute treatment for pulmonary edema. Digoxin can be used to slow the rate of atrial fibrillation.

FURTHER MANAGEMENT OF PULMONARY EDEMA

The vast majority of patients with pulmonary edema will respond to *preload reduction alone* to control the acute symptoms.

In a small number of patients, **acute management with a positive inotrope** will be necessary. There is no evidence that any positive inotrope or contractility inducing agent will lower mortality. They are also the answer on a CCS case of pulmonary edema when furosemide, oxygen, nitrates, and morphine are given and the patient is still short of breath after the clock is moved forward.

Positive Inotropic Agents Used Intravenously in the Intensive Care Unit	
Dobutamine (drug of choice) Amrinone Milrinone	These are used as **further management** of acute pulmonary edema cases after the clock is moved forward 30–60 minutes and there is no response to preload reduction.

An 80-year-old woman is admitted to the intensive care unit for acute pulmonary edema. She has rales to the apices and jugulovenous distention. Her EKG shows ventricular tachycardia. Which of the following is the best therapy?

a. Synchronized cardioversion
b. Unsynchronized cardioversion
c. Lidocaine
d. Amiodarone
e. Procainamide

Answer: The correct answer is **A.** Synchronized cardioversion is used when **ventricular tachycardia is associated with acute pulmonary edema.** The same answer would be used if the acute pulmonary edema was associated with the onset of atrial fibrillation, flutter, or supraventricular tachycardia. Unsynchronized cardioversion is used for ventricular fibrillation or ventricular tachycardia without a pulse. Medical therapy, such as lidocaine, amiodarone, or procainamide, can be used for sustained ventricular tachycardia that is hemodynamically stable.

When is nesiritide the answer?

Answer: Nesiritide is a **synthetic version of atrial natriuretic peptide that is used for acute pulmonary edema as a part of preload reduction.** It decreases symptoms of shortness of breath and is not clearly associated with a reduction in mortality. There is no clear indication that the answer is nesiritide.

When is a BNP level the answer?

Answer: BNP or "brain natriuretic peptide" level is **a blood test that can be used to establish a diagnosis of CHF in a patient who is short of breath.** If the presentation is not clear, a BNP level can be used to help distinguish between pulmonary embolus, pneumonia, asthma, and CHF. BNP level goes up in CHF but is rather nonspecific. A normal BNP level excludes CHF.

A patient comes with pulmonary edema. A right heart catheter is placed. Which of the following readings is most likely to be found?

	Cardiac Output	Systemic Vascular Resistance	Wedge Pressure	Right Atrial Pressure
a.	Decreased	Increased	Increased	Increased
b.	Decreased	Increased	Decreased	Decreased
c.	Increased	Decreased	Decreased	Decreased
d.	Decreased	Increased	Decreased	Increased

Answer:

	Cardiac Output	Systemic Vascular Resistance	Wedge Pressure	Right Atrial Pressure
a.	Decreased	Increased	Increased	Increased

*Pulmonary edema is associated with a **decrease in cardiac output because of pump failure**, which results in the **backup of blood into the left atrium and an increased wedge pressure**. There is also an **increase in right atrial pressure**, which is the same as saying jugular venous distention. Increases sympathetic outflow will increase systemic vascular resistance in an attempt to maintain intravascular filling pressure. Choice **B** represents hypovolemic shock, such as dehydration. Choice **C** represents septic shock, which is driven by massive systemic vasodilation, such as from gram-negative sepsis. Choice **D** represents pulmonary hypertension.*

CHRONIC MANAGEMENT OF CONGESTIVE HEART FAILURE

All patients, having been stabilized from acute pulmonary edema, should have an **echocardiogram** to establish whether there is systolic dysfunction with a low ejection fraction or diastolic dysfunction with a normal ejection fraction. Long-term management of dilated cardiomyopathy or systolic dysfunction is based on the use of **ACE inhibitors, beta blockers,** and **spironolactone.** Diuretics are also used but have not been proven to lower mortality. **Digoxin** is used to decrease symptoms and decrease the frequency of hospitalization but has *not* been shown to decrease mortality in congestive failure. **ARBs** can be used interchangeably with **ACE inhibitors.** The two **beta blockers** with evidence for lowering mortality in CHF are metoprolol and carvedilol. ACE inhibitors and beta blockers are indicated for CHF patients with systolic dysfunction at any stage of disease. **Spironolactone** lowers mortality but has only been proven to do so for more advanced, symptomatic disease; any patient originally presenting with pulmonary edema should get spironolactone.

Diastolic dysfunction is reliably treated with beta blockers and diuretics. However, you have to be careful *not* to overuse. The benefit of ACE inhibitors for diastolic dysfunction is not clear. Digoxin and spironolactone definitely do *not* help diastolic dysfunction.

Further management of CHF calls for the following treatments:

> The single most important fact about the "further management" of CHF is that **mortality is decreased by ACE/ARB, beta blockers, and spironolactone.** Digoxin decreases symptoms but does *not* lower mortality.

Systolic Dysfunction (Low Ejection Fraction)	Diastolic Dysfunction (Normal Ejection Fraction)
• ACEI or ARB • Metoprolol or carvedilol • Spironolactone • Diuretics • Digoxin	• Metoprolol or carvedilol • Diuretic

A 69-year-old man is seen in the office for further management of this congestive heart failure. He currently has no symptoms and good exercise tolerance. He has been on lisinopril, metoprolol, spironolactone, and furosemide for the last 6 months. His ejection fraction is 23 percent. Which of the following is most likely to benefit this patient?

a. Intermittent dobutamine therapy

b. Digoxin

c. Cardiac transplantation

d. Implantable cardioverter/defibrillator

e. Chlorthaladone

*Answer: The correct answer is **D.** Implantable cardioverter/defibrillators are indicated in dilated cardiomyopathy. The most common cause of death in CHF is sudden death from arrhythmia. Those with an **ejection fraction below 35 percent that persists** are candidates for implantable defibrillator placement.*

When is a biventricular pacemaker the answer for CHF?

*Answer: Biventricular pacemaker is associated with a decrease in mortality in those with **severe congestive failure and a QRS duration > 130 mSec**. This is also referred to as "cardiac resynchronization therapy."*

When is warfarin the answer for CHF?

Answer: There is no place for routine anticoagulation with warfarin, no matter how low the ejection fraction may be in CHF in the absence of a clot or chronic atrial fibrillation. Warfarin is generally a wrong answer for CHF.

Which of the following is an absolute contraindication to the use of beta blockers?

a. Symptomatic bradycardia

b. Peripheral arterial disease

c. Asthma

d. Emphysema

e. Diabetes

*Answer: The correct answer is **A.** Symptomatic bradycardia is an absolute contraindication for the use of beta blockers. The overwhelming majority of patients with peripheral arterial disease can still use beta blockers. In a patient with a myocardial infarction, the mortality benefit of metoprolol far exceeds the risk of its use when asthma, emphysema, or peripheral arterial disease is present. Two thirds of asthma patients can tolerate beta blockers.*

VALVULAR HEART DISEASE

PRESENTATION

All valvular heart disease presents with **shortness of breath** as the chief complaint. Look for the phrase "**worse with exertion or exercise.**" Hypertension, myocardial infarction, ischemia, increasing age, and rheumatic fever will be in the history but, with the exception of rheumatic heart disease, are probably too nonspecific to give you the diagnosis. Young patients with valvular heart disease will have mitral valve prolapse, hypertrophic obstructive cardiomyopathy, mitral stenosis, or bicuspid aortic valves.

Following are clues to the diagnosis:

Clue to Diagnosis	Diagnosis
Young female, general population	Mitral valve prolapse
Healthy young athlete	Hypertrophic obstructive cardiomyopathy (HOCM)
Immigrant, pregnant	Mitral stenosis
Turner's syndrome, coarctation of aorta	Bicuspid aortic valve
Palpitations, atypical chest pain not with exertion	Mitral valve prolapse

PHYSICAL FINDINGS

All valvular heart disease can be expected to have the following:

- Murmur
- Rales on lung exam

Possible findings on exam are as follows:

- Peripheral edema
- Carotid pulse findings
- Gallops

Therefore, when you suspect valvular disease, select the cardiovascular, chest, and extremities portion of the physical exam.

Murmurs

The most difficult important aspect for the exam is the part of the valvular heart disease section that concerns understanding auscultation, particularly the effects of various maneuvers on these murmurs. **Systolic murmurs** are most commonly aortic stenosis, mitral regurgitation, mitral valve prolapse, and hypertrophic obstructive cardiomyopathy (HOCM). **Diastolic murmurs** are most commonly aortic regurgitation and mitral stenosis. All **right-sided murmurs** increase in intensity with inhalation. All **left-sided murmurs** increase with exhalation.

R	Tricuspid valve both
Inspiration	Stenosis and Regurgitation
G	Pulmonic valve
H	
T	
L	Mitral and aortic valve
Exhalation	lesions
F	
T	

Effects of Valsalva, Standing, Squatting, and Leg Raise

Maneuvers predominantly affect the volume of blood entering the heart. **Squatting and lifting the legs in the air** increase venous return to the heart. **Valsalva maneuver and standing up** suddenly decrease venous return to the heart.

Valsalva maneuver is exhaling against a closed glottis, like bearing down during a bowel movement or blowing against a thumb stuck in the mouth. This **increases intrathoracic pressure,** which decreases blood return to the heart.

When you **suddenly squat,** you are squeezing the veins of the legs, which are rather large. This essentially **squeezes blood up into the heart** like squeezing on a tube of toothpaste. For those too weak to squat suddenly, the physician can **lift up the legs.** This has the same effect as squatting, which is to drain blood into the chest from the lower extremities.

The majority of murmurs increase in intensity with squatting and leg raise. Aortic stenosis (AS), aortic regurgitation (AR), mitral stenosis (MS), mitral regurgitation (MR), and all right-sided heart lesions will become **louder** with squatting and leg raising. The only two murmurs that become **softer** with these maneuvers are mitral valve prolapse (MVP) and hypertrophic obstructive cardiomyopathy (HOCM).

Valvular Lesion	Squatting/Leg Raise (Increase Blood Return)	Standing/Valsalva (Decreased Blood Return)
Aortic stenosis (AS)	Increase	Decrease
Aortic regurgitation (AR)	Increase	Decrease
Mitral stenosis (MS)	Increase	Decrease
Mitral regurgitation (MR)	Increase	Decrease
Ventricular septal defect (VSD)	Increase	Decrease
Hypertrophic obstructive cardiomyopathy (HOCM)	Decrease	Increase
Mitral valve prolapse (MVP)	Decrease	Increase

Effects of Handgrip and Amyl Nitrate

Handgrip is a maneuver that increases afterload by compressing the arteries of the arm by contracting the muscles of the arm. Handgrip does *not* significantly increase venous return to the heart: the veins of the arms are not as large as those of the legs, so compressing them does not make much difference in venous return to the heart. Handgrip, because it increases afterload, essentially functions as the **opposite of an ACE inhibitor,** worsening the murmurs of conditions that would get better with an ACE inhibitor. For instance, AR and MR are treated with ACE inhibitors, because afterload reduction increases the forward flow of blood into the aorta. **Handgrip will, therefore, worsen AR and MR murmurs** by pushing blood backwards into the heart. Handgrip will make the murmurs of AR and MR louder and more intense. The same is true for VSD. **Handgrip worsens the murmur of VSD,** because more blood now goes from the left ventricle into the right ventricle.

Amyl nitrate is a vasodilator that decreases afterload by dilating peripheral arteries. Amyl nitrate has the **opposite effect of handgrip.** Giving amyl nitrate is like giving an ACE inhibitor or ARB. If handgrip worsens AR and MR, then amyl nitrate **improves AR and MR.**

Handgrip improves or lessens the murmurs of MVP and HOCM. The murmurs of MVP and HOCM lessen when the left ventricular chamber is larger or more full. What happens to the size of the left ventricular (LV) chamber if there is increased afterload? The LV chamber will not empty and, therefore, the LV will be larger. A larger LV chamber relieves or lessens the obstruction in HOCM.

Amyl nitrate will do the opposite. It increases ventricular emptying and, therefore, decreases the size of the LV. **Amyl nitrate worsens the murmurs of MVP and HOCM** by increasing the obstruction and the degree of prolapse of the valves in MVP.

The effect of handgrip and amyl nitrate on aortic stenosis can be hard to understand. **Handgrip softens the murmur of aortic stenosis.** This happens by preventing blood from leaving the ventricle; you can't have a murmur if blood is not moving. If afterload goes up, blood can't eject from the LV, and the AS murmur will soften. Another way of saying it is that the murmur of AS is based on the **gradient** between the LV and the aorta. If the LV pressure is greater than the aorta pressure, then the gradient or difference is high. The higher the gradient, the louder the murmur and the more severe the AS is considered. Handgrip increases pressure in the aorta; therefore, the gradient or difference between the LV and aorta decreases. Handgrip is like covering up a trombone or trumpet. You can't produce music if you put a hand over the front of a wind instrument.

Amyl nitrate has exactly the opposite effect on AS compared to handgrip. **Amyl nitrate decreases afterload and decreases the pressure in the aorta, thus increasing the gradient between LV and aorta and worsening (making louder) the murmur of AS.**

Mitral stenosis (MS) is little affected by either handgrip or amyl nitrate. These generally do not affect ventricular filling, which is the major component of MS. ACE inhibitors, likewise, have very little effect on MS.

Valvular Lesion	Handgrip	Amyl Nitrate
Aortic stenosis (AS)	Decrease	Increase
Aortic regurgitation (AR)	Increase	Decrease
Mitral stenosis (MS)	Negligible effect	Negligible effect
Mitral regurgitation (MR)	Increase	Decrease
Ventricular septal defect (VSD)	Increase	Decrease
Hypertrophic obstructive cardiomyopathy (HOCM)	Decrease	Increase
Mitral valve prolapse (MVP)	Decrease	Increase

Location and Radiation of Murmurs

One of the main clues to the identity of a murmur is the location at which the murmur is heard.

- **Aortic stenosis** is heard best at the **second right intercostal space and radiates to the carotid arteries.** It is classically described as a crescendo-decrescendo murmur.
- **Pulmonic valve murmurs** are heard at the **second left intercostal space.**
- **Aortic regurgitation and tricuspid murmurs, as well as VSD murmurs,** are heard at the lower left sternal border.
- **Mitral regurgitation (MR)** is heard at the **apex and radiates into the axilla.** The apex is at the level of the 5th intercostal space, below the left nipple.

Intensity of Murmurs

- I/VI: Only heard with special maneuvers (e.g. Valsalva, handgrip)
- II/VI and III/VI: Majority of murmurs; no objective difference between them
- IV/VI: Thrill present (A thrill is a palpable vibration you can feel from a severe valve lesion.)
- V/VI : Can be heard with stethoscope partially off the chest
- VI/VI: Stethoscope not needed to hear it

> Step 3 USMLE has multimedia—heart sounds are played for you that you must identify.

> USMLE multimedia will show an animation of auscultation at a particular location on the chest wall and then play the sound for you.

DIAGNOSTIC TESTING

The best initial diagnostic test for valve lesions on single best answer questions is an **echocardiogram.** The most accurate test is a **left heart catheterization.** This can also measure pressure gradients, such as in aortic stenosis, most accurately. On CCS cases, you should also add an **EKG and chest X-ray** for valvular lesion assessment.

> Order transthoracic echocardiography (TTE) first on CCS. Then order a transesophageal echocardiogram (TEE) if the TTE is not fully diagnostic.

TREATMENT

Regurgitant lesions are best treated with **vasodilator therapy,** such as ACE inhibitors, ARBs, or nifedipine. Afterload reduction will slow the progression of regurgitant lesions. If handgrip makes it worse, then ACE inhibitors are the "most effective medical therapy." If the patient still progresses despite medical therapy, then surgical replacement of the valve should be performed.

Stenotic lesions are best treated with **anatomic repair.** Mitral stenosis should undergo balloon valvuloplasty, even if the patient is pregnant. Aortic stenosis that is severe must be surgically replaced. Aortic valve replacement is well tolerated even in the very old. Diuretics can decrease pulmonary vascular congestion with stenotic lesions, but they are not as effective or important as anatomic repair.

> - Valsalva improves murmur = diuretics indicated
> - Amyl nitrate improves murmur = ACE inhibitor indicated

Valvular Lesion	Standing/Valsalva	Diuretics Indicated
Aortic stenosis (AS)	Decrease	Yes (replace best)
Aortic regurgitation (AR)	Decrease	Yes
Mitral stenosis (MS)	Decrease	Yes (balloon best)
Mitral regurgitation (MR)	Decrease	Yes
Ventricular septal defect (VSD)	Decrease	Yes
Hypertrophic obstructive cardiomyopathy (HOCM)	Increase	No
Mitral valve prolapse (MVP)	Increase	No

Valvular Lesion	Amyl Nitrate	ACE Inhibitor Indicated
Aortic stenosis (AS)	Increase	No
Aortic regurgitation (AR)	Decrease	Yes
Mitral stenosis (MS)	Negligible effect	No
Mitral regurgitation (MR)	Decrease	Yes
Ventricular septal defect (VSD)	Decrease	Yes
Hypertrophic obstructive cardiomyopathy (HOCM)	Increase	No
Mitral valve prolapse (MVP)	Increase	No

AORTIC STENOSIS (AS)

Aortic stenosis most commonly presents with **chest pain.** Syncope and CHF are less common presentations. The patient will be **older** and often has a history of **hypertension.** Coronary artery disease will be present in as many as 50 percent of patients.

> On CCS, the intensity, radiation, and location of the murmur will automatically be given to you with the cardiovascular examination. You do *not* need to ask for them separately.

Prognosis

- **Coronary disease:** 3- to 5-year average survival
- **Syncope:** 2- to 3-year average survival
- **CHF:** 1.5- to 2-year average survival

Physical Exam

Choose the cardiovascular exam (CV), chest, and extremities.

AS gives a crescendo-decrescendo systolic murmur. The murmur will be heard best at the second right intercostal space and radiate to the carotid arteries. The murmur will increase in intensity with leg raising, squatting, and amyl nitrate. The murmur will decrease with Valsalva, standing, and handgrip. The case may describe delayed carotid upstroke as well.

Diagnostic Testing

The **transthoracic echocardiogram (TTE)** is the best initial diagnostic test. A **transesophageal echocardiogram (TEE)** is more accurate. **Left heart catheterization** is the most accurate diagnostic test and allows the most accurate method of assessing the pressure gradient across the valve. The normal gradient is < 30 mm Hg. Moderate disease is indicated by 30–70 mm Hg, and severe disease is indicated by a gradient > 70 mm Hg. For CCS cases, also choose an **EKG** and a **chest X-ray,** which will show **left ventricular hypertrophy.**

Treatment

Diuretics are the best initial therapy but will not alter long-term prognosis. Further, **overdiuresis is dangerous,** and use of diuretics needs to be very judicious. **The treatment of choice is valve replacement.** Bioprosthetic valves (porcine, bovine) will last 10 years on average, but do *not* require anticoagulation with warfarin. Mechanical valves do *not* have to be replaced but must be also treated with warfarin to an INR of 2–3. Valve replacement is well tolerated, even in the elderly.

AORTIC REGURGITATION (AR)

Hypertension, rheumatic heart disease, endocarditis, and cystic medial necrosis cause AR. Rarer causes are Marfan's syndrome, ankylosing spondylitis, syphilis, and reactive arthritis. Reactive arthritis is an inflammatory arthritis of large joints, inflammation of the eyes (conjunctivitis and uveitis), and urethritis, previously commonly referred to as Reiter's syndrome. **Shortness of breath and fatigue are the most common presentation.**

Physical Exam

Choose the cardiovascular exam (CV), chest, and extremities.

The murmur of AR is a **diastolic decrescendo murmur heard best at the left sternal border.** There are several unique physical findings that are rarely seen with AR. The murmur will increase in intensity with leg raising, squatting, and handgrip.

- **Quinke pulse:** Arterial or capillary pulsations in the fingernails
- **Corrigan's pulse:** High bounding pulses (also known as a "water-hammer pulse")
- **Musset's sign:** Head bobbing up and down with each pulse
- **Duroziez's sign:** Murmur heard over the femoral artery
- **Hill sign:** Blood pressure gradient much higher in the lower extremities

Diagnostic Testing

TTE is the best initial diagnostic test. **TEE** is more accurate. **Left heart catheterization** is the most accurate test. For CCS cases, also choose an EKG and a chest X-ray, which will show left ventricular hypertrophy.

Treatment

ACE inhibitors, ARBs, and nifedipine are the best initial therapy. For CCS cases, you should add a **loop diuretic,** such as furosemide. **Surgery** is the answer when the ejection fraction drops below 55 percent or the left ventricular end systolic diameter goes above 55 mm; surgery should be done in patients with these criteria even if they are asymptomatic.

MITRAL STENOSIS (MS)

Rheumatic fever is the most common cause of MS. Look for an **immigrant patient** because of the low rates of rheumatic fever in the United States. Also look for a **pregnant patient** because of the large increase in plasma volume with pregnancy. Special features of MS are as follows:

- **Dysphagia:** Large left atrium pressing on the esophagus
- **Hoarseness:** Pressure on recurrent laryngeal nerve
- **Atrial fibrillation** leading to stroke

Physical Exam

Choose the cardiovascular exam (CV), chest, and extremities.

The murmur of MS is a **diastolic rumble after an opening snap,** which can be described as an "extra sound" in diastole. The S1 is louder. As the mitral stenosis worsens, the opening snap moves closer to S2. The murmur will increase in intensity with leg raising, squatting, and expiration.

Diagnostic Testing

TTE is the best initial diagnostic test. **TEE** is more accurate. **Left heart catheterization** is the most accurate test. For CCS cases, also choose an **EKG and a chest X-ray,** which will show left atrial hypertrophy. On chest X-ray, there is **straightening of the left heart border and elevation of the left mainstem bronchus.** There may also be a description of a double density in the cardiac silhouette (from left atrial enlargement).

Treatment

Diuretics are the best initial therapy. They do *not* alter progression. **Balloon valvuloplasty** is the most effective therapy. Pregnant women can and should be readily treated with balloon valvuloplasty. Pregnancy is *not* a contraindication to valvuloplasty.

MITRAL REGURGITATION (MR)

MR is caused by **hypertension, ischemic heart disease, and any other condition that leads to dilation of the heart.** You cannot have dilation of the heart without the mitral valve leaflets separating. **Dyspnea on exertion** is the most common complaint.

Physical Exam

Choose the cardiovascular exam (CV), chest, and extremities.

The murmur of MR is **holosystolic and obscures both S1 and S2.** MR is **heard best at the apex and radiates to the axilla.** The murmur increases in intensity with leg raising, squatting, and handgrip. Standing, Valsalva, and amyl nitrate decrease the intensity. S3 gallop is often present.

Diagnostic Testing

TTE is the best initial diagnostic test. **TEE** is more accurate

Treatment

ACE inhibitors, ARBs, and nifedipine are the best initial therapy and the medications must likely to decrease the rate of progression of the disease. For CCS cases, you should add a loop diuretic, such as furosemide. **Surgery** is the answer when the left ventricular ejection fraction drops below 60 percent or the left ventricular end systolic diameter goes above 45 mm. Surgery should be done in patients with these criteria even if they are asymptomatic.

The operative criteria for regurgitant lesions in asymptomatic patients are as follows:

	Aortic Regurgitation	Mitral Regurgitation
Ejection fraction	< 55%	< 60%
Left ventricular end systolic diameter	> 55 mm	> 45mm

VENTRICULAR SEPTAL DEFECT (VSD)

Asymptomatic patients may present with only a **holosystolic murmur at the lower left sternal border.** Larger defects leads to **shortness of breath.** The murmur worsens with exhalation, squatting, and leg raise.

Diagnostic Testing

Echocardiography is the diagnostic test to use first, but **catheterization** is used to determine the degree of left-to-right shunting most precisely.

Treatment

Mild defects can be left without mechanical closure.

ATRIAL SEPTAL DEFECT (ASD)

Small ASDs are **asymptomatic.** Larger ones may lead to **shortness of breath** or signs of right ventricular failure, such as **shortness of breath and a parasternal heave.** The most frequently tested knowledge is that **ASD is associated with fixed splitting of S2.**

Treatment

Percutaneous or catheter devices are the best therapy. **Repair** is most often indicated when the shunt ratio exceeds 1.5 to 1.

S3 gallop is associated with fluid overload states, such as congestive heart failure or mitral regurgitation. An S3 can be normal in patients under the age of 30.

SPLITTING OF S2

Wide, P2 Delayed	Paradoxical, A2 Delayed	Fixed
• Right bundle branch block • Pulmonic stenosis • Right ventricular hypertrophy • Pulmonary hypertension	• Left bundle branch block • Aortic stenosis • Left ventricular hypertrophy • Hypertension	ASD

CARDIOMYOPATHY

DILATED CARDIOMYOPATHY

Dilated cardiomyopathy presents and is managed **in the same way as the case of CHF** described above.

Diagnostic Testing

Echocardiography is the best initial test to determine the ejection fraction and look for wall motion activity. MUGA or nuclear ventriculography is the most accurate method of determining ejection fraction.

Treatment

Besides **ischemia,** the most common causes of dilated cardiomyopathy are **alcohol, adriamycin, radiation, and Chagas's disease.** The treatment for *all* forms of dilated cardiomyopathy, no matter their cause, is with **ACE inhibitors, ARBs, beta blockers, and spironolactone.** Digoxin decreases symptoms but does *not* prolong survival.

HYPERTROPHIC CARDIOMYOPATHY

This condition presents with **shortness of breath on exertion and an S4 gallop** on examination.

Diagnostic Testing

Echocardiography shows a normal ejection fraction.

Treatment

The mainstay of therapy is with **beta blockers and diuretics.** ACE inhibitors can be used, but their benefit is not as clear. Digoxin and spironolactone do *not* benefit hypertrophic cardiomyopathy.

> S4 gallop is a sign of left ventricular hypertrophy and decreased compliance or stiffness of the ventricle. S4 gallop does not automatically indicate the need for additional therapy.

RESTRICTIVE CARDIOMYOPATHY

Restrictive cardiomyopathy presents with a history of **sarcoidosis, amyloidosis, hemochromatosis, cancer, myocardial fibrosis, or glycogen storage diseases. Shortness of breath** is the main presenting complaint in all forms of cardiomyopathy. **Kussmaul's sign** is present: this is an increase in jugular venous pressure on inhalation.

Diagnostic Testing

Cardiac catheterization shows rapid x and y descent. The **EKG** shows low voltage. **Echocardiography** is the mainstay of diagnosis. **Endomyocardial biopsy** is the single most accurate diagnostic test of the etiology.

Treatment

Diuretics and correcting the underlying cause are the best treatments.

PERICARDIAL DISEASE

PERICARDITIS

Chest pain that is **pleuritic** (changes with respiration) and **positional** (relieved by sitting up and leaning forward) is the presentation that is given on Step 3. The pain will be described as **sharp and brief.** Ischemic pain is dull and sore, like being punched. The vast majority of pericarditis cases are viral. Although any infectious agent, collagen-vascular disease, or trauma can be in the history, remember that Step 3 most often hands you a clear diagnosis and asks what you want to do about it, such as testing and treatment.

Physical Exam

The only pertinent positive finding is a **friction rub,** which can have three components. The rub is only present in 30 percent of patients. There is *no* pulsus paradoxus, tenderness, edema, or Kussmaul's sign present. Blood pressure is *normal,* and there is *no* jugular venous distention or organomegaly.

Diagnostic Testing

The best initial test is the **EKG. ST segment elevation** is present everywhere (all leads). **PR segment depression** is pathognomonic but is not always present.

Treatment

The best initial therapy is an **NSAID,** such as indomethacin, naprosyn, aspirin, or ibuprofen. Advance the clock 1–2 days and have the patient visit the office. If the pain persists, add **prednisone orally** to the treatment and advance the clock 1–2 more days.

PERICARDIAL TAMPONADE

Tamponade presents with **shortness of breath, hypotension, and jugular venous distention.** On CCS, also examine the **lungs,** because they will be clear.

Following are the unique features of tamponade:

- **Pulsus paradoxus:** This is a decrease of blood pressure > 10 mm Hg on inhalation.
- **Electrical alternans:** This is alterations of the axis of the QRS complex on EKG, manifested as the height of the QRS complex.

Diagnostic Testing

Echocardiography is the most accurate diagnostic test. The earliest finding of tamponade is **diastolic collapse of the right atrium and right ventricle.** Remember that it is normal to have 50 ml or less of pericardial fluid, but there should be *no* collapse of the cardiac structures.

EKG will show low voltage and electrical alternans. Electrical alternans is variation of the height of the QRS complex from the heart moving backwards and forwards in the chest.

Right heart catheterization will show "equalization" of all the pressures in the heart during diastole. The wedge pressure will be the same as the right atrial and pulmonary artery diastolic pressure.

Treatment

- Best initial therapy: **Pericardiocentesis**
- Most effective long-term therapy: **Pericardial window placement**
- Most dangerous therapy: Diuretics

CONSTRICTIVE PERICARDITIS

Constrictive pericarditis presents with **shortness of breath** and the following **signs of chronic right heart failure:**

- Edema
- Jugular venous distention
- Hepatosplenomegaly
- Ascites

Following are the unique features of contrictive pericarditis:

- **Kussmaul's sign:** Increase in jugular venous pressure on inhalation
- **Pericardial knock:** Extra diastolic sound from the heart hitting a calcified, thickened pericardium

Diagnostic Testing

- **Chest X-ray:** Showing calcification
- **EKG:** Low voltage
- **CT and MRI:** Showing thickening of the pericardium

Treatment

- Best initial therapy: **Diuretic**
- Most effective therapy: **surgical removal of the Pericardium** (i.e., pericardial stripping)

AORTIC DISEASE

DISSECTION OF THE THORACIC AORTA

Dissection of the thoracic aorta presents with the following symptoms:

- Chest pain **radiating to the back between the scapula**
- Pain that can be described as *very* severe and "ripping"
- **Difference in blood pressure between right and left arms**

Diagnostic Testing

- Best initial test: **Chest X-ray showing a widened mediastinum**
- Most accurate test: **CT angiography**

Treatment

When the case describes **severe chest pain radiating to the back and hypertension,** order **beta blockers** with the first screen in addition to an **EKG and chest X-ray.** No matter what the EKG shows, move the clock forward and order either **CT angiography, TEE,** or **magnetic resonance angiography (MRA):** all three are equally accurate.

- CT angiography = TEE = Magnetic resonance angiography (MRA)

After starting beta blockers, order **nitroprusside** to control the blood pressure.

Aortic dissection cases should be placed in the **ICU,** and a **surgical consultation** should be ordered. **Surgical correction** is the most effective therapy.

ABDOMINAL AORTIC ANEURYSM (AAA)

Screening with an **ultrasound** should be ordered in **over-65 men who were smokers.**

PERIPHERAL ARTERIAL DISEASE (PAD)

PAD presents with **claudication** (pain in the calves on exertion). The case may also describe **"smooth, shiny skin"** with **loss of hair and sweat glands,** as well as **loss of pulses in the feet.**

Diagnostic Testing
- Best initial test: **Ankle: brachial index (ABI)** (A normal ABI should be ≥ 0.9. Blood pressure in the legs should be equal to or greater than the pressure in the arms. If there is > **10 percent difference,** then an obstruction is present.)
- Most accurate test: **Angiography**

Treatment
- Best initial therapy:

  - **Aspirin**
  - **Blood pressure control with ACE inhibitors**
  - **Exercise as tolerated**
  - **Cilostazol**
  - **Lipid control with statins to a target LDL < 100**

- Marginally effective therapy: **Pentoxyfilene**
- Ineffective therapy: Calcium channel blocker

- Pain + Pallor + Pulseless = Arterial Occlusion

On CCS, move the clock forward several weeks. PAD is *not* an emergency! If initial therapies do *not* work and the pain progresses, *or* there are signs of ischemia such as gangrene or pain at rest, then perform surgical bypass.

RHYTHM DISORDERS

ATRIAL FIBRILLATION (A-FIB)

A-fib presents with **palpitations and an irregular pulse** in a person with a history of hypertension, ischemia, or cardiomyopathy.

Spinal stenosis will give pain that is worse with walking downhill and less with walking uphill or while cycling or sitting. Pulses and skin exam will be normal with spinal stenosis.

Abdominal aortic aneurysm is detected by ultrasound first. AAAs are repaired when they are > 5 cm. Smaller ones are monitored.

Acute arterial embolus will be very **sudden in onset** with **loss of pulse and a cold extremity.** It is also quite painful. AS and atrial fibrillation are often in the history for arterial embolus.

Beta blockers are *not* contraindicated with PAD. If the patient needs them for ischemic disease, they should be used.

Diagnostic Testing

If the initial EKG does not show the answer, a patient in the hospital should be placed on **telemetry monitoring.** Outpatients who are hemodynamically stable should undergo **Holter monitoring,** which is continuous, ambulatory cardiac rhythm monitoring for 24 hours or longer.

For CCS cases, other tests to order once A-fib is found on EKG are the following:

- **Echocardiography:** Looking for clots, valve function, and left atrial size
- **Thyroid function testing:** T4 and TSH levels
- **Electrolytes:** Potassium, magnesium, and calcium levels
- **Troponin or CK-MB levels:** These may be appropriate to test in some acute-onset cases.

Treatment

Unstable patients should undergo immediate **synchronized electrical cardioversion.** Unstable patients should be cardioverted with the **first screen,** without waiting for TEE or anticoagulation with heparin or warfarin. *Instability* is defined as a systolic blood pressure < 90, congestive failure, confusion related to hemodynamic instability, or chest pain.

Stable patients should have their ventricular heart rate slowed if it is > 100 per minute.

Rate control medications are **beta blockers** (metoprolol, esmolol), **calcium channel blockers** (diltiazem), or **digoxin.** In the acute setting, such as the emergency department, these agents should be given intravenously.

Once the rate has been controlled, **anticoagulation with warfarin to a target INR of 2–3** is the next best step in all patients with an atrial arrhythmia persisting beyond two days. If the question does not state the duration, you are to treat it as if it were persisting for longer than 2 days.

Routine cardioversion of atrial fibrillation is *not* indicated.

The long-term use of **rate control medications,** such as metoprolol, diltiazem, or digoxin, **combined with anticoagulation** is equal or better than cardioversion with electricity or medications.

ATRIAL FLUTTER (A-FLUTTER)

Atrial flutter is managed **in the same way as atrial fibrillation.** The only difference is that the **rhythm is regular** on presentation.

The following table shows how to choose the right rate control medication for a-fib and a-flutter.

Beta Blockers (Metoprolol)	Calcium Channel Blockers (Diltiazem)	Digoxin
• Ischemic heart disease • Migraines • Graves's disease • Pheochromocytoma	• Asthma • Migraine	• Borderline hypotension

MULTIFOCAL ATRIAL TACHYCARDIA (MAT)

This condition presents like an **atrial arrhythmia in association with COPD/ emphysema.** EKG will show **polymorphic P waves,** revealing different atrial foci for the QRS complexes. As the name implies, patients with MAT have **tachycardia** (heart rate > 100). MAT manifests as an **irregular chaotic rhythm** on EKG. DO NOT USE BETA BLOCKERS OR DIGOXIN.

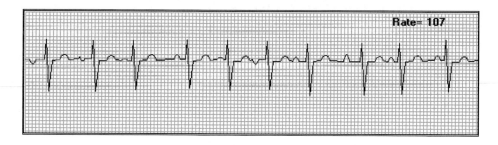

SUPRAVENTRICULAR TACHYCARDIA (SVT)

SVT presents with **palpitations and tachycardia** and occasionally syncope. It is *not* associated with ischemic heart disease. SVT has a **regular rhythm with a ventricular rate of 160–180.**

Diagnostic Testing

If the EKG does not show SVT, order **Holter monitor** or **telemetry** to increase the sensitivity of detection.

On CCS, all cases of dysrhythmia should undergo **echocardiography (TTE)** after the initial set of orders.

Treatment

- Best initial management for *unstable* patients: **Synchronized cardioversion**
- Best initial management for *stable* patients: **Vagal maneuvers** (carotid sinus massage, ice immersion of the face, Valsalva)
- Next best step in management if vagal maneuvers do *not* work: **Intravenous adenosine** (Note: This is the most frequently asked SVT question.)
- Best long-term management: **Radiofrequency catheter ablation**

WOLFF-PARKINSON-WHITE SYNDROME (WPW)

WPW presents as **SVT that can alternate with ventricular tachycardia** (VT). The other main clue to the diagnosis is **worsening of SVT after the use of calcium blockers or digoxin.**

Diagnostic Testing

WPW is diagnosed with finding a **delta wave on the EKG.** The most accurate test is **electrophysiologic studies.**

Treatment

Treatment is as follows:

- Best initial therapy *if* the patient is described as being in SVT or VT from WPW: **Procainamide**
- Best long-term therapy: **Radiofrequency catheter ablation**

VENTRICULAR TACHYCARDIA (VT)

VT can present as **palpitation, syncope, chest pain, or sudden death.**

Diagnostic Testing

You cannot determine that VT is present without an **EKG.** If the EKG does not detect VT, then **telemetry monitoring** should be ordered. The most accurate diagnostic test is **electrophysiologic studies.**

Treatment

The table below shows therapy options for persistent VT:

Hemodynamically Stable	Hemodynamically Unstable
• Amiodarone • Lidocaine • Procainamide • Magnesium	• Synchronized cardioversion

VENTRICULAR FIBRILLATION (V-FIB)

V-fib presents as **sudden death.**

Diagnostic Testing

You cannot tell what caused the loss of pulse without an **EKG.**

Treatment

Treatment of V-fib is *always* with **unsynchronized cardioversion** first. Do *not* answer intubation first. Dead people are never breathing. If you shock them back to life, they are more likely to breath!

Unsynchronized	Synchronized
anywhere in EKG	"no shock T"
Indication: VFIB	*Indication:* AFIB

> **Torsade de pointe** is ventricular tachycardia with an undulating amplitude. **Magnesium** should always be given in addition to **medical or electrical therapy.**

Unsynchronized cardioversion (defibrillation) is administered as follows:

1. Continue CPR
2. Reattempt defibrillation
3. Administer IV epinephrine or vasopressin
4. Reattempt defibrillation
5. Administer IV amiodarone or lidocaine
6. Reattempt defibrillation
7. Repeat several cycles of CPR between each shock

SYNCOPE EVALUATION

The management of syncope is based on three criteria:

1. Was the loss of consciousness sudden or gradual?

Sudden Loss of Consciousness	Gradual Loss of Consciousness
• Cardiac etiology • Neurologic (seizures)	• Toxic-metabolic problems • Hypoglycemia • Drug toxicity/intoxication • Anemia • Hypoxia

2. Was the regaining of consciousness sudden or gradual?

Sudden Regaining of Consciousness	Gradual Regaining of Consciousness
• Cardiac etiology • Rhythm disorder versus structural disease	• Neurologic (seizures)

3. Cardiac exam

Cardiac Exam Normal	Cardiac Exam Abnormal

• Ventricular arrhythmia	• Structural heart disease
	  - Aortic stenosis
	  - HOCM
	  - Mitral stenosis
	  - Mitral valve prolapse (rare)

DIAGNOSTIC TESTING

On the initial screen, order the following:

- Cardiac and neurological examination
- EKG
- Chemistries (glucose)
- Oximeter
- CBC
- Cardiac enzymes (CK-MB, troponin)

Treat special circumstances as follows:

- If a murmur **is present,** order an echocardiogram.
- If the **neurological exam is** focal **or there is a** history of head trauma **due to syncope,** order head CT.
- If a headache **is described,** order head CT.
- If a **seizure is described or suspected,** order head CT and EEG.

On further management, if the diagnosis is not clear after you move the clock forward to obtain the results of initial tests, order the following:

- Holter monitor on outpatients
- Telemetry monitoring for inpatients
- Repeat check of CK-MB and troponin levels 4 hours later
- Urine and blood toxicology screens

On further management, particularly if the etiology is not clear, order the following:

- <u>Tilt table testing</u> to diagnose neurocardiogenic (vasovagal) syncope
- **Electrophysiological testing**

TREATMENT

Treatment of syncope is based on the etiology. The majority of cases never get a specific diagnosis. The *most* important thing to do in syncope is to **exclude a cardiac etiology, such as an arrhythmia.** The majority (> 80 percent) of mortality from syncope involves a cardiac etiology.

If a ventricular dysrhythmia is diagnosed as the etiology of syncope, **an implantable cardioverter/defibrillator** is indicated.

ENDOCRINOLOGY

4

DIABETES

DIAGNOSTIC TESTING

Diagnosis is made with *one* of the following:

1. *Two* **fasting glucose > 126**
2. **One random glucose > 200 with symptoms** (poluyuria, polydipsia, polyphagia)
3. **Abnormal glucose tolerance test** (2-hour glucose tolerance test with 75 g glucose load)

Although an elevated hemoglobin A1c (HgA1c) is consistent with diabetes, an abnormal HgA1c is *not* one of the diagnostic criteria for diabetes.

TYPE 2 DIABETES

Treatment

Diet, exercise, and weight loss are the best initial therapy for type 2 diabetes. Of patients with type 2, 25 percent can be controlled with exercise and weight loss alone.

The best initial medical therapy is **metformin.** Metformin is particularly beneficial in obese patients, because it does not lead to added weight gain. Sulfonylurea medications, because they increase the release of insulin, lead to increased weight gain.

A 65-year-old Hispanic man is seen in the office for follow-up. He was placed on metformin for type 2 diabetes after not responding to modifications of diet and exercise several months ago. Despite maximal doses of metformin, his blood glucose is > 150 mg/dl, and his HgA1c is above 7 percent. What is the next best step in management?

a. Add glyburide
b. Add insulin subcutaneously
c. Add insulin pump
d. Add rosiglitazone
e. Add acarbose or miglitol
f. Switch to a sulfonylurea

*Answer: The correct answer is **A**. If a patient with type 2 diabetes cannot be adequately controlled with metformin, then add a second medication. The greatest efficacy and safety is with a **sulfonylurea**. If the question describes a patient originally placed on a sulfonylurea but not adequately controlled, then add metformin. There are several options before having to start insulin.*

- **Metformin:** This agent works by **blocking gluconeogenesis.** The following are the main advantages of starting with metformin:
  - No risk of hypoglycemia
  - Does not increase obesity

- Metformin is *contraindicated* with the following:
  - **Renal insufficiency:** The metformin may accumulate and increase the risk of lactic acidosis.
  - **Use of contrast agents** for any radiologic or angiographic procedure: The contrast agents may lead to acute renal failure and, therefore, to the accumulation of metformin.

- **Sulfonylureas:** These are **glyburide, glimepiride, and glipizide.** These agents work by causing the **increased release of insulin** from the pancreas. Following are the *adverse effects* of sulfonylureas:
  - Hypoglycemia
  - SIADH

- **Thiazolidinediones:** These are **rosiglitazone and pioglitazone.** These agents work by **increasing peripheral insulin sensitivity.** They may worsen congestive heart failure and must be used with caution.

- **Alpha-glucosidase inhibitors:** These are **acarbose and miglitol.** These agents **block the absorption of glucose at the intestinal lining.** They can lead to diarrhea, abdominal pain, bloating and flatulence in much the same way as lactose intolerance.

- **Insulin secretagogues:** These are **nateglinide and repaglinide.** These agents work in a **very similar fashion as sulfonylureas.** They are short acting and can cause hypoglycemia.

> If other agents do not sufficiently control the level of glucose, then the patient is switched to **insulin**. A **long-acting insulin**, such as insulin glargine, which is a once-a-day injection with an extremely steady-state level of insulin, is used in combination with a **very short-acting insulin** at meal time.

- **Long-acting insulin**
  - **Glargine (Lantus®):** Once a day
  - **NPH:** Twice a day

- **Short-acting insulin:** Both of the following medications are given at mealtime and last about 2 hours. Regular insulin is given at mealtime but lasts longer, as much as 6 hours.
  - **Aspart**
  - **Lispro**

TYPE I DIABETES (JUVENILE ONSET)

Type 1 diabetes always results from **underproduction of insulin**. The **pancreas is destroyed** during childhood on an autoimmune/genetic basis.

These patients are thin and do *not* respond to weight loss, exercise, or oral hypoglycemic agents. Sulfonlyureas do *not* work, because there is no functioning pancreas to stimulate to increase insulin release from.

Type 1 diabetics are more prone to developing **diabetic ketoacidosis** because of severe insulin deficiency.

The table below compares type 1 and type 2 diabetes.

Diabetes	Type 1	Type 2
Onset	Juvenile	Adult
Body type	Thin	Obese
Diabetic Ketoacidosis (DKA)	Frequent	Rare
Treatment	Insulin	Lifestyle management, oral agents, or insulin

DIABETIC KETOACIDOSIS (DKA)

DKA presents as an extremely ill patient with **hyperventilation** as compensation for the **metabolic acidosis** (low bicarbonate). The patient also has a **"fruity" odor of the breath** from acetone and possibly **confusion** from the hyperosmolar state.

Diagnostic Testing

- Best initial test: **Serum bicarbonate** is the best way to determine the severity of illness. If the glucose level is high, this does *not* tell you that the patient has become acidotic. The patient may just have hyperglycemia. A **low serum bicarbonate** implies an elevated anion gap, and this is the marker for severe DKA.
- **Beta hydroxybutyrate** can also be obtained as a marker of ketone production. As you correct the ketoacidosis, the betahydroxybutyrate level should decrease.

Lab findings in DKA are as follows:

- **Hyperglycemia (> 250)**
- **Hyperkalemia:** Initially there will be *hyper*kalemia. This is from transcellular shift of potassium out of the cell in exchange for Hydrogen ions going into the cell. The cells "suck up acid" as a way of compensating for the severe metabolic acidosis and release potassium in exchange. Also, insulin drives potassium into cells with glucose. If there is no insulin, potassium builds up outside the cell. The hyperkalemia will quickly translate into *hypo*kalemia as you treat the DKA. So it is very important to make sure you **supplement with potassium.**
- **Decreased serum bicarbonate**
- **Low pH,** with low pCO2 as respiratory compensation
- **Acetone, acetoacetate, and beta hydroxybutyrate levels elevated**
- **Elevated anion gap**

- Acidosis = Hyperkalemia
- Alkalosis = Hypokalemia

Treatment

On this initial screen, order both the **labs** (chemistry, arterial blood gas, acetone level) and **fluids** (bolus of normal saline).

Once the high glucose and the low serum bicarbonate are found, order **IV insulin.** CCS does not require you to know doses, and, in fact, there is no way for you to write in a dose.

- **High glucose + Low bicarb = DKA** → Give bolus saline and IV insulin

---

As you move the clock forward, you will notice that the potassium level drops into the normal range. Insulin drives potassium into cells, and as the acidosis corrects, the potassium level drops. At this point, you should **add potassium to the IV fluids.**

> In a patient with DKA, the total body level of potassium is low. Chronic hyperkalemia depletes the body of potassium.

COMPLICATIONS OF DIABETES

This is an excellent choice for an "office-based" setting of follow-up management on CCS.

Hypertension

The goal of management of hypertension in diabetes is a **BP < 130/80.** This is less than the usual goal of < 140/90 in the general population. BP control is critical in diabetes to prevent long-term complications to the heart, eye, kidney, and brain.

Lipid Management

Diabetes is a coronary artery disease (CAD) equivalent. The LDL goal in a diabetic is < **100.** When the patient has *both* CAD and diabetes, the LDL goal is < **70.**

Retinopathy

A **dilated eye exam** should occur yearly in diabetics to detect **proliferative retinopathy.** If this is present, **laser photocoagulation** should be performed.

Nephropathy

Order a **urine microalbumin,** which detects minute amounts of albumin in the urine. If *any* form of protein, no matter how small, is present, give **ACE inhibitors.** Use ACE inhibitors for proteinuria even if the blood pressure is normal. ARBs have the same indication. Furthermore, use ACE inhibitors as first-line hypertensive agents in diabetics.

Neuropathy

Foot examination yearly for diabetic neuropathy is indicated. If neuropathy is present, diagnostic testing is *not* necessary; go straight to treatment. Use **gabapentin** or **pregabalin.** Tricyclic antidepressants and carbamazepine are not as effective.

Erectile Dysfunction

There is no routine screening test for this condition except to **ask about its presence.** Treat with sildenafil and other phosphodiesterase inhibitors as usual. Remember: *No* sildenafil with nitrates!

Gastroparesis

The major stimulant for gastric motility is "stretch." In patients with longstanding diabetes, there is impaired ability to perceive stretch in the GI tract and impaired motility. Look for "bloating," constipation, abdominal fullness, and diarrhea. Treat with **metoclopromide** or **erythromycin.** Erythromycin increases the release of "motilin," a promotility GI hormone. You can also confirm the diagnosis with a gastric-emptying scan, but this is often unnecessary.

A 63-year-old man with longstanding diabetes comes to the office with a "pins and needles" sensation in both his feet. He is also chronically bloated and constipated. On review of systems, you find he cannot maintain erection sufficiently to complete intercourse. Urinalysis shows microalbuminuria. His LDL is 147. What is the best management for this patient?

a. HgA1c
b. Nerve conduction studies
c. Hydralazine and sildenafil
d. Ramipril, erythromycin, atorvostatin, and pregabalin
e. Gastric-emptying study and penile tumescence studies

*Answer: The correct answer is **D:** prescribe ACE inhibitors for the proteinuria, erythromycin for the diabetic gastroparesis and to increase GI motility, atorvostatin to decrease the LDL level to < 100 for a patient, and pregabalin for diabetic neuropathy. No further specific diagnostic tests are required when you see this collection of abnormalities.*

THYROID DISEASE

The following table shows the clinical presentation of hypo- and hyperthyroidism.

	Hypothyroidism	Hyperthyroidism
Weight	Gain	Loss
Intolerance	Cold	Heat
Hair	Course	Fine
Skin	Dry	Moist
Mental	Depressed	Anxious
Heart	Bradycardia	Tachycardia, tachyarrhythmias such as atrial fibrillation
Muscle	Weak	Weak
Reflexes	Diminished	
Fatigue	Yes	Yes
Menstrual changes	Yes	Yes

HYPOTHYROIDISM

This condition arises most often from "burnt out" Hashimoto's thyroiditis. It presents as a slow, tired, fatigued patient with weight gain.

Following are the best initial tests:

- **T4:** Decreased
- **Thyroid-stimulating hormone (TSH):** Increased

Treat with **T4** or **thyroxine replacement.** T4 will be converted in the local tissues to T3 as needed.

HYPERTHYROIDISM

All forms of hyperthyroidism give an **elevated T4 level.** Almost all give a **suppressed TSH level.**

The table below summarizes the presentation and treatment of four forms of hyperthyroidism.

	Grave's	Silent	Subacute	Pituitary adenoma
Physical findings	Eye, skin, and nail findings	None	Tender gland	None
RAIU	Elevated	Low	Low	Elevated
Treatment	Radioactive iodine ablation	None	Asprin	Surgical removal

Grave's Disease

In addition to the findings of hyperthyroidism described above, Grave's disease has several unique physical findings:

- **Ophthalmopathy:** The symptoms of ophthalmopathy include exophthalmos (eyes are bulging) and proptosis (lid is retracted).

- **Dermopathy:** This is thickening and redness of the skin just below the knee.
- **Onycolysis:** Occurring in only 10 percent of cases, this is separation of the nail from the nailbed.

The radioactive iodine uptake (RAIU) level is elevated.

Treatment is as follows:

- Use **propylthiouracil (PTU)** or **methimazole** acutely to bring the gland under control.
- Then use **radioactive iodine** to ablate the gland.
- Use **propranolol** to treat sympathetic symptoms, such as tremors, palpitations, etc.

"Silent" Thyroiditis

This condition is an autoimmune process with a **nontender gland and hyperthyroidism.** There are *no* eye, skin, or nail findings.

Unlike Grave's disease, the radioactive iodine uptake (RAIU) test is normal, since this is not a hyperfunctioning gland; it is just "leaking." **Antibodies to thyroid peroxidase and antithyroglobulin antibodies** may be present. There is *no* treatment.

Subacute Thyroiditis

This condition has a viral etiology (we think!) and presents with a **tender gland.**

Diagnostic testing shows the following:

- **RAIU is low.**
- **T4 is high.**
- **TSH is low,** but that is not specific to this form of hyperthyroidism.

Treat with **aspirin** to relieve pain.

Pituitary Adenoma

This condition is rare. It is the *only* cause of hyperthyroidism with an **elevated TSH.**

Treat as follows:

- **MRI** the brain.
- **Remove adenoma.**

Exogenous Thyroid Hormone Abuse

The **T4 is up** and the **TSH suppressed.** However, the **thyroid gland will atrophy** to the point of nonpalpability on examination.

Thyroid "Storm"

Acute severe, life-threatening hyperthyroidism is also known as "thyroid storm."

Treat as follows:

- **Iodine:** Blocks uptake of iodine into the thyroid gland.
- **Propylthiouracil or methimazole:** Blocks production of thyroxine.
- **Dexamethasone:** Blocks peripheral conversion of T4 to T3.
- **Propranolol:** Blocks target organ effect.

GOITER

You *cannot* determine etiology only from the presence of a goiter. An enlarged gland can be associated with hyperthyroidism, hypothyroidism, or normal function of the thyroid.

SOLITARY THYROID NODULE

Perform a **fine needle aspiration.** The *wrong* answers are ultrasound, radioactive iodine scan, or anything that is not a "fine needle aspiration" or something that says "sample" the gland.

If the nodule is cancer, the patient must have it removed surgically by an expert.

CALCIUM DISORDERS

HYPERCALCEMIA

The most common cause of hypercalcemia, by far, is **primary hyperparathyroidism.** An enormous number of people are walking around with hyperparathyroidism with no symptoms. Other causes of hypercalcemia are the following:

- **Malignancy:** Produces a parathyroid hormone–like particle.
- **Granulomatous disease:** Sarcoid granulomas actually make vitamin D.
- **Vitamin D intoxication**
- **Thiazide diuretics:** These increase tubular **reabsorption of calcium.**
- **Tuberculosis**
- **Histoplasmosis**
- **Berylliosis**

Hyperparathyroidism

The vast majority of cases present as **asymptomatic hypercalcemia.** Target organ damage is as follows:

- **Kidney stones**
- **Osteoporosis/osteomalacia/fractures**
- **Confusion**
- **Constipation and abdominal pain**

Diagnostic testing shows an **increased parathyroid hormone (PTH) level with hypercalcemia.**

Treatment is by **surgical removal.** Remember: Hyperparathyroidism may be a part of multiple endocrine neoplasia (MEN) syndrome. The nature of cases is as follows:

- Solitary adenoma: 80 percent
- Four-gland hyperplasia: 19 percent
- Cancer: 1 percent

When is the answer to a question about hyperparathyroidism surgical removal of the parathyroid gland?

Answer: Remove the gland under any of the following circumstances:
- *Any symptomatic disease ("stones, bones, psychic moans, GI groans")*
- *Renal insufficiency, no matter how slight*
- *Markedly elevated 24-hour urine calcium*
- *Very elevated serum calcium (> 12.5)*

Acute, Severe Hypercalcemia

This condition presents with the following:

- **Confusion**
- **Constipation**
- **Polyuria and polydipsia** from nephrogenic diabetes insipidus
- **Short QT syndrome** on the EKG
- **Renal insufficiency, ATN, kidney stone**

Treatment is as follows:

1. **Hydration:** High volume (3–4 liters) of normal saline
2. **Furosemide:** Only *after* hydration has been given. Loop diuretics increase calcium excretion by the kidney.
3. **Bisphosphonate** (pamidronate) is very potent but slow, taking a *week* to work.

4. **Calcitonin:** *If* hydration and furosemide do not control the calcium and you need something faster than a bisphosphonate, then calcitonin is the answer.

5. **Steroid:** Use if the etiology is **granulomatous disease.**

HYPOCALCEMIA

Hypocalcemia may be caused by the following:

- **Surgical removal of parathyroid glands**
- **Hypomagnesemia:** Magnesium is needed to release PTH from the gland.
- **Vitamin D deficiency**
- **Acute hyperphosphatemia:** Phosphate binds with the calcium and lowers it.
- **Fat malabsorption:** This binds calcium in the gut.
- **PTH resistance:** Pseudohypoparathyroidism that accompanies short fourth finger, round face, and mental retardation

Diagnostic Testing

Severe hypocalcemia presents with the following:

- **Seizures**
- **Neural twitching** (Chvostek's sign, Trousseau's sign)
- **Arrhythmia-prolonged QT** on EKG

Treatment

Replace the calcium. If there is vitamin D deficiency or hypoparathyroidism, then **give vitamin D and calcium.**

ADRENAL DISORDERS

CUSHING'S SYNDROME

Any form of hyperadrenalism or hypercortisolism, no matter what the cause, has a common clinical presentation consisting of the following:

- **Fat redistribution:** Truncal obesity, "moon face," buffalo hump, thin arms and legs
- **Easy bruising and striae:** Loss of collagen from the cortisol thins the skin
- **Hypertension:** From fluid and sodium retention (look for hypokalemia in hyperaldosteronism)
- **Muscle wasting**
- **Hiruitism:** From increased adrenal androgen levels

The following table summarizes the characteristics of the three sources of Cushing's disease.

	Pituitary Tumor	Ectopic ACTH Production	Adrenal Adenoma
ACTH	High	High	Low
High-dose dexamethasone	Suppression	No suppression	No suppression
Specific test	MRI Petrossal vein sampling	Scan chest and abdomen	Scan adrenals
Treatment	Removal	Removal	Removal

Diagnostic Testing and Treatment

Lab abnormalities are as follows:

- **Hyperglycemia, hyperlipidemia**
- **Osteoporosis**
- **Leukocytosis**
- **Metabolic alkalosis** from increased urinary loss of H+

Following are the best initial diagnostic tests:

- **One mg overnight dexamethasone suppression testing:** A normal person will suppress the 8:00 AM level of cortisol if given dexamethasone at 11 PM the night before. A normal 1 mg overnight dexamethasone suppression test excludes hypercortisolism of all kinds. An abnormal test can still be falsely elevated from various stresses, such as these:
  - Depresssion
  - Alcoholism
  - Emotional or physical stress

- **24-hour urine cortisol:** This test is done to confirm that an overnight dexamethasone suppression test is not falsely abnormal. The 24-hour urine cortisol adds specificity to the overnight test. If the overnight dexamethasone test is abnormal (fails to suppress), then get the 24-hour urine cortisol to confirm hypercortisolism (Cushing's syndrome).

The overnight dexamethasone suppression and the 24-hour urine cortisol test are to **diagnose** the presence of Cushing's syndrome. They do *not* determine the etiology or cause.

If high-dose dexamethasone suppresses the ACTH, the origin is the pituitary. Scan the pituitary. Remove the adenoma if it is visible.

If high-dose dexamethasone does not suppress the ACTH, the origin is an ectopic production of ACTH or a cancer that is making ACTH. Scan the chest for lung cancer or carcinoid. Remove the cancer if possible.

"I have Cushing's syndrome. Where is it coming from?"

"After the 1 mg overnight test and the 24-hour urine test confirm the presence of hyper-cortisolism, then we must determine the location or origin to treat it."

Following are indicators of the source of the hypercortisolism:

- **ACTH level low:** This means the origin is in the **adrenal gland. Scan the gland** with a CT or MRI and **remove the adenoma** that you find.
- **ACTH level high:** This means the origin is either in the **pituitary gland** or from the **ectopic production of ACTH.**

The next step is a high-dose dexamethasone suppression test.

To diagnose the presence of Cushing's syndrome, perform the following tests:

- 1 mg overnight dexamethasone test
- 24-hour urine cortisol

To diagnose the location or origin of Cushing's syndrome, look at the ACTH level:

- ACTH level high: Pituitary or ectopic source
- ACTH level low: Adrenal source

Why bother with all this complex testing for Cushing's syndrome? Why not just scan the brain and adrenals and remove what you find?

Answer: Many people have incidental adrenal and pituitary lesions. If you start with a scan, you might remove the wrong part of the body, and you cannot put it back!

A man with hypercortisolism is found to have an elevated ACTH level that suppresses with high-dose dexmethasone. MRI of this pituitary shows no visible lesion. What is the next best step in management?

a. Remove the pituitary

b. Repeat the dexamethasone suppression test

c. Use ketoconazole

d. Do petrosal venous sinus sampling

e. Order a PET scan of the brain

*Answer: The correct answer is **D**. MRI and CT of the brain lack both sensitivity and specificity in diagnosing endocrine disorders. It is important to confirm the identity of an adrenal disorder functionally prior to scanning the patient. This patient has high cortisol with a high ACTH, indicating either the pituitary or an ectopic source of hyperadrenalism. The fact that the ACTH levels suppress with high-dose dexamethasone indicates a **pituitary adenoma**, which is the cause of Cushing's syndrome in about 45 percent of patients. If the tests point to a pituitary source but the scanning is indeterminant, inferior petrosal sinus sampling is used to confirm it. Petrosal sinus sampling is also used **to localize the lesion**, as well to see which half of a pituitary should be removed.*

ADDISON'S DISEASE (ADRENAL INSUFFICIENCY)

The majority of cases of Addison's are of autoimmune origin. It presents with the following:

- **Fatigue, anorexia, weight loss, weakness with hypotension**
- **Thin patient with hyperpigmented skin**

Diagnostic Testing

Laboratory abnormalities are as follows:

- **Hyperkalemia** with a **mild metabolic acidosis** from the inability to excrete either H^+ or K^+ because of the loss of aldosterone.
- **Hyponatremia**
- May have hypoglycemia and neutropenia: Glucocorticoids increase glucose and white cell levels.

The most accurate diagnostic tests are these:

- **Cosyntropin (synthetic ACTH) stimulation test:** You measure the level of cortisol before and after the administration of cosyntropin. If there is adrenal insufficiency, there will be no rise in cortisol level.
- **CT scan of the adrenal gland**

Treatment

1. **Steroid replacement:** For **acute** Addisonian (hypoadrenal) crisis, draw a cortisol level and give fluids and hydrocortisone.
2. **Prednisone: Stable** (nonhypotensive) patients are treated with prednisone.
3. **Fludrocortisone** is the steroid highest in mineralocorticoid content. Fludrocortisone is used for patients with adrenal insufficiency who are still hypotensive *after* initial replacement with prednisone.

- Hypertension + Low renin + Low potassium = Hyperaldosteronism

HYPERALDOSTERONISM

This condition presents with **hypertension, hypokalemia, and metabolic alkalosis.** The hypokalemia may lead to **motor weakness** from the inability to have normal motor contraction with the low potassium level. **Nephrogenic diabetes insipidus** can occur from hypokalemia. Hence, the case may feature "polyuria and polydipsia"; however, in primary hyperaldosteronism, the glucose level will be normal.

Diagnostic Testing

- **Low renin**
- **Hypertension**
- **Elevated aldosterone level** *despite* salt loading with normal saline

Confirm the diagnosis with a **CT scan** of the adrenal glands.

Treatment

- Solitary adenoma: **Surgical resection**
- Hyperplasia **Spironolactone**

- Pheochromocytoma = Episodic hypertension

PHEOCHROMOCYTOMA

The patient presents with headache, palpitations, tremors, anxiety, and flushing. However, these symptoms are relatively nonspecific. Blood pressure that goes up in episodes is as close a clue as we get to knowing the diagnosis prior to testing.

Diagnostic Testing

- Best initial tests:
    - **High plasma and urinary catecholamines levels**
    - **Plasma-free metanephrine and VMA levels**
- Most accurate test:
    - **CT or MRI of the adrenal glands**
    - Metastatic disease is detected with an **MIBG scan,** which is a nuclear isotope scan to detect occult collections of pheochromocytoma.

Treatment

1. **Phenoxybenzamine (alpha blockade)** *first* to control blood pressure

Without alpha blockade, patients' blood pressure can significantly drop intraoperatively.

2. **Propranolol** is used *after* an alpha blocker like phenoxybenzamine.
3. **Surgical or laparoscopic resection**

CONGENITAL ADRENAL HYPERPLASIA (CAH)

All forms of CAH have the following characteristics:

- **Elevated ACTH.**
- **Low aldosterone and cortisol levels.**
- Treatable with **prednisone,** which inhibits the pituitary.

	Hypertension	Virilization
21	No	Yes
11	Yes	Yes
17	Yes	No

The different kinds of CAH:

- **21 hydroxylase deficiency:** This is the most common kind.
  - **Hypotension and hirsuitism** from *increased* adrenal androgens
  - Diagnose with **increased 17 hydroxyprogesterone level**

- **11 hydroxylase deficiency**
  - **Hypertension and hirsuitism** from *increased* adrenal androgens

- **17 hydroxylase deficiency**
  - **Hypertension** with *low* adrenal androgen levels

PROLACTINOMA

Prolactinoma is the most common pituitary tumor. It presents differently in men and women:

- **Men**
  - Presents with **impotence, decreased libido, and occasionally gyneco-mastia.** Presents *late.* No man rushes to the doctor in a panic to yell, "I can't get an erection and my breasts are big, too!"
  - Men are more likely to have the signs of mass effect of a tumor, such as **headache and visual disturbance.**

- **Women**
  - **Amenorrhea and galactorrhea in the absence of pregnancy** has women presenting *early.* Prolactin inhibits GNRH. If there is no GNRH, the body cannot release LH and FSH.

Prolactinoma should *only* be investigated under the following conditions:

- Pregnancy has been excluded.

- Drugs such as metoclopromide, phenothiazines, or tricyclic antidepressants have been excluded as the cause of the high prolactin level.
- Prolactin level is *very* high (> 200).
- Other causes of hyperprolactinemia have been excluded:
  - Hypothyroidism: High thyrotropin-releasing hormone level stimulates prolactin
  - Nipple stimulation, chest wall irritation
  - Stress, exercise

Diagnostic Testing

The most accurate diagnostic test is an **MRI of the brain.**

Treatment

- Best initial therapy: **Dopamine agonist** agents, such as **bromocriptine** or **cabergoline.** Most prolactinomas respond to dopamine agonists.
- **Surgical removal** is performed for the small number of patients in whom medical therapy does *not* work.

ACROMEGALY

Acromegaly is the excess production of growth hormone from a growth hormone-secreting adenoma in the pituitary. It presents with **enlargement of the head** (hat size), **fingers** (ring size), **feet** (shoe size), **nose, and jaw.** In addition, there is **intense sweating** from enlargement of the sweat glands. It also causes the following:

- **Joint abnormalities:** These arise from unusual growth of the articular cartilage.
- **Amenorrhea:** Growth hormone is frequently cosecreted with prolactin.
- **Cardiomegaly and hypertension**
- **Colonic polyps**

Diabetes is common because growth hormone acts as an anti-insulin.

Diagnostic Testing

- Best initial test: **Insulinlike growth factor (IGF)** is done *first* to confirm a diagnosis of acromegaly. Growth hormone (GH) level is *not* done first, because GH has its maximum secretion in the middle of the night during deep sleep. GH also has a short half-life. IGF is the "best initial test" because it has a much longer half-life.
- Most accurate test: Normally GH should be suppressed by glucose. GH raises glucose levels because it is a stress hormone. If the glucose level is high, this should suppress the level of GH. **Suppression of GH by giving glucose excludes acromegaly.**

• MRI will show a lesion in the pituitary, but it is essential to know the function of a pituitary tumor *before* anatomic visualization happens with an MRI.

Treatment

- **Surgical resection with transphenoidal removal** cures 70 percent of cases.
- **Cabergoline or bromocriptine:** Dopamine agonists inhibit growth hormone release.
- **Octreotide:** Somatostatin has some effect in preventing the release of growth hormone.
- **Pegvisomant:** This is a growth hormone receptor antagonist.

HORMONES OF REPRODUCTION

AMENORRHEA

Primary amenorrhea is from a genetic defect, such as the following:

1. **Turner's syndrome:** Look for short stature, webbed neck, wide-spaced nipples, and scant pubic and axillary hair. The **XO karyotype** prevents menstruation.
2. **Testicular feminization:** This is a genetically male patient who looks, feels, and acts as a woman. Socially the patient is female. The absence of testosterone receptors results in no penis, prostate, or scrotum. The patient does not menstruate.

Secondary amenorrhea is caused by the following:

- **Pregnancy, exercise, extreme weight loss, hyperprolactinemia**
- **Polycystic ovary syndrome:** Obesity, amenorrhea, and hirsuitism are associated with large cystic ovaries. There are increased adrenal androgens.

> Testicular feminization presents as a girl who does not menstruate. The girl has breasts but no cervix, tubes, or ovaries, and she is missing the top third of the vagina. She also does not have a penis, prostate, or scrotum.

MALE HYPOGONADISM

Klinefelter's Syndrome

Patients with this syndrome are **tall men** with the following characteristics:

- **Insensitivity of the FSH and LH receptors on their testicles**
- **XXY on karyotype**
- The **FSH and LH levels are very high,** but *no* testosterone is produced from the testicles.

Treatment is with **testosterone.**

Kallman's Syndrome

This syndrome results in **anosmia with hypogonadism.** This is a problem originating at the hypothalamus, so there is **low GnRH, FSH, and LH. Anosmia** is the key to the diagnosis.

PULMONARY

5

ASTHMA

Asthma presents as a patient who is short of breath with **expiratory wheezing.** In severe cases, there is use of accessory muscles, and the patient is unable to speak in complete sentences. Remember: To wheeze, one must have airflow. If the asthma exacerbation is severe, there may *not* be any wheezing. This is an ominous sign.

The most important features of a *severe* asthma exacerbation are the following:

- **Hyperventilation/increased respiratory rate**
- **Decrease in peak flow**
- **Hypoxia**
- **Respiratory acidosis**
- **Possible absence of wheezing**

DIAGNOSTIC TESTING

Patient with Unclear Diagnosis of Asthma

If the question describes a patient admitted with **acute shortness of breath** and it is unclear if the diagnosis is asthma, **pulmonary function testing (PFT)** should be performed before and after inhaled bronchodilators. Asthma and reactive airways disease are confirmed with an **increase in the FEV1 of > 12 percent.**

Diagnosis of Asthma in Currently Asymptomatic Patient

A young man comes to the clinic for evaluation of intermittent episodes of shortness of breath. Currently he is not short of breath. What is the best test to determine a diagnosis of reactive airways disease?

a. Chest X-ray

b. Diffusion capacity of carbon monoxide (DLCO)

c. High-resolution CT scan

d. Methacholine stimulation testing

e. Pre- and postbronchodilation pulmonary function testing (PFT)

*Answer: The correct answer is **D**. Methacholine stimulation testing looks for a decrease in FEV1 in response to synthetic acetylcholine. Methacholine will decrease FEV1 if the patient has asthma. The DLCO is a good test of interstitial lung disease, in which it is decreased. Asthmatic patients may have an increased DLCO from hyperventilation. High-resolution CT scanning is a test for interstitial lung disease and for bronchiectasis. Pre- and postbronchodilation PFTs are an appropriate assessment if the patient is currently short of breath to see if there is improvement, but they are of no value in an asymptomatic patient.*

TREATMENT

The best initial therapies, which should be ordered with the first screen on CCS, are the following:

All patients with shortness of breath should receive the following:
- Oxygen
- Continuous oximeter
- Chest X-ray
- Arterial blood gas (ABG)

- **Inhaled bronchodilators (albuterol):** There is no maximum dose of inhaled bronchodilators.

- **Bolus of steroids (methyl prednisilone):** Steroids need 4–6 hours to be effective.

- **Inhaled ipratropium**

- **Oxygen**

Any patient with asthma and **respiratory acidosis with CO2 retention** should be placed in the **ICU.** *Persistent* respiratory acidosis is an indication for **intubation and mechanical ventilation.**

The following therapies have *no* benefit for acute asthma exacerbation:

- Theophyline
- Cromolyn and nedocromil
- Monteleukast
- Inhaled corticosteroids
- Omalizumab
- Salmeterol and long-acting beta agonists
- Epinephrine: Subcutaneously administered epinephrine has *no* benefit in addition to inhaled bronchodilators.
- Terbutaline: Terubutaline is less efficacious than inhaled albuterol. Terbutaline is always a *wrong* answer choice.

Treatment of Asthma in Nonacute Patients

1. Best initial therapy: **Inhaled bronchodilator**
2. If the patient is not controlled, add a chronic controller medication, such as an **inhaled steroid.**
3. If inhaled albuterol and inhaled steroids do not control symptoms, add a **long-acting inhaled beta agonist,** such as salmeterol.
4. Oral steroids are used *only* as a last resort because of adverse effects.

The following table shows alternate long-term controller medications besides inhaled steroids.

Cause	Medication
Extrinsic allergies, such as hay fever	Cromolyn or nedocromil
Atopic disease	Monteleukast
Chronic obstructive pulmonary disease (COPD)	Tiotropium, ipratropium
High IgE levels, no control with cromolyn	Omalizumab (anti-IgE antibody)

Exercise-Induced Asthma

Exercise-induced asthma is best treated with an **inhaled bronchodialator** prior to exercise.

CHRONIC OBSTRUCTIVE PULMONARY DISEASE (COPD)/EMPHYSEMA

This condition presents in a **long-term smoker with increasing shortness of breath and decreased exercise tolerance.**

Acute episodes of shortness of breath should be handled as follows:

- **Oxygen and arterial blood gas (ABG)**
- **Chest X-ray**
- **Albuterol,** inhaled
- **Ipratropium,** inhaled
- **Bolus of steroids** (e.g., methyl prednisilone)
- **Chest, heart, extremity, and neurological examination**
- If fever, sputum, and/or a new infiltrate is present on chest X-ray, add ceftriaxone and azithromycin for community-acquired pneumonia.

> In cases of COPD, order arterial blood gas (ABG). ABG is critical in acute shortness of breath from COPD because there is no other way to assess for CO2 retention.

For mild respiratory acidosis, answer *CPAP* or *BiPAP* and move the clock forward 30–60 minutes. If the CO2 retention and hypoxia are improved, you can spare the patient intubation.

On CCS, move the clock forward 15–30 minutes and reassess the patient. Oxygen administration in COPD may *worsen* the shortness of breath by eliminating hypoxic drive.

Do *not* intubate patients with COPD for CO2 retention.

These patients often have **chronic CO_2 retention.** *Only* intubate if there is a worsening drop in pH indicative of a worse **respiratory acidosis.** Serum bicarbonate is often elevated due to metabolic alkalosis as compensation for chronic respiratory acidosis.

OFFICE/CLINIC-BASED CASES EMPHASIZING "FURTHER MANAGEMENT"

CCS as well as single best answer questions on Step 3 often emphasize chronic conditions needing "further management." Although one should perform a complete physical examination in all of these cases, the important findings are the following:

- Physical findings:
  - Barrel-shaped chest
  - Clubbing of fingers
  - Increased anterior-posterior diameter of the chest
  - Loud P2 heart sound as a sign of pulmonary hypertension
  - Edema as a sign of decreased right ventricular output (The blood is backing up due to the pulmonary hypertension.)

In moderate to severe cases of COPD, patients may become members of the 50/50 club—the PCO2 is 50 mm Hg and the PO2 is also 50 mm Hg. Here's an example ABG for a patient with COPD:
- pH: 7.35
- PCO2: 49
- PO2: 52
- HCO3: 32

- Laboratory testing:
  - **EKG:** Right axis deviation, right ventricular hypertrophy, right atrial hypertrophy
  - **Chest X-ray:** Flattening of the diaphragm (due to hyperinflation of the lungs), elongated heart, and substernal air trapping
  - **CBC: Increased hematocrit** is a sign of chronic hypoxia. Reactive erythrocytosis from chronic hypoxia is often **microcytic.** An erythropoietin level is not necessary.
  - **Chemistry: Increased serum bicarbonate** is metabolic compensation for respiratory acidosis.
  - **ABG:** Should be done even in office-based cases to assess CO_2 retention and the need for chronic home oxygen based on PO_2 (you expect the PCO_2 to rise and the PO_2 to fall).

- **Pulmonary function testing (PFT):** You should expect to find the following:
  - Decrease in FEV1
  - Decrease in FVC from loss of elastic recoil of the lung
  - Decrease in the FEV1/FVC ratio

- Increase in total lung capacity from air trapping
- Increase in residual volume
- Decrease in DLCO from destruction of lung interstitium

PFT Results: COPD

FEV$_1$	FVC	FEV$_1$/FVC ratio	Total Lung Capacity	Residual Volume	DLCO
↓	↓	↓	↑	↑	↓

CHRONIC MEDICAL THERAPY OF COPD

- **Tiotropium** or **ipratropium inhaler**
- **Albuterol inhaler**
- **Pneumococcal vaccine:** Heptavalent vaccine, Pneumovax®
- **Influenza vaccine:** Yearly
- **Smoking cessation**
- **Long-term home oxygen** if the PO2 < 55 or the oxygen saturation is < 88 percent

Which of the following lowers mortality in COPD?

a. Smoking cessation

b. Home oxygen therapy (continuous)

Answer: Both of these therapies reduce mortality in COPD.

ALPHA 1 ANTITRYPSIN DEFICIENCY

This is a genetic disorder that presents with a combination of cirrhosis and COPD. Look for a case of COPD at an **early age (< 40)** in a **nonsmoker** who has bullae at the bases of the lungs.

DIAGNOSTIC TESTING

- **Chest X-ray:** Findings of COPD (bullae, barrel chest, flat diaphragm)
- **Blood tests:** Low albumin level and elevated prothrombin time (from **cirrhosis**)
- **Alpha 1 antitrypsin level is low**
- **Genetic testing**

TREATMENT

Treatment is with alpha-1 antitrypsin infusion.

BRONCHIECTASIS

Bronchiectasis is caused by an **anatomic defect** of the lungs, usually from an infection in childhood. This results in **profound dilation of bronchi.**

It presents as chronic resolving and recurring **episodes of lung infection** that give a very **high volume of sputum** that can be measured by the cupful. **Hemoptysis and fever** occur as well. Clubbing is often present.

DIAGNOSTIC TESTING

A **chest X-ray** shows dilated bronchi with **"tram tracking,"** which are parallel lines consistent with dilated bronchi. The most accurate diagnostic test is a **high-resolution CT scan of the chest.**

TREATMENT

There is *no* curative therapy. Treat the infectious episodes as they occur.

- **Chest physiotherapy** with "cupping and clapping" will help dislodge secretions.
- **Rotating antibiotics** are tried to avoid the development of resistance.

INTERSTITIAL LUNG DISEASE (ILD)

ILD can be idiopathic, such as a form of pulmonary fibrosis secondary to occupational or environmental exposure and medications (e.g., trimethoprim/sulfamethoxole [Bactrim®]). If no cause is found, the diagnosis is "idiopathic pulmonary fibrosis" by exclusion.

The following table shows the causes of interstitial lung disease:

Cause	Disease
Asbestos	Asbestosis
Glass workers, mining, sandblasting, brickyards	Silicosis
Coal worker	Coal worker's pneumoconiosis
Cotton	Byssinosis
Electronics, ceramics, fluorescent light bulbs	Berylliosis
Mercury	Pulmonary fibrosis

PRESENTATION

ILD presents with **shortness of breath with a dry, nonproductive cough and chronic hypoxia.** ILD is a long-term disease and is often punctuated by episodes of bronchitis and pneumonia.

Physical findings are the following:

- **Dry, "Velcro" rales**
- **Loud P2 heart sound as a sign of pulmonary hypertension**
- **Clubbing**

ILD does *not* give fever or systemic findings.

DIAGNOSTIC TESTING

- **Chest X-ray:** Interstitial fibrosis
- **High-resolution CT scan:** Shows more detail on interstitial fibrosis
- **Lung biopsy**
- **Pulmonary function testing (PFT):** Shows decreased FEV1 and decreased FVC with a normal ratio, decreased total lung capacity, and decreased DLCO. All the measures are decreased, but they are decreased proportionately.

PFT Results: COPD

FEV$_1$	FVC	FEV$_1$/FVC ratio	Total Lung Capacity	Residual Volume	DLCO
↓	↓	Normal / ↑	↓	↓	↓

TREATMENT

There is *no* specific therapy to reverse any of the forms of ILD.

- If the biopsy shows an inflammatory infiltrate, a **trial of steroids** is used. The only form of ILD that definitely responds to steroids is **berylliosis,** because it is a granulomatous disease.
- There is definitely no therapy for silicosis, mercury vapor-induced fibrosis, asbestosis, or byssinosis.

> The most common type of cancer in asbestosis is *lung cancer,* not mesothelioma.

BRONCHIOLITIS OBLITERANS ORGANIZING PNEUMONIA (BOOP), ALSO KNOWN AS CRYPTOGENIC ORGANIZING PNEUMONIA (COP)

BOOP/COP is a rare bronchiolitis or inflammation of small airways with a chronic alveolitis of unknown origin, although a few cases are associated with rheumatoid arthritis.

Although BOOP/COP has many similarities to ILD, the presentation is more acute over weeks to months. In addtion to **cough, rales, and shortness of breath,** there is **fever, malaise, and myalgias.** (These systemic findings are *absent* from ILD.) Also, there is **no occupational exposure** in the history.

DIAGNOSTIC TESTING

- **Chest X-ray:** Shows bilateral patchy infiltrates
- **Chest CT:** Shows interstitial disease and alveolitis
- Most accurate diagnostic test: **Open lung biopsy** is the only definitive way to make the diagnosis of BOOP/COP.

TREATMENT

Treat BOOP/COP with **steroids.** There is *no* response to antibiotics.

The following table compares BOOP/COP and ILD.

BOOP/COP	ILD
Fever, myalgias, malaise (clubbing uncommon)	No fever, no myalgias
Presents over days to weeks	Six months or more of symptoms
Patchy infiltrates	Interstitial infiltrates
Steroids effective	Rarely responds to steroids

SARCOIDOSIS

This condition presents as an **African-American woman** under 40 with **cough, shortness of breath,** and **fatigue** over a few weeks to months. Physical examination shows **rales.** Although sarcoidosis can involve many organs, the vast majority of cases present with lung findings only.

Rare physical findings/presentation include the following:

- **Eye:** Uveitis that can be sight threatening
- **Neural:** Seventh cranial nerve involvement is the most common.
- **Skin:** Lupus pernio (purplish lesion of the skin of the face), erythema nodosum
- **Cardiac:** Restrictive cardiomyopathy, cardiac conduction defects
- **Renal and hepatic involvement:** Occurs without symptoms
- **Hypercalcemia:** This occurs in a small number of patients secondary to vitamin D production by the granulomas of sarcoidosis.

DIAGNOSTIC TESTING

- Best initial test: **Chest X-ray,** which always shows **enlarged lymph nodes.** There may be interstitial lung disease in addition to the nodal involvement.
- Most accurate diagnostic test: **Lung or lymph node biopsy** showing **noncaseating granulomas**
- Calcium and ACE levels may be elevated, but these are not specific enough to lead to a specific diagnosis.
- **Bronchoalveolar lavage** shows increased numbers of helper cells.

TREATMENT

Steroids are the undisputed best therapy.

PULMONARY HYPERTENSION

Primary pulmonary hypertentsion presents as an idiopathic cause of **shortness of breath, more often in young women,** from overgrowth and obliteration of pulmonary vasculature, leading to decreased flow out of the right ventricle. Pulmonary hypertension can occur secondary to the following:

- Mitral stenosis
- COPD
- Polycythemia vera
- Chronic pulmonary emboli
- Interstial lung disease

Physical findings are as follows:

- **Loud P2**
- **Tricuspid regurgitation**
- **Right ventricular heave**
- **Raynaud's phenomenon**

DIAGNOSTIC TESTING

- **Transthoracic echocardiogram (TTE):** Shows right ventricular hypertrophy and enlarged right atrium
- **EKG:** Shows the same findings as well as right axis deviation
- Most accurate test: **Right heart catheterization with increased pulmonary artery pressure**

TREATMENT

- **Bosentan** is an endothelin inhibitor that prevents growth of the vasculature of the pulmonary system.
- **Epoprostanil** and **treprostanil** are prostacyclin analogues that act as pulmonary vasodilators.
- **Calcium channel blockers** (weak efficacy)
- **Sildenafil**

PULMONARY EMBOLISM (PE)

PE presents with the **sudden onset of shortness of breath** and **clear lungs** in patients with risks for deep venous thrombosis (DVT). The following are risk factors for DVT:

- Immobility
- Malignancy
- Trauma
- Surgery, especially joint replacement
- Thrombophilia, such a factor V mutation, lupus anticoagulant, or protein C and S deficiency

There are *no* specific physical findings for PE.

DIAGNOSTIC TESTING

- **Chest X-ray:** The most common result is **normal.** The most common abnormality found is **atelectasis.** Wedge-shaped infarction and pleural-based humps are rare.
- **EKG:** The most common showing is **sinus tachycardia.** The most common abnormality is **nonspecific ST-T wave changes.** Right axis deviation and right bundle branch block are uncommon.
- **ABG:** This shows hypoxia with an increased A-a gradient and mild respiratory alkalosis.

A patient who has recently undergone hip fracture repair develops the sudden onset of shortness of breath. His pulse is 110 per minute. The chest is clear to auscultation. Chest X-ray is normal, and the EKG shows sinus tachycardia. ABG shows pH 7.48, pCO2 28, pO2 75. What is the next best step in management?

a. Heparin
b. V/Q scan
c. Spiral CT scan
d. D-Dimers
e. Lower extremity Dopplers
f. Angiography

*Answer: The correct answer is **A**. When the case so clearly suggests a pulmonary embolus with sudden onset of shortness of breath and clear lungs in a patient with a risk factor, the first thing to do after the chest X-ray and blood gas is to start heparin. Do not wait for the results of V/Q scan or spiral CT to start heparin.*

CONFIRMATORY TESTING

Spiral CT

A spiral CT is standard to confirm the presence of a pulmonary embolus. The spiral CT is excellent if it is positive because of its specificity. The sensitivity of spiral CT may not be ideal, and the test can miss some emboli if they are small and in the periphery. The spiral CT is clearly the **test of choice if the X-ray is abnormal.**

V/Q Scan

For a V/Q scan to be accurate, the chest X-ray *must* be normal. The less normal the X-ray, the less accurate the V/Q scan. This is still a good test for PE. The problem is that *only* a truly normal scan excludes a PE. Of patients with low-probability scans, 15 percent still have a PE, and 15 percent of those with high-probability scans don't have a PE.

Lower Extremity Dopplers

These are excellent tests *if* they are positive; if positive, no further diagnostic testing is necessary. The problem is that 30 percent of PEs originate in pelvic veins, and the Dopplers are normal even in the presence of a PE. Hence, the sensitivity of lower extremity Doppler is about 70 percent.

D-Dimer Testing

This is a very sensitive test with poor specificity. If the D-dimer is negative, PE is extremely unlikely. The best use of D-Dimer testing is in a patient with a **low probability of PE in whom you want a single test to exclude PE.**

Angiography

Angiography is the single most accurate test for PE. Unfortunately, angiography is **invasive with a significant risk of death** of about 0.5 percent.

> *A 45-year-old man comes to the emergency department after a motor vehicle accident resulting in a liver hematoma. On the third hospital day, he becomes suddenly short of breath. His chest X-ray is normal, and he is diagnosed with a pulmonary embolus. What is the next best step in management?*
>
> *a. Angiography*
> *b. Embolectomy*
> *c. Heparin*
> *d. Inferior vena cava filter*
>
> *Answer: The correct answer is **D**. When a patient has a pulmonary embolism and there is a contraindication to anticoagulation, a vena cava interruption filter should be placed. This patient has a liver hematoma, so a filter should be placed.*

TREATMENT

- **Heparin and oxygen:** This is the standard of care in pulmonary embolism.
- **Warfarin:** Should be used for **at least 6 months** *after* the use of heparin.
- **Venous interruption filter:** This should be placed in all patients who have **a contraindication to anticoagulation.**
- **Thrombolytics:** These are used in patients who are **hemodynamically unstable.** Hemodynamic instability can be defined as *hypotension*. Thrombolytics essentially replace embolectomy, which is rarely performed because of the high operative mortality.

PLEURAL EFFUSION

DIAGNOSTIC TESTING

- Best initial test: **Chest X-ray.** Decubitus films with the patient lying on one side should be done next to see if the fluid is freely flowing.
- **Chest CT** may add a little more detail to a chest X-ray.
- Most accurate test: **Thoracentesis**

Exudate	Transudate
Cancer and infection	Congestive failure
Protein level **high** (> 50 percent of serum level)	Protein level **low** (< 50 percent of serum level)
LDH level **high** (> 60 percent of serum level)	LDH level **low** (< 60 percent of serum level)

- Order the following tests on pleural fluid:
  - Gram stain and culture
  - Acid-fast stain
  - Total protein (also order serum protein)
  - LDH (also order serum LDH)
  - Glucose
  - Cell count w/differential
  - Triglycerides
  - pH

TREATMENT

- Small pleural effusions do *not* need therapy. **Diuretics** can be used, especially for those from congestive heart failure (CHF).
- For larger effusions, especially those from infection (empyema), a **chest tube** for drainage is placed.
- If the effusion is large and recurrent from a cause that cannot be corrected, **pleurodesis** is performed. Pleurodesis is the infusion of an irritative agent, such as bleomycin or talcum powder, into the pleural space. This inflames the pleura, causing fibrosis so the lung will stick to the chest wall. When the pleural space is eliminated, the effusion cannot reaccumulate.
- If pleurodesis fails, **decortication** is performed. Decortication is the stripping off of the pleura from the lung so it will stick to the interior chest wall. This is an operative procedure.

SLEEP APNEA

Look for an **obese patient** complaining of **daytime somnolence.** The patient's sleep partner will report **severe snoring.** In addition, there will be hypertension, headache, erectile dysfunction, and a fat neck.

The majority (95 percent) of cases are obstructive sleep apnea from fatty tissues of the neck blocking breathing. A small number of patients will have central sleep apnea, which is decreased respiratory drive from the central nervous system.

DIAGNOSTIC TESTING

Sleep apnea is diagnosed with a sleep study, **polysomnography.** The patient is observed for periods of apnea lasting > 10 seconds each. The patient's oxygen saturation is also monitored. Mild sleep apnea is defined as 5–20 apneic periods an hour. Severe sleep apnea is defined as > 30 periods an hour.

TREATMENT

Obstructive Disease

- Treat with **weight loss** and **continuous positive airway pressure (CPAP)** or **BiPAP.**
- If this is not effective, **surgical resection of the uvula, palate, and pharynx** can be performed.

Central Sleep Apnea

- Central sleep apnea is managed by **avoiding alcohol and sedatives.**
- It may respond to **acetazolamide,** which causes a metabolic acidosis. This may help drive respiration.
- Some patients respond to **medroxyprogesterone,** which is also a central respiratory stimulant.

ALLERGIC BRONCHOPULMONARY ASPERGILLOSIS (ABPA)

This presents as an **asthmatic patient with worsening asthma symptoms** who is coughing up **brownish mucous plugs with recurrent infiltrates.** There is **peripheral eosinophia. Serum IgE is elevated. Central bronchiectasis is visible.**

DIAGNOSE TESTING

- *Aspergillus* **skin testing**
- Masurement of **IgE levels, circulating precipitins, and A.** *fumigatus*-**specific antibodies**

TREATMENT

Treatment is with **corticosteroids** and, in patients with refractory disease, **itraconazole.**

ACUTE RESPIRATORY DISTRESS SYNDROME (ARDS)

ARDS is a **sudden, severe respriratory failure syndrome** occurring from diffuse lung injury secondary to a number of **overwhelming systemic injuries** such as these:

- Sepsis
- Aspiration of gastric contents

- Shock
- Infection: pulmonary or systemic
- Lung contusion
- Trauma
- Toxic inhalation
- Near drowning
- Pancreatitis
- Burns

DIAGNOSTIC TESTING

- **Chest X-ray:** This shows diffuse patchy infiltrates that become confluent. May suggest congestive failure.
- Normal wedge pressure
- **pO_2/FIO_2 ratio < 200,** with the FIO_2 expressed as a decimal (e.g., room air is 0.21). For example, if the pO_2 is 100/0.21, the ratio is 476.

TREATMENT

- **Ventilatory support** with **low tidal volume** of 6 ml per kg
- **Positive end expiratory pressure (PEEP)** to keep the alveoli open
- **Prone positioning** of the patient's body
- Possible use of **diuretics** and **positive inotropes,** such as dobutamine
- Transfer the patient to the **ICU** if not already there

> Steroids are *not* effective in cases of ARDS.

SWAN-GANZ (PULMONARY ARTERY) CATHETERIZATION

Use the measurements below when a case is described and the question says: Which of the following will most likely be found in this patient?

Type	Cardiac Output	Wedge Pressure	Systemic Vascular Resistance (SVR)
Hypovomia	Low	Low	High
Cardiogenic Shock	Low	High	High
Septic Shock	High	Low	Low

Pneumonia

Pneumonia presents with **fever, cough, and often sputum.** Severe illness also presents with **shortness of breath.** Following are the most likely organisms involved:

- **Community-acquired pneumonia (CAP):** *Pneumococcus*
- **Hospital-acquired pneumonia (HAP):** Gram-negative bacilli

What is the strongest indication for admission?

a. Respiratory distress
b. Hypotension, tachycardia
c. Confusion
d. Fever
e. Leukocytosis, hyponatremia, hyperglycemia

*Answer: The answer is **A**. Patients who are older (> 65) with chronic diseases of the lungs, liver, or kidney are more prone to respiratory failure. Other risks for a poor prognosis are diabetes, HIV, steroid use, and lack of a spleen. The pneumonia severity index (PSI) is used to risk-stratify patients with pneumonia. You do not need to memorize the criteria for Step 3, but suffice it to say that **elderly, hypoxic patients with or without a fever should be admitted.** You should consider the ICU, depending on the severity of the hypoxia. Decide whether to use outpatient versus inpatient monitoring; then, if inpatient, ICU or no ICU.*

DIAGNOSTIC TESTING

- Best initial diagnostic test: **Chest X-ray**
- Most accurate test: **Sputum gram stain and culture**

Order tests as follows:

- *All* cases of respiratory disease (fever, cough, sputum) should have a **chest X-ray and oximeter** ordered with the first screen.
- If there is shortness of breath, also order **oxygen** with the first screen.
- If there is shortness of breath and/or hypoxia, order an **ABG.**

Treat outpatient pneumonia with:

- **Macrolide** (azithromycin, doxycycline, or clarithromycin)
- **Respiratory fluoroquinolone** (levofloxacin, gatifloxacin, moxifloxacin)
- **Inpatient pneumonia** is treated with the following:
  - **Ceftriaxone and azithromycin**
  - **Fluoroquinolone** as a single agent

Treat ventilator-associated pneumonia with:

- Imipenem or meropenem, piperacillin/tazobactam or cefepime;
- Gentamicin; *and*
- Vancomycin or linezolid

SPECIFIC ASSOCIATIONS

Presentation	Cause
Recent viral syndrome	*Staphylococcus*
Alcoholics	*Klebsiella*
Gastrointestinal symptoms, confusion	*Legionella*
Young, healthy patients	*Mycoplasma*
Animals present at the time of birth of the animal	*Coxiella burneti*
Arizona construction workers	Coccidioidomycosis
HIV with < 200 CD4 cells	Pneumocystis (PCP)

An HIV-positive man comes to the emergency department with shortness of breath and a dry cough. His LDH is elevated and the chest X-ray shows bilateral interstitial infiltrates. His pO_2 is 65. What is the next best step in management?

a. Sputum induction

b. Respiratory isolation

c. Trimethoprim/sulfamethoxazole and prednisone

d. Pentamidine

e. Bronchoalveolar lavage

*Answer: The correct answer is **C**. PCP is best managed with trimethoprim/sulfamethoxazole. This has better efficacy than pentamidine. Bronchoalveolar lavage needs to be done and is the most accurate test, but It is more important to start specific therapy. Steroids are indicated if the pO_2 < 70 or the A-a gradient > 35.*

TUBERCULOSIS (TB)

TB occurs in **specific risk groups,** such as immigrants, HIV-positive patients, homeless patients, prisoners, and alcoholics. TB presents with **fever, cough, sputum, weight loss, and night sweats.**

DIAGNOSTIC TESTING

- Best initial test: **Chest X-ray**
- **Sputum acid-fast stain and culture** should be done to confirm the presence of TB.

TREATMENT

Once the acid-fast stain is positive, treatment with 4 antituberculosis medications should be started. Six months of therapy is the standard of care.

1. Isoniazid: Six months
2. Rifampin: Six months
3. Pyrizinamide: Stop after two months
4. Ethambutal: Stop after two months

All of these medications can lead to **liver toxicity.** TB medications should be stopped if the transaminases reach 5 times the upper limit of normal. Specific toxicities are the following:

- Isoniazid-peripheral neuropathy
- Rifampin-red/orange-colored bodily secretions
- Pyrizinamide-hyperuricemia
- Ethambutal-optic neuritis

The following conditions require treatment for **more than 6 months:**

- Osteomyelitis
- Meningitis
- Miliary tuberculosis
- Cavitary tuberculosis
- Pregnancy

LATENT TUBERCULOSIS (THE PPD)

The **PPD is a screening test for those in risk groups,** such as the homeless, immigrants, alcoholics, health care workers, and prisoners. A **positive test** is as follows:

- 5 mm: Close contacts, steroid users, HIV-positive
- 10 mm: Those in the risk groups described above
- 15 mm: Those without an increased risk

If a patient has never been tested or it has been several years since the last test, **two-stage testing** is recommended. This means that if the first test is negative, a second test should be performed in 1–2 weeks to make sure the first test was truly negative.

If the PPD is **positive,** proceed as follows:

1. A **chest X-ray** should be performed to make sure occult active disease has not been detected.
2. If the chest X-ray is abnormal, **sputum staining for tuberculosis** is performed.
3. If this is positive, then **full-dose, four-drug therapy** is used.

Bacille–Calmette Guerin (BCG) administration in the past has *no* effect or influence on these recommendations for treatment of latent TB. It does not matter if a patient has had BCG in the past; the patient must still take isoniazid if the PPD is positive. If you see BCG as an answer choice, it is *always* wrong according to current guidelines.

Isoniazid alone is used for 9 months to treat a positive PPD. This reduces the 10 percent lifetime risk of developing tuberculosis to 1 percent. Once a PPD is positive, the test should never be repeated.

RHEUMATOLOGY

6

RHEUMATOID ARTHRITIS (RA)

Rheumatoid arthritis presents most often in **women > 50.** Patients have **joint pain and morning stiffness** that is **symmetrical** and in **multiple joints of the hands** lasting for **more than 1 hour in the morning** with the symptomatic episode going on for **at least 6 weeks.** There is often a prodrome of malaise and weight loss, but this is *not* enough to make a clear diagnosis.

RA is defined as having 4 or more of the following present for diagnosis:

- **Morning stiffness lasting more than 1 hour**
- **Wrist and finger** involvement (MCP, PIP)
- **Swelling of at least 3 joints**
- **Symmetric** involvement
- Rheumatoid **nodules**
- **X-ray abnormalities showing erosions**
- **Positive rheumatoid factor**

Rheumatoid arthritis is diagnosed with a **constellation of physical findings, joint problems, and lab tests.** There is *no* single diagnostic criteria to confirm the diagnosis. There is *no* single therapy to control and treat the disease.

> Other findings in RA include the following:
> - **Cardiac:** Pericarditis, valvular disease
> - **Lung:** Pleural effusion with a very low glucose level, lung nodules
> - **Blood:** Anemia with normal MCV
> - **Nerve:** Mononeuritis multiplex
> - **Skin:** Nodules

A 34-year-old woman presents with pains in both hands for the last few months and stiffness that improves as the day goes on. Multiple joints are swollen on exam. X-rays of the hands show some erosion. What is the single most accurate test?

a. Rheumatoid factor
b. Anticitrullinated cyclic peptide (anti-CCP)
c. Sedimentation rate
d. ANA
e. Joint fluid aspirate

*Answer: The correct answer is **B**. Rheumatoid factor (RF) is only present in 75–85 percent of patients with rheumatoid arthritis (RA). It can also be present in a number of other diseases; hence, the RF is rather nonspecific. Anticitrulinated cyclic peptide (anti-CCP) is the single most accurate test for RA. It is > 95 percent specific for RA, and it appears earlier in the course of the disease than the RF. There is nothing specific on joint aspiration to determine a diagnosis of RA.*

Joint findings in RA are the following:

> Felty's syndrome consists of the following:
> * Rheumatoid arthritis
> * Splenomegaly
> * Neutropenia

* **Metacaparpophalangeal (MCP) swelling and pain**
* **Boutonierre deformity:** Flexion of the PIP with hyperextension of the DIP
* **Swan neck deformity**
* **Baker's cyst** (outpocketing of synovium at the back of the knee)
* **C1/C2 cervical spine subluxation**
* **Knee:** Although the knee is commonly involved, multiple small joints are involved more commonly over time.

Baker's cyst

> Normocytic, normochromic anemia is very characteristic of RA.

In addition to X-rays, RF, and anti-CCP, you should also order a **CBC, sedimentation rate,** and gamma globulin level on an **SPEP.** If the case describes a swollen joint with an effusion, **aspiration of the joint** should also be done. If it is a single best answer question, however, these are not necessary.

Which of the following will have the lowest glucose level on pleural effusion?

a. CHF

b. Pulmonary embolus

c. Pneumonia

d. Cancer

e. Rheumatoid arthritis

f. Tuberculosis

*Answer: The correct answer is **E**. Rheumatoid arthritis has the lowest glucose level of all the causes of pleural effusion described here.*

> The sacroiliac joint is *spared* in rheumatoid arthritis.

TREATMENT

NSAIDs and a **disease-modifying antirheumatic drug (DMARD)** is the standard of care in patients with RA. There is *no* therapeutic difference among NSAIDs, and you may use ibuprofen for any of the rheumatological diseases described.

DMARDs

The following are DMARDs (often used in combination):

- **Methotrexate:** This is the best-tolerated and most widely used DMARD. There is *no* point in waiting to use a DMARD in a patient with severe RA or anyone with joint erosions. NSAIDs will *not* delay the progression of the disease. Adverse effects are bone marrow suppression and pneumonitis.
- **Biological agents (infliximab, adalimumab, etanercept):** All of these block the activity of tumor necrosis factor (TNF). Methotrexate *and* these biological agents can be used in combination.
- **Hydroxychloroquine:** Use with **mild disease.** The patient will need a regular **eye exam** to check for retinopathy.
- **Sulfasalazine:** This is the same drug that was used in the past for ulcerative colitis. It can suppress the bone marrow.

The following are alternate DMARDs:

- **Anakinra:** IL-1 receptor antagonist
- **Leflunamide:** Pyrimidine antagonist that is similar in effect to methotrexate with less toxicity
- **Abatacept:** Inhibits T-cell activation
- **Gold salts:** Rarely used because of toxicity, such as nephrotic syndrome

Steroids

Glucocorticoids, such as prednisone, are *not* disease modifying. However, steroids do quickly allow control of the disease and allow time for the other DMARDs to take effect. Long-term glucocorticoid use should be avoided if at all possible. Steroids are a **bridge to DMARD therapy.** They are the answer for an **acutely ill patient with severe inflammation.**

SERONEGATIVE SPONDYLOARTHROPATHIES

These conditions are the following:

- **Ankylosing spondylitis**
- **Reactive arthritis** (formerly known as Reiter's syndrome)
- **Psoriatic arthritis**
- **Juvenile rheumatoid arthritis** (adult-onset Still's disease)

This group of inflammatory arthritic condition all have the following characteristics:

- **Negative test for rheumatoid factor**
- Predilection for the **spine**
- **Sacroiliac joint** involvement
- Association with **HLA B27**

ANKYLOSING SPONDYLITIS (AS)

AS presents in a **young (< 40) male patient with spine or back stiffness.** Peripheral joint involvement is less common. The pain is **worse at night** and is **relieved by leaning forward.** This can lead to **kyphosis** and **diminished chest expansion.** Rare findings are these:

- Uveitis (30 percent)
- Aortitis (3 percent)

A 27-year-old man presents with months of back pain that is worse at night. He has diminished expansion of this chest on inhalation and flattening of the normal lumbar curvature. What is the most accurate of these tests?

a. X-ray
b. MRI
c. HLA-B27
d. ESR
e. Rheumatoid factor

Answer: The correct answer is B. MRI of the SI joint is more sensitive than an X-ray, detecting edematous, inflammatory changes years before an X-ray in ankylosing spondylitis (AS). HLA B27 can be present in 8 percent of the general population and is not necessary to confirm a diagnosis of AS. The ESR is not always elevated and is a nonspecific test. The rheumatoid factor will be negative in AS. In a CCS case, all of these tests should be performed, with the X-ray done first and then going on to the MRI if the X-ray is negative.

Treatment

Treat with the following:

- NSAIDs
- Sulfasalazine
- Biological agents, such as infliximab or adalimumab

REACTIVE ARTHRITIS (FORMERLY KNOWN AS REITER'S SYNDROME)

Reactive arthritis presents with an **asymmetric arthritis with a history of urethritis or gastrointestinal infection.** There may be constitutional symptoms, such as **fever, fatigue, or weight loss.**

- **Arthritis:** May be monoarticular, oligoarticular, or more diffuse
- **Genital lesions:** Circinate balanitis (around head of penis); urethritis or cervicitis in women
- **Conjunctivitis**
- **Keratoderma blenorhagicum:** A skin lesion characteristic of reactive arthritis

Diagnostic Testing and Treatment

There is *no* specific diagnostic test. Look for the triad of **knee (joint), pee (urinary), and see (eye)** problems with a history of *Chlamydia, Shigella, Salmonella, Yersinia,* or *Campylobacter.*

Treat with **NSAIDs.**

PSORIATIC ARTHRITIS

Psoriatic arthritis presents as **joint involvement with a history of psoriasis.** Rheumatoid factor is absent. The **sacroiliac spine is involved,** as it is in all seronegative sponyloarthropaties. The following are key features of psoriatic arthritis:

- **Nail pitting**
- **Distal interphalangeal (DIP) involvement** (Remember: RA involves the proximal joint.)
- **"Sausage-shaped" digits**

FIGURE 3: Psoriasis involvement of the nail produces pitting and yellowing, which can be mistaken for onychomycosis.

Treatment

Treat with the following medications:

- **NSAIDs** are the initial therapy.
- **Infliximab and the other biologic agents** are effective.
- **Methotrexate** is used for resistant disease.

JUVENILE RHEUMATOID ARTHRITIS (JRA) OR ADULT-ONSET STILL'S DISEASE

JRA presents with the following:

- **Fever**
- **Salmon-colored rash**
- **Polyarthritis**
- **Lymphadenopathy**
- **Myalgias**

This can be a *very* difficult diagnosis to recognize. Additional minor criteria are the presence of **hepatosplenomegaly and elevated transaminases.**

Diagnostic Testing

There is *no* specific diagnostic test. JRA is characterized by the following:

- **Very high ferritin level**
- **Elevated white cell count**
- **Negative rheumatoid factor and negative ANA** are *essential* to establishing the diagnosis.

Treatment

Treat with **NSAIDs.** Unresponsive cases can be treated with **methotrexate.**

WHIPPLE'S DISEASE

Although it causes **diarrhea** and **fat malabsorption,** the most common presentation of Whipple's disease is with **joint pain.**

Biopsy of the bowel is the most specific test, and treatment with **TMP/SMX** is curative.

OSTEOARTHRITIS (OA)

Osteoarthritis, the most common joint abnormality, is associated with aging and increased use of a joint. The **morning stiffness is < 30 minutes** in duration and there is **crepitus** on moving the joint. OA affects the **distal interphalangeal (DIP) joints** (RA does *not* affect the DIPs). Note the following:

- Heberden's nodes: DIP osteophytes
- Bouchard's nodes: PIP osteophytes

Heberden's Nodes

DIAGNOSTIC TESTING

The best initial test is **X-ray of the joint.**

For CCS, *all* of the following should be ordered; there is *no* specific diagnostic test:

- **ANA**
- **ESR**
- **Rheumatoid factor**
- **Anti-CCP**

All other inflammatory markers will be normal. Joint fluid will have a *low* leukocyte count, $< 2,000/mm^3$.

TREATMENT

Treatment is with **NSAIDS. Glucosamine sulfate and chondroitin sulfate** are used to slow joint deterioration.

The following table compares osteoarthritis with rheumatoid arthritis.

	OA	RA
Morning stiffness	< 30 minutes	> 1 hour
DIP	Yes	No
PIP	Yes	Yes
MCP	No	Yes
RF, anti-CCP	No	Yes
Joint fluid	< 2,000	5,000–50,000

SYSTEMIC LUPUS ERYTHEMATOSUS (SLE)

- Rash + Joint pain + Fatigue = Lupus

As shown in the following table, there are 11 criteria for lupus; **4 are needed** to confirm the diagnosis.

Skin	• Malar rash • Photosensitivity rash • Oral ulcers rash • Discoid rash
Arthralgias	Present in 90 percent of patients
Blood	Leukopenia, thrombocytopenia, hemolysis; Any blood involvement counts as *1 criteria*
Renal	Varies from benign proteinuria to end stage renal disease
Cerebral	Behavioral change, stroke, seizure, meningitis
Serositis	Pericarditis, pleuritic chest pain, pulmonary hypertension, pneumonia, myocarditis
Serology	• ANA (95 percent sensitive) • Double-stranded (DS) DNA (60 percent sensitive) Each of the serologic abnormalities counts as 1 criteria. Hence, if the person has joint pain, a rash, and both an ANA and DS DNA, that patient would have 4 criteria.

Malar Rash

DIAGNOSTIC TESTING

- Best initial test: **ANA**
- Most specific test: **Anti-DS DNA or anti-Sm** (Smith)

> *What is the best test to follow the severity of a lupus flair-up?*
>
> *Answer:* **Complement levels** *(drop in flair-up) and* **anti-DS DNA** *(rise in flair-up).*

> *As part of prenatal care, a woman with lupus is found to have a negative test for anti-cardiolipin antibodies, but she is positive for anti-Ro (SSA) antibody. What is the baby at risk for?*
>
> *Answer: Heart block. The presence of anti-Ro or anti-SSA antibodies is a risk for the development of heart block.*

The following are other findings in lupus that are *not* part of specific diagnostic criteria:

- **Fatigue**
- **Hair loss**
- **Antiphospholipid syndrome**
- **Elevated sedimentation rate**

> **SLE on CCS:** Complement levels, anti-Sm, and anti-DS DNA should be performed on *all* patients.

TREATMENT

Treatment is as follows:

- **Acute flair-ups:** Prednisone and other glucocorticoids
- **Joint pain:** NSAIDs
- **Rash and joint pain not responding to NSAIDs:** Hydroxychloroquine and antimalarials
- **Severe disease relapsing with stopping steroids:** Azathioprine and cyclophosphamide
- **Nephritis:** Steroids and mycophenolate mofetil (Mycophenolate is superior to cyclophosphamide.)

DRUG-INDUCED LUPUS

The most common causes of drug-induced lupus are **hydralazine, procainamide, and isoniazid.** Keep the following in mind:

- ALWAYS gives **anti-HISTONE antibodies**
- NEVER gives renal or CNS involvement
- Complement level and anti-DS DNA are normal

SJÖGREN'S SYNDROME

Look for a **woman** (9:1 female predominance) with **dry eyes, dry mouth, and a sensation of "sand under the eyelid."** There is often **loss of taste and smell** from profound mouth dryness. (You need saliva to wet the food so you can taste it.) Look for **loss of teeth at an early age,** because saliva is critical to preventing dental cavities.

DIAGNOSTIC TESTING

- Most accurate test: **Lip biopsy**
- **Schirmer test:** Decreased wetting of paper held to the eye shows decreased lacrimation.
- Serologic testing:
    - **ANA:** 95 percent sensitive but least specific
    - **RF:** 70 percent sensitive
    - **Anti-Ro/SSA:** 50–65 percent sensitive but fairly specific
    - **Anti-La/SSB:** 30–65 percent sensitive but fairly specific

When you see **anti-Ro(SSA) or La (SSB)**, think **Sjögren's syndrome. They are present in a small number of people with lupus, and can help diagnose ANA-negative lupus.**

TREATMENT

- **Keep the eyes and mouth moist.**
- **Pilocarpine and cevimiline** increase acetylcholine, which increases oral and ocular secretions.

SCLERODERMA (SYSTEMIC SCLEROSIS)

Scleroderma presents with three main symptoms:

- Tight Skin + Heartburn + Raynaud's = Scleroderma

1. **Skin:** Look for a **woman** with **tight, fibrous thickening of the skin** that gives a tight face and tight, immobile fingers known as **"sclerodactyly."**

2. **Raynaud's phenomenon:** This is a three-phase **vascular hyperreactivity,** with the skin of the fingers becoming white, then blue, then red; it can be quite painful. **Digital ulceration** may occur from infarction of the skin. There might also be abnormal **giant capillaries in the nailfolds.**

3. **Joint pain:** The pain is **mild and symmetrical.**

Diffuse scleroderma also presents with the following:

- **Lung: Fibrosis and pulmonary hypertension** (These are the leading cause of death.)
- **GI:** Wide-mouthed colonic diverticula and esophageal dysmotility, leading to reflux and Barrett's esophagus. There is primary biliary cirrhosis in 15 percent of patients.
- **Heart:** Restrictive cardiomyopathy
- **Renal:** May lead to malignant hypertension

DIAGNOSTIC TESTING

There is *no* single diagnostic test.

- ANA is present in 95 percent of cases but is nonspecific.
- **Antitopoisomerase (anti-Scl 70)** is only present in 30 percent of patients.

TREATMENT

No treatment has been proven effective in stopping scleroderma. Penicillamine is *not* effective in delaying progression of this disease. One can use the following therapies:

- **Renal involvement and hypertension:** Use ACE inhibitors.
- **Pulmonary hypertension:** Use **bosentan** (endothelin antagonist), **protsacyclin analogs** (epoprostanil, treprostanil, iloprost), or **sildenafil.**
- **Raynaud's:** Use alcium channel blockers.

"CREST" SYNDROME, OR LIMITED SCLERODERMA

This form of scleroderma presents with the following:

- Calcinosis of the fingers
- Raynaud's
- Esophageal dysmotility
- Sclerodactyly
- Telangiectasia

It does *not* present with the following:

- Joint pain
- Heart involvement
- Lung involvement
- Kidney involvement

DIAGNOSTIC TESTING

CREST syndrome does *not* involve anti-Scl70.

> CREST is characterized by **anticentromere antibodies.**

EOSINOPHILIC FASCIITIS

Eosinophilic fasciitis presents with **thickened skin that looks like scleroderma.** However, the following are *not* present:

- Hand involvement
- Raynaud's
- Heart, lung, or kidney involvement

There is **marked eosinophilia** and the appearance of an **"orange peel" (peau d'orange).**

Treatment is with **corticosteroids.**

POLYMYOSITIS (PM) AND DERMATOMYOSITIS (DM)

In both conditions, the patient **cannot get up from a seated position** without using the arms. There can also be **muscle pain and tenderness.**

For **polymyositis,** look for the following:

- **Proximal muscle weakness**
- Signs of **muscle inflammation** on blood tests, electromyography, and biopsy

For **dermatomyositis,** you find the same thing and **various rashes.**

- **Gottron's papules:** Over metocarpophalangeal joint surfaces
- **Heliotrope rash:** Periorbital and purplish lesion around the eyes
- **Shawl sign:** Shoulder and neck erythema

> - Weakness + ↑CPK + ↑Aldolase + Biopsy = Polymyositis
> - Weakness + ↑CPK + ↑Aldolase + Biopsy + Skin rash = Dermatomyositis

DIAGNOSTIC TESTING

Testing reveals **elevated CPK and aldolase** with an **abnormal electromyogram (EMG).** For CCS, order **all the liver function tests** as well as **ANA.**

> **Biopsy** is the single most accurate test of PM/DM.

A 50-year-old patient presents with muscle weakness of the girdle with an increased CPK and aldolase. Her anti-Jo-1 antibody is positive. Which of the following is most likely to happen to her?

a. Stroke

b. Myocardial infarction

c. Septic arthritis

d. DVT

e. Interstitial lung disease

*Answer: The correct answer is **E**. PM/DM presents with weakness and increased markers of muscle inflammation. The presence of **anti-Jo 1** indicates a markedly increased risk of interstitial lung disease.*

What is the most common serious complication of PM/DM?

a. Rhabdomyolysis

b. Hyperkalemia

c. Metabolic acidosis

d. Malignancy

*Answer: The correct answer is **D**. For unclear reasons, the most common serious threat to life from PM/DM is malignancy. DM has a greater risk than PM.*

TREATMENT

Treat polymyositis and dermatomyositis with glucocorticoids.

FIBROMYALGIA

Look for a **woman** (10 times more common in females) with **muscle aches and stiffness with trigger points on palpation and nonrefreshing sleep. Depression and anxiety** are common.

DIAGNOSTIC TESTING

All blood tests are normal. There is *no* objective evidence of disease. This is a pain syndrome with tender trigger points.

Fibromyalgia trigger points

TREATMENT

Treat symptoms with the following:

- **Exercise**
- **Tricyclic antidepressants,** such as amitriptyline, pregabalin, or gabapentin

POLYMYALGIA RHEUMATICA (PMR)

Presents with a **person > 50 years old** with **profound pain and stiffness of the proximal muscles,** such as shoulders and pelvic girdle. The stiffness is **worse in the morning** and is **localized to the muscles** rather than to the joints. The **ESR is elevated,** and there is an amazing response to steroids.

> Pain is much more prominent than weakness in PMR.

> Age > 50 + Proximal muscle pain + ↑ESR = PMR

Nonspecific features of PMR are the following:

- Fever, weight loss, and malaise
- Normocytic anemia
- *Normal* CPK, EMG, aldolase, and muscle biopsy
- *No* muscle atrophy

The following table compares chronic fatigue syndrome, fibromyalgia, and polymyalgia rheumatica.

	Chronic Fatigue Syndrome	Fibromyalgia	Polymyalgia Rheumatica
Fatigue/malaise	+++++ > 6 months	++	++
Nonrefreshing sleep	+++++	++	No
Trigger points	No	Yes	No
Blood tests	All normal	All normal	↑ESR
Treatment	None	Pain relief	Prednisone

VASCULITIS

All forms of vasculitis have some features in common:

- On presentation, they can all have these features:
  - **Fatigue, malaise, weight loss**
  - **Fever:** May present as a fever of unknown origin (FUO)
  - **Skin lesions:** Palpable purpura, rash
  - **Joint pain**
  - **Neuropathy:** Mononeuritis multiplex
- Common laboratory features are these:
  - **Normocytic anemia**
  - **Elevated ESR**
  - **Thrombocytosis**

DIAGNOSTIC TESTING

Biopsy is the most accurate test for vasculitis. See also the lab features noted above.

TREATMENT

Best initial therapy: **Prednisone and glucocorticoids**

If steroids are not effective, alternate and/or additional therapies are the following:

- **Cyclophosphamide**
- **Azathioprine/6-Mercaptopurine**
- **Methotrexate**

POLYARTERITIS NODOSA (PAN)

PAN has **all of the features of vasculitis** described above. What is different or unique enough about PAN to allow you to establish the diagnosis is:

- **Abdominal pain** (65 percent)
- **Renal involvement** (65 percent)
- **Testicular involvement** (35 percent)
- **Pericarditis** (35 percent)
- **Hypertension** (50 percent)

> PAN does **not** affect the lungs.

DIAGNOSTIC TESTING

- Best initial test: **Angiography of abdominal vessels**
- Most accurate test: **Biopsy (of skin, muscle, or sural nerve)**

There is *no* good blood test for PAN.

> Hepatitis B surface antigen is found in 30 percent of patients with PAN.

TREATMENT

Therapy is with **prednisone and cyclophosphamide.**

WEGENER'S GRANULOMATOSIS

This disorder, like PAN, can affect the majority of the body. However, look for **upper and lower respiratory findings and c-ANCA.**

The most accurate test is **biopsy.** Treatment is with **prednisone and cyclophosphamide.**

> - Upper and lower respiratory findings + c-ANCA = Wegener's

CHURG-STRAUSS

Although Churg-Strauss can affect any organ in the body, the key to recognizing it is that it involves **vasculitis, eosinophilia, and asthma.** Although the p-ANCA and anti-myeloperoxidase can be positive, too, these findings are not as different and unique as the presence of eosinophilia and asthma.

Biopsy is the most accurate test, and there is an excellent response to **steroids.**

> - Vasculitis + Eosinophilia + Asthma = Churg-Strauss

TEMPORAL ARTERITIS

Temporal arteritis is a type of **giant cell arteritis.** It is related to polymyalgia rheumatica.

Fever, weight loss, malaise, and fatigue can be present, as they are in all forms of vasculitis.

The most accurate test is a **biopsy.**

A patient presents with headache, jaw claudication, visual disturbance, and tenderness of the scalp. The ESR is elevated. What is the next best step in management?

Answer: **Treatment with steroids** *is more important than getting a specific diagnostic test in temporal arteritis.*

TAKAYASU'S ARTERITIS

- Young Asian female + Diminished pulses = Takayasu's arteritis

Half of patients with Takayasu's arteritis have the usual **vasculitis** findings present *before* the **loss or decrease of pulse:**

- **Fatigue, malaise, weight loss, arthralgia**
- **Anemia, increased ESR**

The special features of this vasculitis are **TIA and stroke** from vascular occlusion.

Takayasu's is also distinctive in that it is diagnosed with **aortic arteriography** or **magnetic resonance angiography (MRA).**

Takayasu's is treated with **steroids** like all vasculitis.

> The most accurate test for Takayasu's is *not* a biopsy.

CRYOGLOBULINEMIA

Cryoglobulinemia has all the usual features of vasculitis, such as **fatigue, malaise, skin lesions, and joint pain.** There is an association with **hepatitis C and renal involvement.**

Treat the hepatitis C with **interferon and ribavirin.** (Note that Step 3 loves this question!)

BEHCET DISEASE

This condition presents in patients of Middle Eastern or Asian ancestry. Features are the following:

- **Oral and genital ulcers**
- **Ocular involvement** (uveitis, optic neuritis): Can lead to blindness.
- **Skin lesions:** "Pathergy," which is **hyperreactivity to needle sticks,** resulting in sterile skin abscesses.

There is *no* specific test for Behcet disease. Use the features described above.

Treatment is with **prednisone and colchicines.**

INFLAMED JOINTS

To diagnose inflamed joints, you need to look at the fluid. Inflamed joints will generally have effusions. **Joint aspiration** is the most accurate test for gout, pseudogout, and septic arthritis.

The gram stain lacks sensitivity and, even in bacterial septic arthritis, will only detect 50–60 percent of infections. The best initial test for septic arthritis is the **cell count.** There is still overlap. Infectious septic arthritis could be present with as few as 20,000 white cells, although most cases have > 50,000–100,000.

SYNOVIAL FLUID CELL COUNT

Normal	Inflammatory (Gout/Pseudogout)	Infectious
< 2,000 WBCs	2,000–50,000 WBCs	> 50,000 WBCs

GOUT

Look for a **man** with a **sudden onset** of **severe pain** in the **toe at night.** The toe will be red, swollen, and tender, and it can look very similar to a toe with an infection.

The following can precipitate acute gouty attacks:

- **Binge drinking of alcohol**
- **Thiazides**
- **Nicotinic acid**

Diagnostic Testing

- Best initial test: **Arthrocentesis** (aspiration of joint fluid)
- Most accurate test: **Polarized light examination** of the fluid will show **negatively birefringent needles.**

> - Gout = Negative birefringence
> - Pseudogout = Positive birefringence

For CCS, also do the following:

- **Joint fluid examination for cell count, culture, and protein level**
- **Serum uric acid level:** However, do *not* rely on uric acid level to make an accurate diagnosis.
- **X-ray of the toe:** May show "punched-out" lesions
- **Extremity examination for tophi**

Of all gout patients, 30 percent can have at least one *normal* uric acid level, especially during the attack, because the uric acid is being deposited into the joints from the blood. An elevated uric acid level alone is *not* an indication for treatment in an asymptomatic patient. You *must* tap the joint.

TREATMENT

- Best initial therapy: **NSAIDs** are the best initial therapy for an acute gouty attack.
- If there is insufficient response to NSAIDS, use **steroids** to treat acute gouty attacks.
- **Colchicine** is useful under the following conditions:
  - In the **first 24 hours** of an attack
  - When there is a **contraindication to the use of NSAIDs,** such as renal insufficiency
  - As part of **preventive therapy** to decrease the risk of a gouty attack
- Colchicine has the following adverse effects:
  - Nausea and diarrhea
  - Bone marrow suppression
- Prevention:
  - **Allopurinol, probenecid, and sulfinpyrazone** lower the level of uric acid. Allopurinol has the following adverse effects: rash, allergic interstitial nephritis, and hemolysis.

  - **Weight loss**
  - **Avoiding alcohol**
  - See the previous information about colchicine.

Do *not* start allopurinol during an acute attack of gout.

CALCIUM PYROPHOSPHATE DEPOSITION DISEASE (PSEUDOGOUT)

In a case of pseudogout, expect hemochromatosis, hyperparathyroidism, acromegaly, or hypothyroidism in the history.

In pseudogout, the **knee and wrist are involved** but *not* the toes. Pseudogout is much slower in onset than gout, and the patient will *not* wake up with severe pain.

Tap the joint and look for **positively birefringent rhomboid-shaped crystals.**

NSAIDS are the best initial therapy. Colchicine is used but is not as effective.

SEPTIC ARTHRITIS

The more abnormal the joint, the more likely a patient is to have septic arthritis. **Any arthritic joint or prosthetic joint** is a risk factor:

- Osteoarthritis is more of a risk than having normal joints.
- Rheumatoid arthritis is more of a risk than osteoarthritis.
- Prosthetic joints are more of a risk than anything else.

Septic arthritis presents with a **swollen, red, immobile, tender joint.**

The etiology is as follows:

- *Staphylococcus aureus* (40 percent)
- *Streptococcus* (30 percent)
- Gram-negative bacilli (20 percent)

Call an **orthopedic surgery consult** when you suspect a septic joint. The consultation won't offer much on the CCS, but it needs to be done.

DIAGNOSTIC TESTING
- Best initial test: **Tap the joint (arthrocentesis).** A finding of > 50,000 white cells is consistent with infection.
- Gram stain has a 50–60 percent sensitivity.
- Most accurate test: **Culture** is > 90 percent sensitive but is *never* available when you must make an acute treatment decision.

TREATMENT
Empiric therapy with **ceftriaxone and vancomycin intravenously** is effective. This is the choice for CCS when you have to write in one answer.

The following table shows other possible answers for multiple-choice questions. These are used **in combination:** one for *Staph/Strep* and one for gram-negative bacilli.

Staph and Strep Drug	Gram-Negative Bacilli Drug
• Oxacillin • Nafcillin • Cefazolin	• Ceftriaxone • Ceftazidime • Gentamicin
Penicillin allergy: Anaphylaxis • Vancomycin • Linezolid • Daptomycin • Clindamycin	Penicillin allergy: Anaphylaxis • Aztreonam • Fluoroquinolone

PAGET'S DISEASE OF BONE

This condition is often **asymptomatic.** It may lead to **pain, stiffness, aching, and fractures.** Soft bones lead to **bowing of the tibias. Sarcoma** arises in 1 percent of patients.

> In cases of Paget's, osteolytic lesions will be found initially. These may be replaced with osteoblastic lesions. So on Step 3,
> • If you see osteo*lytic*, then think Paget's or osteoporosis; *but*
> • if you see osteo*blastic*, think about metastatic prostate cancer in your differential.

DIAGNOSTIC TESTING

- Best initial test: **Alkaline phosphatase level.** It will be elevated.
- Most accurate test: **X-ray**
- For CCS, also order the following:
  - **Urinary hydroxyproline**
  - **Serum calcium level**—It will be normal.
  - **Serum phosphate level**—It will be normal.
  - **Bone scan**

TREATMENT

Treat with **bisphosphonates and calcitonin.**

BAKER'S CYST

A Baker's cyst is a **posterior herniation of the synovium of the knee.** Look for a patient with **osteoarthritis or rheumatoid arthritis** with a **swollen calf.** A ruptured Baker's cyst is a "pseudo-phlebitis." Unruptured cysts can be palpated.

Exclude a deep vein thrombosis with **ultrasound.**

Treat with **NSAIDs** and, occasionally, with steroid injection.

Plantar Fasciitis and Tarsal Tunnel Syndrome

The following table compares these two conditions.

Plantar Fasciitis	Tarsal Tunnel Syndrome
Pain on bottom of foot	Pain on bottom of foot
Very severe in the morning, better with walking a few steps	More painful with more use; like carpal tunnel of the foot; may have numbness of the sole, too
Stretch the foot and calf	Avoid boots and high heels; may need steroid injection
Resolves spontaneously over time	May need surgical release

Morton Neuroma

This condition presents with the following:

- **Painful burning sensation** in the interdigital web space between the 3rd and 4th toes
- **Tenderness** when pressure is applied between the heads of the 3rd and 4th metatarsals
- **Sharp, intermittent pain** radiating into the toes that feels better when shoes are taken off

HEMATOLOGY

7

ANEMIA

PRESENTATION

All forms of anemia lead to **fatigue** and a subjective sense of **loss of energy.** The case will use words such as *tired, fatigue, malaise,* or *loss of energy.* You will be able to recognize more severe anemia when the question says *short of breath, lightheadedness,* or *confusion.* Other diseases may also present with fatigue or shortness of breath, similar to anemia.

> If the question describes a **craving for ice or dirt** (i.e., forms of pica), think anemia. Step 3 loves to use pica as a lead in to anemia.

Diseases with presentations similar to those of anemia are the following:

- Hypoxia
- Carbon monoxide poisoning
- Methemoglobinemia
- Ischemic heart disease

PHYSICAL EXAMINATION

On CCS, choose the following physical exams: general appearance, CV, chest, extremities, and HEENT.

Potential positive findings are **pallor, flow murmur** described as I/VI or II/VI systolic murmur, and **pale conjunctiva.** Hemolysis will also give jaundice and sclera icterus (yellow eyes). The chest exam is chosen routinely in any patient with shortness of breath, even though there are no positive findings in anemia, to exclude other causes of shortness of breath.

There are *no* unique physical findings in anemia to allow you a specific diagnosis. For CCS cases, you find one anyway. For single best answer questions, go straight for the CBC.

LABORATORY TESTING

- Best initial test: **CBC with peripheral smear** (Pay special attention to the MCV/MCHC.)
- Additional initial tests: **Reticulocyte count, haptoglobin, LDH, total and direct bilirubin, TSH with T4, B12/folate levels, iron studies**
- Also order **urinalysis with microscopic analysis**

CATEGORIZING ANEMIA

Based on the MCV, you determine whether the anemia is microcytic, macrocytic, or normocytic. The MCHC may tell you if there is a problem with the synthesis of hemoglobin. Based on this measurement, you can further categorize anemia as hypochromic, hyperchromic, or normochromic.

MICROCYTIC ANEMIA

Diagnostic Testing and Treatment

Specific Diagnostic Tests and Treatments				
When this is in the history/physical...	Blood loss, elevated platelet count	Rheumatoid arthritis; end stage renal disease or any chronic infectious, inflammatory, or connective tissue disease	Very small MCV with few or no symptoms; Target cells	Alcoholic, isoniazid, lead exposure
...this is the diagnosis.	Iron deficiency	Anemia of chronic disease	Thalasemia	Sideroblastic anemia
What is the best initial diagnostic test?	Iron studies: • Low ferritin • High TIBC • Low Fe • Low Fe sat • Elevated RDW	Iron studies: • High ferritin • Low TIBC • Low Fe • Low Fe sat	Iron studies: • Normal	Iron studies: • High Fe
What is the most accurate diagnostic test?	Bone marrow biopsy (do not do this on CCS)		Hemoglobin Electrophoresis Beta: Elevated HgA2, HgF Alpha: Normal	Prussian blue stain
What is the best initial therapy?	Prescribe ferrous sulfate orally	Correct the underlying disease	No treatment	Minor: Prescribe pyridoxine replacement Major: Remove the toxin exposure

A 62-year-old-man with a history of anemia from a bleeding peptic ulcer comes for evaluation. He is constipated and has black stool. His medications are omeprazole, oral ferrous sulfate, and occasional liquid antacids. What would you do next?

a. EGD

b. Colonoscopy

c. Guaiac testing/hemoccult

d. Discontinue omeprazole

e. Increase the dose of ferrous sulfate

*Answer: The correct answer is **C**, heme testing of the stool. Oral ferrous sulfate can turn the stool black, but elemental iron such as this does not make the stool guiac positive. Only the iron in hemoglobin or myoglobin can make the stool guaiac card positive.*

Diagnostic testing is as follows:

- Most important test: **Iron studies/profile** (Fe level, Fe saturation, ferritin, TIBC)
- Most accurate test: **Bone marrow biopsy**

Only iron deficiency is associated with an elevated red cell distribution of width (RDW). This is because the newer cells are progressively smaller and smaller; therefore, the red cell width changes over time. **Prussian blue** is an iron stain. **Sideroblastic anemia** is associated with iron building up inside the mitochondria of the red cell.

A 68-year-old woman is found on routine CBC to have a hematocrit of 32 percent (normal 37–42) and an MCV of 70 (normal 80–100). Her stool is heme negative. What should you do next?

a. Colonoscopy
b. Sigmoidoscopy
c. Barium enema
d. Upper endoscopy
e. Two more stool tests now
f. Repeat the stool testing in a year
g. Capsule endoscopy

*Answer: The correct answer is **A**. Colonoscopy is indicated in all patients > 50 simply as routine screening. Hence, in this case, the patient needs colonoscopy anyway, regardless of what the stool tests show. Another reason to go straight to endoscopy is the presence of microcytic anemia. Unexplained microcytic anemia in a patient above 50 is most likely caused by colon cancer. Sigmoidoscopy will do nothing to evaluate the right side of the colon and would miss nearly 40 percent of cancers. No matter what a sigmoidoscopy showed, you would need to inspect the right side of the colon. Capsule endoscopy is done to evaluate bleeding when the upper and lower endoscopy are normal and the source of bleeding is likely to be in the small bowel.*

A patient comes with end stage renal disease for evaluation of shortness of breath. After dialysis, he is found to have a hematocrit of 28 with an MCV of 68. Iron studies are performed. What do you expect to find?

	Iron	Total Iron Binding Capacity	Ferritin	RDW
a.	Low	High	Low	High
b.	Low	Low	Normal	Normal
c.	Normal	Normal	Normal	Normal
d.	High	High	Normal	Normal

*Answer: The correct answer is **C**. The anemia of chronic disease, such as that found in patients with end stage renal disease, is associated with normal or increased amounts of iron in storage (ferritin/TIBC) but the inability to process the iron into usable cells and hemoglobin. The only form of anemia of chronic disease that reliably responds to erythropoietin is from end stage renal disease.*

MACROCYTIC ANEMIA

> **"Extravascular" hemolysis** occurs in spleen and liver, so you **cannot** see it on the smear.

Presentation

All anemia presents with **fatigue**. The same is true of microcytic anemia, which is caused by **vitamin B12 or folate deficiency.**

- **Vitamin B12 deficiency** presents with **neurological findings** as well.
  - The most common is **peripheral neuropathy,** but *any* form of neurological abnormality can develop at any part of the peripheral or central nervous system.
  - The least common neurological problem is dementia.
  - Neurological problems resolve with treatment if they have been present for a short period of time.

- **B12 deficiency** also causes a **smooth tongue (glossitis) and diarrhea.**
- **Folate deficiency:** This does not present with neurological problems.

Diagnostic Testing

- Best initial test: **CBC with peripheral blood smear** (look for hypersegmented neutrophils and oval cells). The average number of lobes in the normal white cell is 3.5. If the average is > 4 or more than 5 percent of the cells have > 5 lobes, the patient has **megaloblastic anemia** as well as *macrocytosis.* Macrocytosis means "big cells" (i.e., large MCV). Megaloblastic anemia means the presence of hypersegmented neutrophils as well. For CCS cases you should also order a **bilirubin level and LDH,** which are commonly elevated. The **reticulocyte count will be decreased. Oval cells** will be visible on the peripheral smear as well.

- Most accurate tests: **Low B12 level** (for B12 deficiency) and **folate level** (for folate deficiency). Note: Up to 30 percent of those with B12 deficiency can have a *normal* B12 level, because transcobalamin is an acute phase reactant and any form of stress can cause its elevation. If you suspect B12 deficiency but the B12 level is normal, order a **methylmalonic acid level.** Homocysteine levels go up in *both* vitamin B12 deficiency and folate deficiency.

- When asked, *after* finding a low B12 level or elevated methylmalonic acid level, "What is the next best test to confirm the etiology of the B12 deficiency," answer **antiparietal cell antibodies** and **anti-intrinsic factor antibodies.** Antiparietal cell antibodies and anti-intrinsic factor antibodies confirm pernicious anemia as the etiology of the B12 deficiency. Essentially, **pernicious anemia** is an allergy to parietal cells; it is a kind of autoimmune disorder against this part of the stomach.

- Schilling's test is an older, rarely done method of confirming the etiology and is not necessary if the antibodies are present.

Treatment
B12 deficiency and folate deficiency are treated with **replacement.**

HEMOLYTIC ANEMIA
All forms of hemolytic anemia present **with the sudden onset of weakness and fatigue** associated with anemia.

Diagnostic Testing
Hemolysis shows the following:

- Elevated indirect bilirubin level
- Elevated reticulocyte count
- Elevated LDH level
- Decreased haptoglobin level

With hemolysis, order a peripheral smear, LDH, bilirubin level, reticulocyte count, and haptoglobin level on the first CCS screen.

Intravascular hemolysis *also* shows the following:

- Abnormal peripheral smear (schistocytes, helmet cells, fragmented cells)
- Hemoglobinuria
- Hemosiderinuria (metabolic, oxidized product of hemoglobin in the urine)

Intravascular Hemolysis

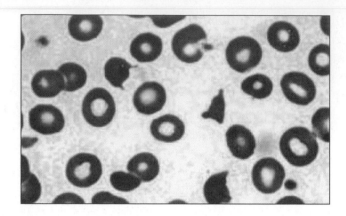

SICKLE CELL ANEMIA

The *most* likely hemolysis question to be asked will concern sickle cell anemia. The question will describe **pain in the chest, back, and thighs that is *very* severe.**

Physical Exam

A **complete physical examination** is *very* important for the sickle cell case. *After* you give oxygen, fluids, analgesics, and antibiotics, then if there is a fever, perform a complete physical examination.

Possible findings of the physical include the following:

- HEENT: Retinal infarction
- CV: Flow murmur from anemia
- Abdomen: Splenomegaly in children; absence of spleen in adults
- Chest: Rales or consolidation from infection or infarction
- Extremities: Skin ulcers (unclear etiology in sickle cell) and aseptic necrosis of hip
- Neurological: Stroke, current or previous

Treatment

- Next best step: **Oxygen, hydration** with normal saline continuously, and **pain medications**
- If a fever is present: Give **ceftriaxone, levofloxacin,** or **moxifloxacin** with the first screen. Fever in a patient with sickle cell disease is an *emergency* because the patient has *no* spleen.
  - Hence, for a question of "Most urgent next step?" answer **antibiotics** when fever is present. This is *more* important than waiting for results of testing.
  - If it is a CCS question, answer **blood cultures, urinalysis, reticulocyte count, CBC, and chest X-ray** with the first screen as well, but if fever is present, do not wait for results.

When do I answer "exchange transfusion" in sickle cell disease?

Answer:
- *Eye: Visual disturbance from retinal infarction*
- *Lung: Pulmonary infarction leading to pleuritic pain and abnormal X-ray*
- *Penis: Priapism from infarction of prostatic plexus of veins*
- *Brain: Stroke*

A patient admitted for sickle cell crisis has a drop from her usual hematocrit of 34 to 26 over 2 days in the hospital. The reticulocyte count is 2 percent. What is the diagnosis? What is the most accurate test? What is the treatment?

*Answer: Sudden drops in the hematocrit in sickle cell patients or those with hemoglobinopathy can be from **parvovirus B19** or **folate deficiency**. Sickle cell patients should universally be on **folate replacement**.*

If the patient is on replacement, then the diagnosis shifts to parvovirus B19, which is an **infection that invades the marrow** and stops production of cells at the level of the pronormoblast. The most accurate diagnostic test is **PCR for DNA of the parvovirus.** This is more accurate than IgM or IgG antibody testing or bone marrow.

Treat with **transfusions and intravenous immunoglobulins.**

When a patient with sickle cell anemia is ready for discharge, prescribe the following:

- Folate replacement
- Pneumococcal vaccination
- Hydroxyurea to prevent further crises if they happen > 4 times per year

HEMOGLOBIN SICKLE CELL (SC) DISEASE

This condition is like a **mild version of sickle cell disease** with fewer crises. Visual disturbance is frequent. Painful crises do not occur. Renal problems are the only significant manifestation, including the following:

- Hematuria
- Isosthenuria (inability to concentrate or dilute the urine)
- Urinary tract infections

There is no specific therapy for hemoglobin SC disease.

Sickle cell trait: Renal manifestations are the only findings. They are hematuria and a concentrating defect.

AUTOIMMUNE HEMOLYSIS

Look for **other autoimmune diseases in the history,** such as SLE or rheumatoid arthritis. Other clues are a history of chronic lymphocytic leukemia (CLL), lymphoma, or medications such as penicillin, alphamethyldopa, quinine, or sulfa drugs.

Diagnostic Testing

The **LDH, indirect bilirubin level, and reticulocyte count will be elevated** as with all forms of hemolysis. The **haptoglobin level can be decreased** in both intravascular and extravascular forms of hemolysis.

- Peripheral smear: May show **spherocytes**
- Most accurate diagnostic test: **Coomb's test**

Treatment

- Best initial therapy: **Steroids,** such as prednisone
- If the case describes recurrent episodes of hemolysis, **splenectomy** is the most effective therapy.

These antibodies are also called **"warm antibodies,"** which are IgG. *Only* IgG antibodies respond to steroids and splenectomy.

If the case describes **severe hemolysis** not responsive to prednisone or repeated blood transfusion, use **intravenous immunoglobulins** as the best therapy to stop acute episodes of hemolysis.

COLD-INDUCED HEMOLYSIS (COLD AGGLUTININS)

Look for the following:

- **Mycoplasma** or **Epstein-Barr virus** is in the history.
- Standard **Coomb's test is negative.**
- **Complement test is positive.**
- There is **no response to steroids, splenectomy, or intravenous immunoglobulins.**

CCS does *not* require you to know dosing. Do not memorize doses. There is no way to order doses on CCS.

GLUCOSE 6 PHOSPHATE DEHYDROGENASE (G6PD) DEFICIENCY

Sudden onset of hemolysis, which can be quite severe, is seen. As an **X-linked disorder,** hemolysis from G6PD deficiency is much more often described in **males.**

The most common form of oxidant stress to cause acute hemolysis with G6PD deficiency is an **infection. Oxidizing drugs,** such as sulfa medication, primiquine or dapsone, are frequently in the history. **Fava bean ingestion** may also be in the history.

Diagnostic Testing

- Best initial test: **Heinz body test, bite cells. Heinz bodies** are collections of oxidized, precipitated hemoglobin embedded in the red cell membrane. **Bite cells** appear when pieces of the red cell membrane have been removed by the spleen.

Heinz bodies

Bite cells

Most accurate diagnostic test: The **level of G6PD**—but *only* after 2 months have passed. A normal level of G6PD immediately after an episode of hemolysis does *not* exclude G6PD deficiency. On the day of the hemolysis, the most deficient cells have been destroyed, and the level of G6PD is normal.

Treatment

There is *no* specific therapy for G6PD deficiency. **Avoid oxidant stress.**

PYRUVATE KINASE DEFICIENCY

Presents the **same way as G6PD deficiency in terms of hemolysis.** However, pyruvate kinase deficiency is *not* provoked by medications or fava beans; what precipitates the hemolysis with pyruvate kinase deficiency is *not* clear.

HEREDITARY SPHEROCYTOSIS

This condition presents with the following:

- **Recurrent episodes**
- **Splenomegaly**
- **Bilirubin gallstones**
- **Elevated mean corpuscular hemoglobin concentration** (MCHC)

The most accurate test for hereditary spherocytosis is an **osmotic fragility test.**

Splenectomy will prevent hemolysis since the cells are destroyed in the spleen. **Splenectomy** helps in these patients.

HEMOLYTIC UREMIC SYNDROME (HUS) AND THROMBOTIC THROMBOCYTOPENIC PURPURA (TTP)

Look for *E. coli* **0157:H7** in the history for HUS. Medications such as **ticlopidine** predispose to TTP.

Diagnostic Testing

There is *no* specific diagnostic test for these. Rather, the diagnosis is based on the following:

- **HUS triad: ART**
  - **Intravascular hemolysis** with abnormal smear (**A:** Autoimmune hemolysis)
  - **Elevated BUN and creatinine** (**R:** Renal failure)

- **Thrombocytopenia** (**T:** Thrombocytopenia)
  - **TTP pentad (FAT RN)** *also* has the following
  - **Fever** (**F:** Fever)
  - **Neurological abnormalities** (**N:** Neurological issues)

Treatment

Most cases **resolve on their own.** Severe cases of either TTP or HUS should be treated with **plasmapheresis.** Steroids will *not* help. Antibiotics for HUS from *E. coli* may make it worse; platelet transfusions for either will *definitely* make it worse.

PAROXYSMAL NOCTURNAL HEMOGLOBINURIA (PNH)

Presents with pancytopenia and recurrent episodes of dark urine, particularly in the morning. The most common cause of death is **large vessel venous thrombosis,** such as portal vein thrombosis.

PNH can transform into the following:

- Aplastic anemia
- Acute myelogenous leukemia (AML)

Diagnostic Testing

- Most accurate test: **CD 55** and **CD 59** antibody (also known as **decay accelerating factor**)
- Older screening tests that are *not* as accurate: the **sugar-water test** and **Ham's test.** These are tests for the activation of complement, which leads to hemolysis.

Treatment

Treatment is with **glucocorticoids,** such as prednisone.

A pregnant woman comes with weakness and elevated liver function tests. She is in her 35th week of pregnancy. The prothrombin time is normal. The smear of blood shows fragmented red cells. Platelet count is low. What is the treatment?

a. Transfuse platelets
b. Plasmapheresis
c. Fresh frozen plasma
d. Delivery of the baby
e. Prednisone

*Answer: The correct answer is **D.** Deliver the baby with the **HELLP syndrome.** HELLP syndrome stands for **hemolysis, elevated liver function tests,** and **low platelets.** This disorder is idiopathic and can be distinguished from DIC by the normal coagulation studies, such as the prothrombin time and aPTT.*

METHEMOGLOBINEMIA

The key to recognizing this condition is that the patient presents with **shortness of breath for no clear reason** with **clear lungs on exam** and a **normal chest X-ray.** Methemoglobinemia is **blood locked in an oxidized state that cannot pick up oxygen.** Look for an **exposure to drugs** such as nitroglycerin, amyl nitrate, nitroprusside, dapsone, or any of the anesthetic drugs that end in *caine* (e.g., lidocaine, bupivicaine, tetracaine). Methemoglobinemia can occur with as little exposure as to a topical anesthetic administered to a mucous membrane. Look for **brown blood** in the case description. Treat with **methylene blue.**

TRANSFUSION REACTIONS

Match the most likely diagnoses with each of the following cases:

a. ABO incompatibility

b. Transfusion-related acute lung injury (TRALI) or "Leukoagglutination reaction"

c. Urticarial reaction

d. IgA deficiency

e. Febrile nonhemolytic reaction

f. Minor blood group incompatibility

Case 1: Twenty minutes after a patient receives a blood transfusion, the patient becomes short of breath. There are transient infiltrates on the chest X-ray. All symptoms resolve spontaneously.

Case 2: As soon as a patient receives a transfusion, he becomes hypotensive, short of breath, and tachycardic. The LDH and bilirubin levels are normal.

Case 3: During a transfusion, a patient becomes hypotensive and tachycardic. She has back and chest pain, and there is dark urine. The LDH and bilirubin are elevated, and the haptoglobin level is low.

Case 4: A few days after a transfusion, a patient becomes jaundiced. The hematocrit does not rise with transfusion, and he is generally without symptoms.

Case 5: A few hours after a transfusion, a patient becomes febrile with a rise in temperature of about 1 degree. There is no evidence of hemolysis.

Answers:

Case 1: The correct answer is B. TRALI presents with acute shortness of breath from antibodies in the donor blood against recipient white cells. There is no treatment, and it resolves spontaneously.

Case 2: The correct answer is D. IgA deficiency presents with anaphylaxis. In the future, use blood donations from an IgA deficient donor or washed red cells.

Case 3: The correct answer is A. ABO incompatibility presents with acute symptoms of hemolysis while the transfusion is occurring.

Case 4: The correct answer is F. Minor blood group incompatibility to Kell, Duffy, Lewis, or Kidd antigens or Rh incompatibility presents with delayed jaundice. There is no specific therapy.

Case 5: The correct answer is E. Febrile nonhemolytic reactions result in a small rise in temperature and need no therapy. These reactions are against donor white cell antigens. They are prevented by using filtered blood transfusions in the future to remove the white cell antigens.

LEUKEMIA

ACUTE LEUKEMIA

Presents with signs of pancytopenia, such as **fatigue, bleeding,** and **infections** from white cells that don't work. Patients have a **functional immunodeficiency.**

Diagnostic Testing

- Best initial test: **Peripheral smear showing blasts**

The most important prognostic finding in acute leukemia is **cytogenetic abnormalities,** such as specific karyotypic abnormalities. Cytogenetics tells who will relapse. If the patient is as high risk for relapse after chemotherapy, **bone marrow transplantation** should be performed as soon as chemotherapy induces remission.

> Auer rods are associated with acute myeloid leukemia (AML).

Treatment

Chemotherapy with **idarubicin** (or **daunorubicin**) and **cytosine arabinoside** is the best initial therapy for acute myelogenous leukemia. Add **all trans retinoic acid (ATRA)** to the treatment of M3 leukemia. Add **intrathecal methotrexate** for acute lymphocytic leukemia (ALL).

> M3, acute promyelocytic leukemia, is associated with disseminated intravascular coagulation (DIC). This is the most frequently tested information about acute leukemia.

A patient presents with shortness of breath, confusion, and blurry vision. His white cell count is over 100,000. What is the best initial therapy?

*Answer: Acute leukemia can sometimes present with an extremely high white cell count. When the count goes above 100,000, these cells result in sludging of the blood vessels of the brain, eyes, and lungs. Chronic lymphocytic leukemia rarely ever does this, because lymphocytes are much smaller and do not occlude vessels. Leukostasis is treated with **leucopheresis**, which removes white cells via centrifugation of blood. **Hydroxyurea** is also added to lower the white cell count.*

MYELODYSPLASIA

This condition presents in elderly patients with **pancytopenia, elevated MCV, low reticulocyte count,** and **macroovalocytes.** There is a special neutrophil with two lobes called a **"Pelger-Huet cell."** Look for a **normal B12 level.** There will be a **small number of blasts** but not enough to be considered acute leukemia. Myelodysplasia is like a **mild, slowly progressive preleukemia syndrome.** Just as cervical dysplasia may sometimes progress to cervical cancer, myelodysplasia may progress to acute leukemia. The most common cause of death is not leukemia; most patients die of **infection** or **bleeding.** Treatment is largely supportive with **transfusions as needed.**

MYELOPROLIFERATIVE DISORDERS

CHRONIC MYELOGENOUS LEUKEMIA (CML)

Look for an **elevated white cell count** that is predominantly neutrophils. **Splenomegaly** is frequent.

Diagnostic Testing

- Best initial test: **Leukocyte alkaline phosphatase (LAP) score.** An elevated neutrophils count with a low LAP score is CML. Reactive high white counts from infection give an elevated LAP score. LAP is up in normal cells, not CML.
- Most accurate test: **Philadelphia chromosome**

Treatment

The best initial therapy is **imatinib** (Gleevec®). **Bone marrow transplantation** is the only way to cure CML, but this is *never* the best initial therapy, because imatinib leads to 90 percent hematologic remission with no major adverse effects.

Following are **wrong** answers for CML treatment:

- Interferon: Much less efficacy; causes uncomfortable, flulike symptoms
- Hydroxyurea: Never makes the Philadelphia chromosome negative
- Busulfan: Never right for anything, unless the exam asks what causes pulmonary fibrosis

> Untreated CML has the highest risk of transformation into acute leukemia of all forms of myeloproliferative disorders.

CHRONIC LYMPHOCYTIC LEUKEMIA (CLL)

CLL exclusively presents in **patients > 50 years old** with an **elevated white cell count** that is described as "normal appearing lymphocytes." CLL is often asymptomatic and is described as being found on "routine" testing.

Diagnostic Testing

- Best initial test: **Peripheral blood smear shows "smudge" cells,** which are ruptured nuclei of lymphocytes. They are like squished jelly donuts.
- Stage 0: Elevated white cell count alone
- Stage 1: Enlarged lymph nodes
- Stage 2: Spleen enlargement
- Stage 3: Anemia
- Stage 4: Low platelets

Treatment for CLL is *entirely* based on the stage of the disease.

Treatment

Early stage disease (Stages 0 and 1) does *not* require therapy. More advanced stages of disease are treated with **fludarabine** or **chlorambucil.** If the question asks, "Which therapy is most likely to extend survival?" the answer is fludarabine for advanced stage disease.

> Do not treat asymptomatic elevations in white count from CLL.

HAIRY CELL LEUKEMIA

This condition presents with the following:

- Pancytopenia
- Middle-aged patient (50s)
- Massive splenomegaly

The most accurate test is **tartrate resistant acid phosphatase (TRAP) smear showing hairy cells.**

The best initial therapy is **cladribine** or **2-CDA.**

MYELOFIBROSIS

Presents in the **same way as hairy cell leukemia** (pancytopenia and spleno-megaly) with a normal TRAP level. A key feature is teardrop-shaped cells on the smear.

There is *no* specific therapy.

POLYCYTHEMIA VERA (PVERA)

PVera presents with **headache, blurred vision, dizziness, and fatigue. Pruritus, described as happening after a hot bath or shower,** also occurs from the release of histamine from basophils. **Splenomegaly** is common.

The key to the diagnosis is a **markedly high hematocrit in the absence of hypoxia with a low MCV. The erythropoietin level will be low.** The white cell count and platelet count can also be elevated. The high hematocrit can lead to thrombosis.

Diagnostic Testing

After the **CBC** shows a high hematocrit, order an **arterial blood gas** to exclude hypoxia as a cause of erythrocytosis. If the case is a CCS, order an **erythropoietin level,** which should be low; hematology consultation; and nuclear red cell mass test.

Treatment

Phlebotomy is the best initial therapy. **Hydroxyurea** is also used to lower the cell count. **Daily aspirin** should also be given. **Anagrelide** is used in the context of thrombocythenia.

ESSENTIAL THROMBOCYTHEMIA (ET)

The key feature of ET is a **markedly elevated platelet count.** ET presents with **headache, visual disturbance, and pain in the hands** referred to as erythromelalgia. The most common causes of death are either **bleeding** or **thrombosis,** with thrombosis being more common.

Therapy is with **hydroxyurea** to lower the platelet count. Anagrelide is an agent specific to the treatment of ET but it is not as strong as hydroxyurea. **Daily aspirin** should also be given if they are thrombosing.

PLASMA CELL DISORDERS

MULTIPLE MYELOMA (MM)

The most frequent presentation of MM is with **bone pain from a fracture occurring under normal use.** The most common causes of death from MM are the following:

- **Infection:** Patients with multiple myeloma are effectively immunodeficient.
- **Renal failure**

Diagnostic Testing

Initial testing is as follows:

- **Skeletal survey** to detect punched out osteolytic lesions. (If you see osteoblastic lesions, think metastatic prostate cancer.)
- **Serum protein electrophoresis (SPEP):** You are looking for elevated levels of monoclonal antibody (usually IgG).
- **Urine protein electrophoresis (UPEP):** Detects Bence-Jones protein.
- **Peripheral smear:** Shows "rouleaux" formation of blood cells.

- **Elevated calcium level:** Makes sense with the osteolytic lesions.
- **Beta 2 microglobulin level:** This is a prognostic indicator.
- **BUN and creatinine:** This is to detect the frequent occurrence of renal insufficiency.

The single most specific test is the **bone marrow biopsy,** which detects high numbers of plasma cells (10 percent).

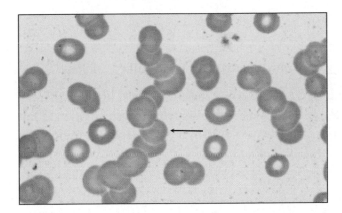

Treatment

Treat with **melphalan and steroids. Thalidomide** may be added: thalidomide is an inhibitor of tumor necrosis factor that has the same efficacy as chemotherapy.

The most effective therapy is an **autologous bone marrow transplantation.** This is reserved for patients who are relatively young with advanced disease.

You should remember *also* to treat the hypercalcemia (hydration/diuresis), bone fractures (bisphosphonates), renal failure (hydration), and anemia (eryhtropoitein) and to prophylax against infections with vaccinations (e.g., flu, pneumovax, tetanus, etc.).

MONOCLONAL GAMMOPATHY OF UNKNOWN SIGNIFICANCE (MGUS)

MGUS presents with an **asymptomatic elevation of IgG** on an SPEP. The SPEP is done because of an elevated total protein level found in an **elderly patient,** typically over 70. There is no treatment for MGUS.

WALDENSTROM'S MACROGLOBULINEMIA

This presents with **hyperviscosity from IgM overproduction.** The question will describe **blurry vision, confusion, and headache. Enlarged nodes and spleen** can be found.

There are *no* specific findings on CBC. The best initial test is a **serum viscosity level,** which will be markedly increased, and an **SPEP,** which will show an elevated IgM level.

Treatment is as follows:

- Best initial therapy: **Plasmapheresis**
- Further treatment: Use the agents you would use for CLL, such as **fludarabine** or **chlorambucil.**

APLASTIC ANEMIA

This condition presents with **pancytopenia** with no identified etiology.

When the patient is young (< 50) and has a match, the best possible therapy is **bone marrow transplantation.** When bone marrow transplantation is not possible (> 50 and/or no match), answer **antithymocyte globulin and cyclosporine.**

> "B" symptoms of lymphoma, which imply more widespread disease, are the following:
> - Fever
> - Weight loss
> - Night sweats

LYMPHOMA

Lymphoma presents with **enlarged lymph nodes,** most commonly in the cervical area. **Hodgkin's disease (HD)** spreads centrifugally away from the center, starting at the neck. **Non-Hodgkin's lymphoma (NHL)** more often presents as widespread disease.

Diagnostic Testing

- Best initial test for both HD and NHL: **Excisional lymph node biopsy.** The most common *wrong* answer is a needle biopsy. Needle biopsy is useful for infections such as tuberculosis but is *not* sufficient to diagnose lymphoma, because the visual appearance of lymphoma cells is normal; they are not grossly abnormal like acute leukemic blasts. The major difference between HD and NHL is that **HD has Reed-Sternberg cells.**
- Next tests: After the initial excisional biopsy shows the abnormal architecture of the cells, further tests **determine the stage** of the lymphoma. Staging is critical to determine therapy.
  - **Stage I:** Single lymph node group
  - **Stage II:** Two lymph node groups on one side of the diaphragm
  - **Stage III:** Lymph node involvement on both sides of the diaphragm
  - **Stage IV:** Widespread disease
- HD and NHL present with stages as follows:
  - **HD:** 80–90 percent present with Stages I and II.
  - **NHL:** 80–90 percent present with Stages III and IV.

- Staging involves the following tests:
  - **Chest X-ray**
  - **CT Scans (with contrast):** Chest, abdomen, pelvis, and head
  - **Bone marrow biopsy**

Treatment

Localized disease **(Stages I and II)** without "B" symptoms is treated predominantly with **radiation.** More advanced stage disease **(Stages III and IV)** is treated with **chemotherapy:**

- HD: **ABVD** (Adriamycin [doxorubicin], bleomycin, vinblastine, dacarbazine)
- NHL: **CHOP** (cyclophosphamide, hydroxyadriamycin, Oncovin [vincristine], prednisone). Also, test for **anti-CD20 antigen;** if present, add **rituximab,** which adds efficacy to CHOP.

> Lymphoma evaluation does *not* need lymphangiogram or exploratory laparotomy of the abdomen. When you see these in the choices, they are *wrong.*

COAGULATION DISORDERS

VON WILLEBRAND'S DISEASE (VWD)

VWD presents with **bleeding from platelet dysfunction**—superficial bleeding from the skin and mucosal surfaces, such as the gingiva, gums, and vagina. **Epistaxis** is consistent with platelet dysfunction. The question may say the bleeding is worse with the use of aspirin. The platelet count is *normal* in VWD.

The **aPTT can be elevated** in up to 50 percent of patients with VWD, because VWF deficiency destabilizes factor VIII.

Whenever there is platelet-type bleeding but the platelet count is normal, the best initial test is a **bleeding time.**

> A case of VWD is likely to present with epistaxis and/or petechiae.

Diagnostic Testing

- Most accurate tests: **Ristocetin cofactor assay** and **Von Willebrand's factor (VWF) level**
- If the level of VWF is normal, **ristocetin testing** will tell if it is working properly.

Treatment

- First-line treatment: **Desmopressin** or **DDAVP.** This will release subendothelial stores of VWF and factor VIII, which will stop the bleeding.
- If DDAVP is not effective, the next best step in management is to use **factor VIII replacement.** Factor VIII replacement has *both* VWF and factor VIII.

Platelet-Type Bleeding	Factor-Type Bleeding
• Petechiae • Epistaxis • Purpura • Gingiva • Gums • Vaginal	• Hemarthrosis • Hematoma

IDIOPATHIC THROMBOCYTOPENIC PURPURA (ITP)

ITP presents with **platelet type of bleeding** if the **platelet count < 50,000.** Following are the tests that diagnose ITP:

- **Antiplatelet antibodies**
- **Sonogram:** To assess for normal spleen size found in ITP
- **Bone marrow:** To find increased numbers of megakaryocytes
- **Antibodies to the glycoprotein IIb/IIIa receptor**

A generally healthy patient comes with epistaxis and petechiae. No spleen is felt on examination. The platelet count is 24,000. What is the next step in management?

a. Prednisone

b. Bone marrow biopsy

c. Antiplatelet antibodies

d. Sonogram

e. Hematology consultation

*Answer: The correct answer is **A**. Prednisone is the most important thing to do first in mild ITP. The main point of most ITP questions is that initiating therapy is more important than determining a specific diagnosis, particularly since ITP is a diagnosis of exclusion. All of the answers listed would be given on a CCS case at the same time. In a single best answer case, however, the most important thing is to start therapy.*

A patient comes in with ITP and a platelet count of 5,000. The patient has epistaxis and petechiae as well as an intracranial hemorrhage and melena. What is the best initial step?

*Answer: **IVIG administration.** The fastest way to raise the platelet count with ITP is to use intravenous immunoglobulins (IVIG) or rhogam. IVIG is the answer when the platelet count is low (< 20,000) and the case describes life-threatening bleeding, such as that into the bowel or brain. Transfusing platelets is wrong; this adds fuel to the fire and will likely make the situation worse.*

Treatment

Case presents with...	Treatment
Platelet count > 50,000	No treatment
Count < 50,000 with minor bleeding	Prednisone
Count < 20,000 with serious bleeding	IVIG or Rhogam (Rho[D] immune globulin)
Recurrent episodes	Splenectomy

UREMIA-INDUCED PLATELET DYSFUNCTION

Uremia by itself prevents platelets from working properly; **they do not degranulate.** Look for a **normal platelet count with platelet-type bleeding in a patient with renal failure.** The ristocetin test and VWF level will be normal.

Treatment is as follows:

- Best initial therapy: **Desmopressin (DDAVP)**

Mixing study is the first test to determine the difference between a clotting factor deficiency and a factor inhibitor antibody. The aPTT will correct to normal with a clotting factor deficiency.

CLOTTING FACTOR DEFICIENCIES

Deficiency	Factor VIII	Factor IX	Factor XI	Factor XII
Presentation	Joint bleeding or hematoma in a male child	Joint bleeding or hematoma; Less common than factor VIII deficiency	Rare bleeding with trauma or surgery	No bleeding
Diagnostic Test	Mixing study first, then specific factor level	Same	Same	Same
Treatment	Factor VIII replacement with severe deficiency (< 1% activity); DDAVP with milder deficiency	Factor IX replacement	Fresh frozen plasma (FFP) with bleeding episodes	No treatment necessary

A woman presents with bleeding into her thigh after minor trauma. The aPTT is prolonged, and the prothrombin time is normal. Mixing study does not correct the aPTT to normal. What is the diagnosis?

*Answer: **Factor VIII antibody** is the most common cause of a prolonged aPTT and bleeding that does not correct with a mixing study.*

HEPARIN-INDUCED THROMBOCYTOPENIA (HIT)

HIT presents with **a drop in platelets** (at least 50 percent) a few days *after* the start of heparin. This can be from any amount of heparin, no matter how small, because HIT is an allergic reaction. **Thrombosis** is the most common clinical manifestation. Venous thromboses are 3 times more common than arterial thromboses. Although low molecular weight heparin is less likely to cause HIT, both types of heparin can do so.

Diagnostic Testing

The best initial diagnostic tests are

- platelet factor 4 antibodies; or
- heparin-induced, antiplatelet antibodies.

Treatment

- Best initial therapy: **Stop the heparin** and use a **direct thrombin inhibitor**, such as argatroban or lepirudin.

If HIT happens with IV unfractionated heparin, do *not* answer "switch to low molecular weight heparin."

THROMBOPHILIA/HYPERCOAGUABLE STATES

Cause	Lupus anticoagulant or anticardiolipin antibodies	Protein C deficiency	Factor V Leiden mutation	Antithrombin deficiency
Presentation	Venous thrombosis; Elevated aPTT with a normal PT Spontaneous abortion; False positive VDRL	Skin necrosis with the use of warfarin	Most common cause of thrombophilia	No change in the aPTT with a bolus of IV heparin
Diagnostic Test	Mixing study first; Russel viper venom test is most accurate for lupus anticoagulant	Protein C level	Factor V mutation test	Level of antithrombin III
Treatment	Heparin followed by warfarin	Heparin followed by warfarin	Heparin followed by warfarin	Large amounts of heparin or direct thrombin inhibitor followed by warfarin

GASTROENTEROLOGY

8

ESOPHAGEAL DISORDERS

In general, esophageal disorders with any degree of anatomic damage leading to narrowing result in **dysphagia** and **weight loss.** All forms of dysphagia can lead to weight loss.

If dysphagia is present and you do not know the diagnosis, then perform a **barium study** first. In the stomach, do **endoscopy** first. The only two esophageal disorders for which endoscopy is indispensible in diagnosis are **cancer** and the precancerous histologic change known as **Barrett's esophagus;** biopsy is necessary to diagnose both of these.

> Remember: Dysphagia (difficulty swallowing) is different from odynophagia (painful swallowing). Odynophagia suggests an infectious process, such as HIV, HSV, or *Candida*.

DYSPHAGIA

Achalasia (failure of GE sphincter to relax)

Achlasia presents in a **young nonsmoker** who has **dysphagia to both solids and liquids** at the same time. There may also be **regurgitation of food particles** and **aspiration of previously eaten material** that is regurgitated and falls into the lungs. This is a nonprogressive form of dysphagia in which the symptoms are already quite bad but do not get worse over time.

Diagnostic testing is as follows:

- Best initial test: **Barium swallow**
- Most accurate test: **Esophageal manometer**

Endoscopy is *not* necessary to diagnose achalasia. Manometry would show absence of esophageal peristalsis (low pressures) and normal or high pressures at the lower esophageal sphincter, since achalasia involves a failure of the gastroesophageal sphincter to relax. There is *no* mucosal abnormality.

Treatment is as follows:

- Best initial therapy: **Pneumatic dilation**
- **Surgery** is the answer when pneumatic dilation is repeatedly unsuccessful.
- **Botulinum toxin injection** is used when the patient refuses surgery or pneumatic dilation.

alt tx:

Esophageal Cancer

Esophageal cancer presents with the following:

- **Dysphagia: Solids first, liquids later**
- May have **heme-positive stool** or **anemia**
- Often in patients > **50** who are **smokers and drinkers of alcohol**

Diagnostic testing is as follows:

- Best initial test: **Endoscopy**
- If endoscopy is not one of the choices, then **barium swallow** can be performed.
- Manometry will *not* be useful, since cancer can *only* be diagnosed with biopsy.

Just order the procedures you think you need on the CCS. Do *not* wait for a consult. If you need a consult for a procedure, the computer will tell you.

Treament involves the following:

- Best initial therapy: **Surgical resection.** Surgery is performed if there are no local or distant metastases.
- Follow surgery with **chemotherapy based on 5-fluorouracil.**

Rings and Webs

These are also known as **"peptic strictures."** They can be caused by the **repetitive exposure of the esophagus to acid,** resulting in scarring and stricture formation. Previous use of **sclerosing agents** for variceal bleeding can also cause strictures, and this is why variceal banding is a superior procedure.

The best initial test is a **barium study.**

Following are the different kinds of strictures:

- **Plummer-Vinson syndrome:** This is a **proximal stricture** found in association with **iron deficiency anemia** and is more common in **middle-aged women.** It is associated with squamous cell esophageal cancer.
  - Best initial therapy: **Iron replacement**

> - Dysphagia + Weight Loss = Esophageal pathology
> - Dysphagia + Weight Loss + Heme-positive stool/ Anemia = Cancer

- **Schatzki's ring:** This is a **distal ring** of the esophagus that presents with **intermittent symptoms of dysphagia.**
  - Best initial therapy: **Pneumatic dilation**

- **Peptic stricture:** This results from **acid reflux.**
  - It is treated with **pneumatic dilation.**

Zenker's Diverticulum

Look for a patient with **dysphagia with horrible bad breath.** There is rotting food in the back of the esophagus from **dilation of the posterior pharyngeal constrictor muscles.**

The best initial test is a **barium study.** The best initial therapy is a **surgical resection.**

> Do *not* do endoscopy or place a nasogastric tube with Zenker's diverticulum to avoid perforation.

Spastic Disorders

Diffuse esophageal spasm and **"nutcracker esophagus"** are essentially the same disease. Look for a case of **severe chest pain,** often without risk factors for ischemic heart disease. The case may describe the pain as **occurring after drinking a cold beverage.** There is *always* pain, but there is *not* always dysphagia. The EKG, stress test, and possibly the coronary angiography will be presented as normal.

Diagnostic testing is as follows:

- Most accurate diagnostic test: **Manometry**
- **Barium studies** may show a **corkscrew pattern,** but *only* during an episode of spasm.

Therapy for esophageal spasm is with **calcium channel blockers and nitrates** (the same treatment as for Prinzmetal's angina).

> Esophageal disorders can mimic **Prinzmetal's variant angina,** because the pain is sudden, severe, and not related to exercise. However, Prinzmetal's will give you ST segment elevation and an abnormality on stimulation of the coronary arteries, while esophageal spasm will not.

Scleroderma (Progressive Systemic Sclerosis)

Scleroderma presents as **symptoms of reflux.** Treat with **proton pump inhibitors.**

An HIV-positive man comes in with progressive dysphagia and odynophagia. He has 75 CD4 cells but no history of opportunistic infections. What is the next best step in management?

a. Fluconazole

b. Amphotericin

c. Barium swallow

d. Endoscopy

e. Antiretroviral therapy

*Answer: The correct answer is **A**. Odynophagia is pain on swallowing. Dysphagia is simply difficulty swallowing (i.e., food getting "stuck" in the esophagus). When odynophagia occurs in an HIV-positive patient, particularly when there are < 100 CD4 cells, the diagnosis is most likely **esophageal candidiasis**, and giving empiric fluconazole is both therapeutic as well as diagnostic. Amphotericin is not necessary.*

ESOPHAGITIS

Esophagitis presents with **pain on swallowing (odynophagia)** as the food rubs against the esophagus.

Diagnostic Testing and Treatment

- In **HIV-negative** patients, **endoscopy** is done first.
- In **HIV-positive** patients with < 100 CD4 cells, give **fluconazole.** Endoscopy in these patients is performed *only* if there is no response to the fluconazole.

Candida esophagitis causes > 90 percent of esophagitis in HIV-positive patients. Other causes of esophagitis are **pills** such as doxycycline or a bisphosphonate such as alendronate. In the case of esophagitis caused by pills, the patient should **sit up and drink more water** when taking pills and **remain upright for at least 30 minutes after taking the pill.**

MALLORY-WEISS TEAR

This is *not* a cause of dysphagia, although Mallory-Weiss tear is clearly an esophageal disorder. It presents as s**udden upper gastrointestinal bleeding** with **violent retching and vomiting** of any cause. There may be either hematemesis or black stool.

Treatment

Most cases resolve **spontaneously.** If bleeding persists, injection of **epinephrine** can be used to stop the bleeding.

Panic avoidance tip: How do I know I am doing the right thing on CCS?

- You may get spontaneous **nurse's notes** telling you whether the patient is doing well or not. You get these automatically as you move the clock forward.
- You can get an "interval history" as a choice under physical exam. This is a two-minute advance of the clock that will "check in" with the patient. This often tells you how the patient is doing and, consequently, how you are doing in management.

GASTROESOPHAGEAL REFLUX DISEASE (GERD)

A patient comes with epigastric pain that is associated with substernal chest pain and an unpleasant metallic taste in the mouth. What is the next best step in management?

a. Endoscopy

b. Barium studies

c. Proton pump inhibitors (PPIs)

d. H2 (histamine) blockers

e. 24-hour pH monitor

*Answer: The correct answer is **C**. Proton pump inhibitors (PPIs) are preferred as the first line of therapy and also serve as a diagnostic test. Using PPIs is far easier than other testing.*

In addition to the epigastric pain and substernal chest pain of GERD, several other symptoms are clearly associated with acid reflux:

- Sore throat
- Metallic or bitter taste
- Hoarseness
- Chronic cough
- Wheezing

As many as 20 percent of those with chronic cough are suffering from GERD.

Diagnostic Testing

PPI administration is both diagnostic and therapeutic. Further diagnostic testing, such as a 24-hour pH monitor, should *only* be done if there is no response to PPIs and the diagnosis is not clear.

Treatment

Mild disease may be controlled with **lifestyle modifications** such as the following:

- Losing weight
- Elevating the head of the bed
- Quitting smoking
- Limiting alcohol, caffeine, chocolate, and peppermint ingestion
- Not eating within 3 hours of going to sleep

If these do not work, **PPIs** are the next best therapy for GERD. They should control 90–95 percent of cases. All PPIs are equal in efficacy.

H2 blockers, such as ranitidine, famotidine, cimetidine, or nizatadine, control GERD in about two thirds of patients. Hence, they are *only* used if a PPI is not available. Promotility agents, such as metoclopromide, are equal to H2 blockers and much less effective than PPIs such as omeprazole; therefore, they would *not* routinely be used.

> When is reflux alarming, and when do I do endoscopy in GERD? When the following symptoms are present:
> - Weight loss
> - Anemia
> - Blood in the stool
> - Dysphagia

Treatment for *Helicobacter pylori* is *not* effective or necessary for GERD. Such treatment will not tighten the LES.

If PPIs are not sufficient to control disease, then a **surgical or endoscopic procedure to narrow the distal esophagus** should be performed, such as a Nissen fundoplication or endoscopically suturing the lower esophageal sphincter (LES) tighter.

BARRETT ESOPHAGUS

Barrett esophagus is a **precancerous lesion.** Approximately 0.5 percent of cases per year will transform into esophageal cancer. This is why **adenocarcinoma** is an increasingly frequent histological type of esophageal cancer.

Diagnostic Testing

This condition can only be diagnosed by **endoscopy** in which you are able to visualize and biopsy the distal esophagus: Barrett esophagus is a **biopsy diagnosis.** Although the color is different, the only way to be certain that the histology has changed from squamous epithelium to columnar epithelium ("Barrett esophagus") is by endoscopy.

Perform endoscopy for all the symptoms described **(weight loss, anemia, heme-positive stool)** and in **anyone with symptoms of reflux disease for more than 5 years.**

Endoscopic Finding	Action
Barrett esophagus	PPI and repeat endoscopy every 2–3 years
Low-grade dysplasia	PPI and repeat endoscopy in 3–6 months
High-grade dysplasia	Distal esophagectomy

EPIGASTRIC PAIN

A 58-year-old man comes to the office for evaluation of epigastric discomfort for the last several weeks. He is otherwise asymptomatic with no weight loss. His stool is heme-negative. What is the next best step in management?

a. Upper endoscopy

b. Serology for Helicobacter pylori

c. Urea breath testing for Helicobacter pylori

d. PPI, amoxicillin, and clarithromycin for 2 weeks

e. Ranitadine empirically

Answer: The correct answer is **A.** *Upper endoscopy should be performed in any patient above the age of 45 with persistent symptoms of epigastric discomfort. This is, essentially, to exclude the possibility of gastric cancer. There is no way to be certain, without endoscopy, who has gastric cancer.*

NON-ULCER DYSPEPSIA

This is the most common cause of epigastric discomfort.

You can only conclude that a person has non-ulcer dyspepsia *after* **endoscopy** has excluded ulcer disease, gastric cancer, and gastritis: this is a diagnosis of exclusion. Treatment consists of symptomatic therapy with **H2 blockers, liquid antacids,** or **PPIs.**

> There is no proven benefit to treating *Helicobacter* for non-ulcer dyspepsia.

PEPTIC ULCER DISEASE

Peptic ulcer disease can be either **duodenal ulcer (DU) or gastric ulcer (GU) disease.** After *Helicobacter,* the most common causes of ulcers are NSAIDs, head trauma, burns, intubation, Crohn's disease, and Zollinger-Ellison syndrome. Gastric cancer occurs in 4 percent of those with GU.

There is *no* way to distinguish DU and GU by symptoms alone. The alteration of pain with food is only suggestive, not definitive. Food more often makes GU pain worse and DU pain better. However, if the patient is **above 45 and has epigastric pain,** you *must* scope to exclude gastric cancer.

GASTRITIS

Gastritis can be associated with *Helicobacter pylori.* If it is present, treat with a **PPI and 2 antibiotics.**

Gastritis can also be **atrophic** from **pernicious anemia** and associated with **vitamin B12 deficiency.** This type of gastritis will *not* improve with treatment for *H. pylori.*

Helicobacter pylori Diagnostic Tests

Testing for this bacteria is as follows.

- Most accurate test: **Endoscopy with biopsy.** If this is done, no further testing is necessary for *Helicobacter.*
- **Serology: Very sensitive but not specific.** If the serology is negative, this excludes *Helicobacter.* A positive test *cannot* distinguish between new and previous infection.
- **Breath testing and stool antigen testing:** These are *not* standard or routinely used. They can, however, distinguish between new and old disease.

Treatment of *Helicobacter pylori*

Treat for this bacteria with **PPI** and **clarithromycin and amoxicillin.** *Only* treat *Helicobacter* if it is associated with gastritis or ulcer disease.

> There is *no* need for routine posttreatment testing of *Helicobacter.* You only test if symptoms or the ulcer persists despite treatment for *Helicobacter.*

If treatment for *H. pylori* fails, proceed as follows:

1. Repeat treatment with **2 new antibiotics and a PPI.** Try **metronidazole and tetracycline** instead of clarithromycin and amoxicillin.
2. If repeat treatment fails, then **evaluate for Zollinger-Ellison syndrome** (gastrinoma).

STRESS ULCER PROPHYLAXIS

Routine prophylactic use of a PPI or H2 blocker or sucralfate should *only* be used if one of the following is present:

- Head trauma
- Intubation and mechanical ventilation
- Burns
- Coagulopathy and steroid use in combination

NSAID or steroid use alone is *not* an indication for routine stress ulcer prophylaxis.

A 52-year-old man has epigastric discomfort. He is seropositive for Helicobacter pylori. *Upper endoscopy reveals no gastritis and no ulcer disease. Biopsy of the stomach shows* Helicobacter. *What should you do?*

a. Breath testing
b. PPI alone as symptomatic therapy
c. Repeat endoscopy after 6 weeks of PPIs
d. PPI, amoxicillin, and clarithromycin

Answer: The correct answer is **B.** *You do* not *need to treat* H. pylori *unless there is gastritis or ulcer disease. This patient has epigastric pain and* Helicobacter *but no ulcer or gastritis. This is* **non-ulcer dyspepsia.** *Treat it symptomatically with a PPI. Enormous numbers of people are colonized with* H. pylori; *you do* not *need to eradicate it from the world without evidence of disease.* Helicobacter pylori *is* not *the cause of non-ulcer dyspepsia.*

A man is found to have ulcer disease. There are 3 ulcers in the distal esophagus 1–2 cm in size. The ulcers persist despite treatment for Helicobacter. *What should you do next?*

a. Switch antibiotics
b. Breath testing
c. Gastrin level and gastric acid output
d. CT scan of the abdomen
e. ERCP

Answer: The correct answer is **C.** *Gastrin level and gastric acid output testing should be done when there is the possibility of* **Zollinger-Ellison syndrome.** *ERCP will only show the ducts of the pancreas and gallbladder; it will not reveal gastrinoma.*

ZOLLINGER-ELLISON SYNDROME (ZES) OR GASTRINOMA

ZES is diagnosed by finding an **elevated gastrin level and an elevated gastric acid output.** Remember: *Everyone* on an H2 blocker or PPI has an elevated gastrin level.

When should I test the gastrin level and gastric acid output?

Test when the following present:
- *Large ulcer (> 1 cm)*
- *Multiple ulcers*
- *Distal location near the ligament of Treitz*
- *Recurrent or persistent despite* **Helicobacter** *treatment*

If the gastrin and acid output level are both elevated, then localization of the gastrinoma is next.

> Most ulcers have the following characteristics:
> - Single
> - < 1 cm
> - Proximal near the pylorus
> - Easily resolve with treatment

Diagnostic Testing

Following are the most accurate tests of ZES:

- **Endoscopic ultrasound:** An endoscopic ultrasound is like performing a transesophageal echocardiogram. It is much more sensitive than a surface ultrasound.

- **Nuclear somatostatin scan:** The nuclear somatostatin scan is very sensitive, because patients with ZES have an enormous increase in the number of somatostatin receptors.

What is the normal effect of infusing secretin intravenously?

- *Normal people decrease gastrin levels and acid output.*
- *Patients with ZES show no change or an increase in gastrin levels and no decrease in acid levels.*

The Effect of Infusing IV Secretin		
	Normal	Zollinger-Ellison
Gastrin secretion	Decreases	No change
Gastric acid output	Decreases	No change

Treatment

- **Local disease:** Surgical resection
- **Metastatic disease:** Lifelong PPIs

When should I look for multiple endocrine neoplasia (MEN) syndrome?

Answer: **Hypercalcemia** *is the clue to the presence of a parathyroid problem with ZES and, therefore, is the clue to a MEN syndrome.*

INFLAMMATORY BOWEL DISEASE (IBD)

Both **Crohn's disease (CD) and ulcerative colitis (UC)** can present with **fever, abdominal pain, diarrhea, blood in the stool, and weight loss.** UC most often presents with abdominal pain and bloody diarrhea.

The **extraintestinal manifestations of IBD** are as follows:

- Joint paint
- Eye findings (iritis, uveitis)
- Skin findings (pyoderma gangrenosum, erythema nodosum)
- Sclerosing cholangitis

Features more common to **Crohn's disease** are the following:

> *Both* Crohn's disease (CD) and ulceratative colitis (UC) can lead to **colon cancer** if CD involves the colon. **Screening colonoscopy** should be performed every 1–2 years after 8–10 years of colonic involvement.

- Masses
- Skip lesion
- Involvement of the upper GI tract
- Perianal disease
- Transmural granulomas
- Fistulae
- Hypocalcemia from fat malabsorption
- Obstruction
- Calcium oxalate kidney stones
- Cholesterol gallstones
- Vitamin B12 malabsorption from terminal ileum involvement

DIAGNOSTIC TESTING

Endoscopy is diagnostic in both CD and UC. **Barium studies** are also diagnostic in both. When the diagnosis is *not* clear from endoscopy or barium studies, **blood tests** are helpful.

Crohn's Disease

- Antisaccharomyces cerevesiae (ASCA): **Positive**
- Antineutrophil cytoplasmic antibody (ANCA): **Negative**

Ulcerative Colitis

- ASCA: **Negative**
- ANCA: **Positive**

	CD	UC
ASCA	Positive	Negative
ANCA	Negative	Positive

TREATMENT

Treatment for inflammatory bowel disease is as follows:

- Best initial therapy for *both* CD and UC: **Mesalamine**
- Sulfasalazine is *not* the best initial therapy for either CD or UC because of the following adverse effects:
  - Rash
  - Hemolytic anemia

- Interstitial nephritis
- **Steroids: Budesonide** is a glucocorticoid that can be used to control acute exacerbations of IBD. It has extensive first-pass effect in the liver and, therefore, has limited systemic adverse effects.
- **Azathioprine and 6-mercaptopurine:** These are used in those with **severe disease** who have **recurrent disease when the steroids are stopped.** Azathioprine and 6MP are used to wean a patient off of steroids.
- **Infliximab:** This is a **TNF inhibitor** that is most useful in controlling CD that is associated with fistula formation. TNF is what maintains a granuloma in place. Plant a PPD and give isoniazid if the PPD is positive prior to the use of infliximab. Remember to **screen for tuberculosis;** infliximab can reactivate tuberculosis by releasing dormant TB from granulomas.
- **Metronidazole and ciprofloxacin:** These antibiotics are used for **perianal involvement in CD.**
- **Surgery:** This can be **curative in UC by removing the colon.** However, CD will recur at the site of the surgery. Occasionally, you must do surgery in CD, despite the risk of recurrence, *if* there is a stricture and obstruction.

> **Infliximab** reactivates tuberculosis. Screen with a PPD prior to its use in fistulizing CD.

DIARRHEA

INFECTIOUS DIARRHEA

The most important feature of infectious diarrhea on presentation is the **presence of blood.** Blood means the presence of invasive bacterial pathogens, such as the following:

- *Campylobacter:* This is the most common cause of food poisoning. It can be associated with Guillain-Barre syndrome and reactive arthritis.
- *Salmonella:* This is transmitted by chickens and eggs.
- *Vibrio parahemolyticus:* This is associated with seafood.
- *E. coli:* This can have several variants, some of which are associated with blood.
  - *E. coli* 0157:H7 is most commonly associated with **hemolytic uremic syndrome** (via effects of verotoxin). Look for undercooked beef in the history. Do not give platelet transfusions or antibiotics, which can make it worse.
- *Vibrio vulnificus:* Look for shellfish (oysters, clams) in a person with liver disease and skin lesions.
- *Shigella:* Secretes Shiga toxin. This bacteria is also associated with reactive arthritis.
- *Yersinia:* Rodents (rarely other mammals) are the natural reservoir of this bacteria. Transmission occurs via vegetables, milk-derived products, and meat (case may describe pork) that is contaminated with infected urine or feces.
- **Amebic:** Perform three-stool ova and parasite examinations or serologic testing. Treat with metronidazole. May be associated with liver abscesses.

If blood is not described in the case, **fecal leukocytes** should be tested. Fecal leukocytes tell you that an invasive pathogen is present and indicate the same diseases described above that are associated with the presence of blood.

- Best initial test: **Fecal leukocytes**
- Most accurate test: **Stool culture**

Treatment
- **Mild disease:** This will resolve on its own, and the patient should be hydrated only.
- **Severe disease: Fluoroquinolones,** such as **ciprofloxacin,** are the best initial therapy. Severe disease is defined as the presence of the following:
  - Blood
  - Fever
  - Abdominal pain
  - Hypotension and tachycardia

NONBLOODY DIARRHEA

All of the pathogens described above **can present without blood as well as with blood.** The presence of blood does *exclude* the following pathogens, which *never* result in blood:

- **Viruses:** Rotavirus, norovirus (also called "Norwalk virus")
- *Giardia:* Look for camping/hiking and men who have sex with men. Stool ELISA antigen is > 90 percent sensitive and specific and is more accurate than three-stool ova and parasite exams. Look for bloating, flatus, and signs of steatorrhea. Treat with metronidazole or tinidazole.
- **Staphylococcus aureus:** Presents with vomiting in addition to diarrhea. It will resolve spontaneously.
- **Bacillus cereus:** Associated with refried Chinese rice and vomiting. It resolves spontaneously.
- **Cryptosporidiosis:** Look for an HIV-positive patient with < 100 CD4 cells. Diagnose with a modified acid-fast stain. There is *no* proven effective therapy besides using antiretroviral medications to raise the CD4 count. Paromomycin is only partially effective.
- **Scombroid:** This is histamine fish poisoning. This has the fastest onset of diarrhea; within 10 minutes of eating an infected tuna, mackerel, or mahi-mahi, the patient has vomiting, diarrhea, wheezing, and flushing. Treat with antihistamines, such as **diphenhydramine.**

ANTIBIOTIC-ASSOCIATED DIARRHEA/*CLOSTRIDIUM DIFFICILE* (*C-DIFF*)

This develops several days to weeks after the use of antibiotics. Although **clindamycin** is the most common cause, antibiotic-associated diarrhea can be caused by **any antibiotic.** Recently **fluoroquinolones** have also come to be associated with *Clostridium difficile.* There can be both blood and fecal leukocytes with *Clostridium difficile* colitis.

The best initial test is a **stool toxin assay.**

Treatment
- Best initial therapy: **Metronidazole**
- **Oral vancomycin** is used only if there is no response to metronidazole. (IV Vancomycin is *not* useful).
- If antibiotic-associated diarrhea resolves with metronidazole and then recurs later, the patient should be **retreated with metronidazole,** not treated with vancomycin.

When treating antibiotic-associated diarrhea, *only* use oral vancomycin if metronidazole fails.

CHRONIC DIARRHEA

Lactose Intolerance

This is probably the most common cause of chronic diarrhea and flatulence.

Diagnose and treat by **removing all milk and milk-related products** from the diet with the *exception* of yogurt. A lactose-intolerance test may also be performed.

Carcinoid Syndrome

This is associated with **flushing and episodes of hypotension.**

Diagnose with a **urinary 5-HIAA level.** Treat with the somatostatin analogue **octreotide.**

Inflammatory Bowel Disease

Look for blood, fever, and weight loss. (This is discussed in more detail earlier in this chapter.)

MALABSORPTION

This type of chronic diarrhea is always associated with **weight loss. Fat malabsorption** is associated with **steatorrhea,** which leads to **oily, greasy stools** that float on the water in the toilet. There is a particularly **foul smell to the stool.**

The causes of fat malabsorption are as follows:

- **Celiac disease** (gluten sensitive enteropathy) or **nontropical sprue**
- **Tropical sprue**
- **Chronic pancreatitis**
- **Whipple's disease**

All forms of fat malabsorption are associated with the following:

- **Hypocalcemia** from vitamin D deficiency, which may lead to osteoporosis
- **Oxalate overabsorption and oxalate kidney stones**
- **Easy bruising and elevated prothrombin time/INR** from vitamin K malabsorption
- **Vitamin B12 malabsorption** from either destruction of the terminal ileum or loss of the pancreatic enzymes that are necessary for B12 absorption

Diagnostic Testing

- Best initial test: **Sudan black stain of stool** to test for the presence of fat.
- Most sensitive test: **72-hour fecal fat**

CELIAC DISEASE (GLUTEN-SENSITIVE ENTEROPATHY)

Celiac disease can also present with **malabsorption of iron** and **microcytic anemia.** This does *not* happen with pancreatic insufficiency, since pancreatic enzymes are not necessary for iron absorption. **Folate malabsorption** also occurs from destruction of villi. Celiac disease is associated with a vesicular skin lesion not present on mucosal surfaces. This is called **dermatitis herpetiformis.**

Diagnostic Testing

- Best initial test: **Antigliadin, antiendomyseal, and antitissue transglutaminase antibodies**
- Most accurate test: **Small bowel biopsy**
- **D-xylose testing** is abnormal in celiac disease, Whipple's disease, and tropical sprue, because the villous lining is destroyed and D-xylose cannot be absorbed. However, this test is *rarely necessary*, because the specific antibody tests eliminate the need for it.
- **Bowel biopsy** is always necessary for celiac disease, even if the diagnosis is confirmed with antibody testing, to exclude bowel wall lymphoma.

Treatment

Eliminate wheat, oats, rye, and barley from the diet. It may take several weeks for symptoms to resolve.

TROPICAL SPRUE

This presents in the **same way as celiac disease.** There will be a history of the patient being in the **tropics.** The serologic tests, such as antitissue transglutaminase, will be negative.

The most accurate test is a **small bowel biopsy showing microorganisms.** Treatment consists of **tetracycline** or **trimethoprim/sulfamethoxazole** (TMP/SMX) for 3–6 months.

WHIPPLE'S DISEASE

Whipple's disease has several additional findings on presentation, such as the following:

- **Arthralgia**
- **Neurological abnormalities**
- **Occular findings**

Diagnostic Testing

- Most accurate test: **Small bowel biopsy showing PAS positive organisms**
- An alternate test is **PCR of the stool** for *Trophyrema whippelei.*

Treatment

Treat with **tetracycline** or **trimethoprim/sulfamethoxazole** (TMP/SMX) for 12 months.

CHRONIC PANCREATITIS

Look for a **history of alcoholism** and **multiple episodes of pancreatitis.** The amylase and lipase levels will most likely be normal, since the fat malabsorption does not develop until the pancreas is burnt out and largely replaced by calcium and fibrosis. Malabsorption of fat-soluble vitamins, such as vitamin K and vitamin D, is less common than with celiac disease.

Diagnostic Testing

- Best initial tests:
  - **Abdominal X-ray** is 50–60 percent sensitive for the detection of **pancreatic calcifications.**
  - **Abdominal CT scan** (without contrast) is 60–80% sensitive.
- Most accurate test: **Secretin stimulation testing.** A normal person should release a large volume of bicarbonate-rich pancreatic fluid in response to the intravenous injection of secretin.
- Iron and folate levels will be normal, since pancreatic enzymes are not necessary to absorb these. D-xylose testing will be normal.

Treatment

Replace the pancreatic enzymes chronically by mouth. Amylase, lipase, and trypsin can be combined in one pill for chronic use.

IRRITABLE BOWEL SYNDROME

Irritable bowel syndrome is a **pain syndrome with altered bowel habits.** This condition presents with the following symptoms:

- Abdominal pain relieved by a bowel movement
- Abdominal pain that is less at night
- Abdominal pain with diarrhea alternating with constipation

Diagnostic Testing

All the diagnostic tests will be normal. On CCS, you should order the following:

- **Stool guiac, stool white cells, culture, ova, and parasite exam**
- **Colonoscopy**
- **Abdominal CT scan**

> Irritable bowel syndrome presents with pain. There is *no* fever, *no* weight loss, and *no* blood in the stool.

Treatment

- Best initial therapy: **Fiber.** Bulking up the stool helps relieve the pain. Fiber gives the guts a stretch, like sending the colon to yoga class!
- If there is no relief of pain with fiber, then you should add **antispasmodic/ anticholinergic agents,** such as **dicyclomine** or **hyoscyamine,** which "relax" the bowel.
- If there is no response to the antispasmodic/anticholinergic agents, you should add a **tricyclic antidepressant,** such as **amytriptyline.** Tricyclic antidepressants help IBS because they
    - are anticholinergic;
    - relieve neuropathic pain; and
    - are antidepressant.

COLON CANCER

The most important thing for you to know about colon cancer, by far, is what **screening** to perform.

DIAGNOSTIC TESTING

General Population

- Begin screening at **age 50.**
- Screen with the following:
    - **Colonoscopy every 10 years**
    - **Sigmoidoscopy every 3–5 years**
    - **Fecal occult blood testing yearly**
    - **Barium enema**

> - Hamartomas and hyperplastic polyps: Benign
> - Dysplastic polyps: Malignant

What is the best method of screening for colon cancer?

*Answer: **Colonoscopy every 10 years** is the best method by far. All other methods are less accurate.*

When is a "virtual colonoscopy" by CT scan the answer?

Answer: This is the answer when you are asked what colon cancer screening test not to do. It lacks both sensitivity and specificity, because you cannot biopsy and it misses small lesions.

One Family Member with Colon Cancer

- Colonoscopy starting at **age 40 *or* 10 years before the age of the family member** who had cancer

Three Family Members, Two Generations, One Premature (< 50)

- Colonoscopy every **1–2 years starting at age 25.** This is a "Lynch syndrome" or hereditary nonpolyposis colon cancer syndrome.

Familial Adenomatous Polyposis (FAP)

- Start screening sigmoidscopies at age 12.
- Perform a colectomy once polyps are found.

Gardner's Syndrome

This presents with **benign bone tumors known as osteomas,** as well as other soft tissue tumors. There is *no* additional screening indicated.

Peutz-Jeghers Syndrome

This presents with **melanotic spots on the lips.** There are **hamartomatous polyps** throughout the small bowel and colon. The lifetime risk of colon cancer is about 10 percent, only slightly higher than the 6–8 percent risk of colon cancer in the general population. There is *no* extra screening recommended.

Juvenile Polyposis

There are multiple extra hamartomas in the bowel. Hamartomas do not bring a significant increase in the risk of colon cancer. There is *no* extra screening recommended. This is markedly different from FAP.

Dysplastic Polyp Found

Repeat colonoscopy **3–5 years after the polyp was found.**

On routine X-ray, a man is found to have several osteomas. What do you recommend?

*Answer: Perform a **colonoscopy** to screen for cancer. This is **Gardner's syndrome.***

The following table summarizes the recommendations for colon cancer screening:

General Population	Single Family Member with Colon Cancer	Three Family Members, Two Generations, One < 50	Familial Adenomatous Polyposis	Gardner's, Peutz-Jeghers, Juvenile Polyposis, Turcot's Syndrome
Start screening at age 50. Colonoscopy every 10 years.	Start screening at age 40 or 10 years earlier than the age at which the family member contracted cancer.	Colonoscopy every 1–2 years starting at age 25.	Sigmoidoscopy every 1–2 years starting at age 12.	No extra screening recommendations.

Carcinoembryonic antigen (CEA) is *never* a screening test. CEA is used to follow response to therapy.

DIVERTICULAR DISEASE

DIVERTICULOSIS AND DIVERTICULITIS

Diverticulosis

Diverticulosis is incredibly common in older Americans due to a low-fiber, high-fat, hamburger-filled, low-residue diet. They often present as follows:

- Left lower quadrant (LLQ) abdominal pain
- Lower GI bleeding

Diagnostic testing is as follows:

- Most accurate test: **Colonoscopy**
- Best diagnostic test: **Abdominal CT scan**

Treat with a high-fiber diet.

Diverticulitis

Diverticulitis is a complication of diverticulosis. It presents as follows:

- Left lower quadrant (LLQ) abdominal pain
- Tenderness
- Fever
- Elevated white cell count in blood

> Colonoscopy and barium enema are *contraindicated* in diverticulitis because of an increased risk of perforation.

- LLQ Pain + Tenderness + Fever + Leukocytosis = Diverticu*litis*

Antibiotics are the mainstay of treatment for diverticulitis. Combine agents against **gram-negative bacilli,** such as a quinolone or cephalosporin, with an agent against **anaerobes,** such as metronidazole. **Ciprofloxacin and metronidazole** are a standard combination.

Gastrointestinal (GI) Bleeding

GI bleeding presents in various ways:

- **Red blood:** Usually indicates **lower GI bleeding.** In about 10 percent of cases, extremely brisk/rapid or high-volume upper GI bleeding leads to red blood from the rectum.
- **Black stool:** Indicates **upper GI bleeding,** which is usually defined as that occurring proximal to the ligament of Treitz (demarcation between the duodenum and the jejunum). Black stool usually results from at least 100 ml of blood loss.

- **Heme-positive brown stool:** This can occur from as little as 5–10 ml of blood loss.
- **Coffee ground emesis:** Needs very little gastric, esophageal, or duodenal blood loss—as little a 5–10 ml.

A 74-year-old man with a history of aortic stenosis comes to the emergency department having had 5 red/black bowel movements over the last day. His pulse is 112, blood pressure 96/64. What is the next best step in management?

a. Colonoscopy

b. Consult gastroenterology

c. CBC

d. Bolus of normal saline

e. Transfer to the intensive care unit

*Answer: The correct answer is **D**. The most urgent step in severe gastrointestinal (GI) bleeding is **fluid resuscitation**. When the systolic blood pressure is low or the pulse high, there has been at least a 30 percent volume loss. Step 3 does not allow you to order specific doses; hence, all you can order is a "bolus." It is fortunate that you do not have to spend a lot of time calculating or memorizing specific doses of fluids or specific medications. Although endoscopy is important, it is not as important as fluid resuscitation.*

> **Orthostasis** presents with one of the following:
> - Systolic blood pressure < 100
> - Heart rate > 100
> Either of these implies more than 30 percent volume loss.

The *most* important thing to do in acute GI bleeding is to determine if there is **hemodynamic instability.** Orthostatic hypotension means a drop in blood pressure or rise in pulse when going from a lying to a standing or seated position. **Orthostasis** is defined as a drop in systolic pressure of > 20 mm hg or a rise in pulse of > 10 beats per minute.

On CCS with large-volume GI bleeding, order the following:

- Bolus of normal saline or Ringer's lactate
- CBC
- Prothrombin time/INR
- Type and cross
- Consultation with gastroenterology
- EKG

As you move the clock forward on CCS, the results of all tests will automatically pop up. You do not have to do anything for them to come. Test results on CCS are like your phone bill: you do not have to do anything for your bills to arrive; they automatically show up as time passes.

Test	Route of Administration	Time Ordered	Report Available
CBC	Applies to medications ordered	09:00	09:15

When do I transfuse packed red blood cells?

Answer:

- *Hematocrit < 30 in an older person*
- *Hematocrit < 20–25 in younger patients with no heart disease*

When do I transfuse fresh frozen plasma?

Answer: When there is elevated prothrombin time/INR and vitamin K is too slow.

When do I transfuse platelets?

Answer: If the patient is bleeding or to undergo surgery, transfuse platelets when they are < 50,000.

What is the most common cause of death in GI bleeding?

Answer: **Myocardial ischemia.** *That is why you should get an EKG in older patients with severe GI bleeding. The myocytes to the left ventricle cannot distinguish between ischemia, anemia, carbon monoxide poisoning, or coronary artery stenosis. All of these lead to myocardial infarction.*

When is "nasogastric tube" the answer?

Place a nasogastric (NG) tube in the occasional patient when you are not clear as to whether the source of bleeding is from an upper or lower gastrointestinal source. The nasogastric tube has no therapeutic benefit; it will not stop bleeding. Iced saline lavage is worthless and is always wrong.

TREATMENT

Gastrointestinal bleeding of large volume is managed first with **fluid resuscitation.** The most important measures of severity are the **pulse and blood pressure.** If the pulse is elevated or the blood pressure is decreased, you can always give more fluid. If you must give so much fluid to maintain blood pressure that the patient becomes **hypoxic,** then give the fluid and increase **oxygenation,** even if it means intubating the patient. **Hypotension** supersedes all other therapeutic priorities. Fluid resuscitation is *more important* than determining the specific etiology of the source of bleeding.

Correcting anemia, thrombocytopenia, or coagulopathy is *more* important than **endoscopy.** If the platelets are low, then giving platelets is *more* important than consulting gastroenterology or moving the patient to the ICU. Note that 80 percent of GI bleeding stops with adequate fluid resuscitation even *without* endoscopy. If you scope the patient but do *not* correct anemia, thrombocytopenia, or elevated prothrombin time/INR, the bleeding will *not* stop.

> Fluid resuscitation beats scoping!

ULCER DISEASE

Add a **proton pump inhibitor** to the initial resuscitation of fluids, blood, platelets, and plasma.

VARICEAL BLEEDING

Look for an **alcoholic with hematemesis and/or liver disease (cirrhosis)**. The other clues to the presence of esophageal varices are the presence of **splenomegaly, low platelets,** and **spider angiomata** or **gynecomastia**.

Treatment

Treat variceal bleeding as follows:

- Add **octreotide** to the initial orders. This is a somatostatin analogue and it decreases portal hypertension.
- **Upper endoscopy** should be performed promptly to do banding of the varices.
- If the bleeding persists with moving the clock forward, a **transjugular intra-hepatic portosystemic shunt (TIPS)** procedure should be performed. This is using a catheter to place a shunt between the portal vein and hepatic vein. This essentially replaces the need for surgical shunt placement. The most common complication of a TIPS procedure is **hepatic encephalopathy.**
- **Blakemore gastric tamponade balloon:** This procedure will *temporarily* stop bleeding from varices. It is rarely performed and is only a temporary measure to stop bleeding to allow a shunt to be placed.

SOURCES OF BLEEDING

Bleeding in the **upper GI** can have the following causes:

- **Ulcer disease**
- **Esophagitis, gastritis, duodenitis**
- **Varices**
- **Cancer**

Bleeding in the **lower GI** can have the following causes:

- **Angiodysplasia**
- **Diverticular disease**
- **Polyps**
- **Ischemic colitis**
- **Inflammatory bowel disease**
- **Cancer**

Diagnostic Testing

- **Technitium bleeding scan ("tagged red cell scan"):** This test is performed to detect the site of bleeding *if* endoscopy does not reveal the source. It will let you know the location but *not* the exact cause.
- **Angiography:** This test tells you the **precise vessel that is bleeding.** It can be done preoperatively in massive GI bleeding to let you know which part of the colon to resect.
- **Capsule endoscopy:** Swallowing a capsule with a camera in it can detect the **location of GI bleeding from the small bowel,** *if* upper and lower endoscopy do not reveal the answer. It gives an enormous quantity of pictures but does *not* allow a biopsy or therapeutic intervention such as you can do with endoscopy.

ACUTE MESENTERIC ISCHEMIA

This is an **embolus from the heart** resulting in an **infarction of the bowel.** There is a **sudden onset of extremely severe abdominal pain** and possible bleeding as well. Physical examination shows a relatively benign abdomen. Look for an **older patient** with a history of **valvular heart disease** and the very sudden onset of pain.

Diagnostic Testing

Look for **metabolic acidosis (elevated lactic acid)** on blood testing and an **elevated amylase level.** The most accurate test is **angiography.**

Treatment

Treatment is **surgical resection of the bowel.** Very ill patients should go *straight* to the operating room for surgical resection. This is a surgical emergency. If left undetected and untreated, the patient will die quickly.

> - Abdominal pain out of proportion to physical exam = Mesenteric ischemia

CONSTIPATION

The vast majority of cases have **no clear etiology.** Although Step 3 seldom asks specifically for the diagnosis, the management of constipation involves correcting the underlying cause. Therefore, knowing the etiology is the key to determining the treatment. Following are possible causes of constipation:

- **Dehydration:** Look for decreased skin turgor in an elderly patient with an increased BUN-to-creatinine ratio (> 20:1).
- **Calcium channel blockers**
- **Narcotic medication use**
- **Hypothyroidism**

- **Diabetes:** Loss of sensation in the bowels leads to decreased detection of stretch in the bowel, which is one of the main stimulants of GI motility.
- **Ferrous sulfate iron replacement:** The stool is **black** and can look as though there is upper GI bleeding. Blood is cathartic and will usually produce **rapid bowel movement.** Ferrous sulfate is constipating and is also heme-negative when one tests for occult blood.
- **Anticholinergic medication:** This includes tricyclic antidepressants.

Treatment with **hydration and increased fiber** is always a good option. You may consider prescribing a bowel regimen with Senokot® and docusate.

Dumping Syndrome

Dumping syndrome is a relatively rare disorder related to **prior gastric surgery,** usually done for ulcer disease. Treatment and eradication of *Helicobacter pylori* has made surgery for ulcer disease rare.

The patient presents with **shaking, sweating, and weakness.** There may be hypotension resulting from the rapid release of the gastric contents into the duodenum, which causes an osmotic draw into the bowel. The other reason is a rapid rise in blood glucose resulting in a reactive hypoglycemia.

Dumping syndrome is managed with **frequent small meals.**

Diabetic Gastroparesis

Longstanding diabetes impairs the neural supply of the bowel. There is impairment of normal motility. Patients present with **bloating and constipation as well as diarrhea.**

Treat with **erythromycin** or **metoclopromide.** Erythromycin increases motilin in the gut, a hormone that stimulates gastric motility.

Acute Pancreatitis

This condition presents as **severe midepigastric abdominal pain and tenderness** in an **alcoholic** or someone with **gallstones.** Other causes are the following:

- Hypertriglyceridemia
- Trauma
- Infection
- ERCP
- Medications such as thiazides, didanosine, stavudine, or azathioprine

Other symptoms include the following:

- Vomiting without blood
- Anorexia
- Tenderness in the epigastric area

Severe cases involve these symptoms:

- Hypotension
- Metabolic acidosis
- Leukocytosis
- Hemoconcentration
- Hyperglycemia
- Hypocalcemia from fat malabsorption
- Hypoxia

Diagnostic Testing

- Best initial test: **Amylase and lipase** (Lipase has higher specificity.)
- Most accurate test: **Abdominal CT scan.** A CT scan can detect dilated common bile ducts and even comment on intrahepatic ducts.
- If there is dilation of the common bile duct *without* a pancreatic head mass, consider **endoscopic retrograde cholangiopancreatography (ERCP).** The ERCP can be used to detect the presence of stones or strictures in the pancreatic duct system. ERCP can also remove stones and dilate strictures.
- **Trypsinogen activation peptide:** This is a **urinary test** that can be used to determine the severity of pancreatitis. Pancreatitis seems to arise from the **premature activation of trypsinogen** while it is still within the pancreas instead of when it reaches the duodenum. Hence, the trypsin starts to digest and inflame the pancreas.

Treatment

Therapy consists of the following:

- No feeding (bowel rest)
- Hydration
- Pain medications

We do *not* have a medication to reverse pancreatitis.

NECROTIC PANCREATITIS

In the past, Ranson's criteria were the major method of determining the severity of pancreatitis. **Ranson's criteria** are operative criteria to see **who needs pancreatic debridement.** The **CT scan** effectively replaces Ranson's criteria as the most precise method of determining severity.

Treatment

When the **CT shows > 30 percent necrosis** of the pancreas, the patient should

- receive antibiotics such as imipenem; and
- undergo CT-guided biopsy.

If the biopsy shows **infected, necrotic pancreatitis,** the patient should have **surgical debridement** of the pancreas.

ACUTE HEPATITIS

All patients with acute hepatitis will present is a very similar way. You *cannot* accurately determine the etiology of acute hepatitis only from history and presentation. All patients present with the following:

- **Jaundice**
- **Fatigue**
- **Weight loss**
- **Dark urine from bilirubin in the urine**

Hepatitis B and C are more likely to present with **serum sickness-phenomena** like joint pain, urticaria, and fever.

No treatment is available for any form of *acute* hepatitis.

> - Hepatitis B is associated with polyarteritis nodosa (PAN) in 30 percent of cases.
> - Hepatitis C is associated with cryoglobulinemia.

DIAGNOSTIC TESTING

- *All* patients with acute hepatitis will give an **elevated conjugated (direct) bilirubin.** This will lead to bilirubin in the urine or urobilinogen. Unconjugated bilirubin, such as that associated with hemolysis, is not water soluble and will not go into the urine. Unconjugated bilirubin is attached to albumin.
- **Viral hepatitis** gives an **elevated ALT level.**
- **Drug-induced hepatitis** is associated with an **increased AST.**

```
        A                          A
     ViraL                      DrugS
        T                          T
```

Hepatitis E is the worst in pregnancy. It can be fatal.

- Most accurate tests:
  - For **hepatitis A, C, D, and E**, the confirmatory test is **serology.** IgM levels acutely rise, and IgG levels rise in the recovery phase.
  - **Surface antigen, core antibody, e-antigen, or surface antibodies** are not present in hepatitis A, C, D, or E. These tests are associated with **hepatitis B.**

Hepatitis B Testing

The *first* test to become abnormal in acute Hepatitis B infection is the **surface antigen.** Elevation in ALT, e-antigen, and symptoms all occur *after* the appearance of hepatitis B surface antigen. The following table shows the appearance of the antigens and antibodies through the course of the disease:

	Surface Antigen	e-Antigen	Core Antibody	Surface Antibody
Acute disease	+ +	+ +	+ +	−
Window period (recovering)	−	−	+ +	−
Vaccinated	−	−	−	+ +
Healed/recovered	−	−	+ +	+ +

Chronic hepatitis B gives the same serologic pattern as acute hepatitis B, but it is based on **persistence of the surface antigen beyond six months.**

	Surface Antigen	Core Antibody	E Antigen	Surface Antibody
Acute Hepatitis	Positive	Positive	Positive	Negative
Chronic Hepatitis	Positive	Positive	Positive	Negative
Resolved Infection	Negative	Positive	Negative	Positive
Window Period	Negative	Positive	Negative	Negative

> • Hepatitis B DNA polymerase = e-Antigen = Hepatitis B PCR for DNA

These three tests are essentially *equal* in meaning. They all indicate **active viral replication.**

Hepatitis C Testing

- Best initial test: **Hepatitis C antibody.** This test *cannot,* however, tell the level of activity of the virus.
- Most accurate tests:
  - **Hepatitis C PCR** for RNA is the most accurate method of determining the degree of viral replication and activity of the disease. PCR RNA is also the most accurate way of determining response to therapy.
  - **Liver biopsy** is the most accurate way of determining the seriousness of the disease. The patient can have 10 years of active viral replication with relatively little liver damage. Use the biopsy to determine how much damage there has been to the liver.

TREATMENT OF CHRONIC HEPATITIS

Chronic Hepatitis B

The patient with surface antigen, e-antigen, and DNA polymerase or PCR for DNA is the patient who is most likely to benefit from **antiviral therapy.** Look for **> 6 months of positive serology.** Chronic hepatitis B is treated with the following single agents:

- **Lamivudine**
- **Adefovir**
- **Entecavir**
- **Telbivudine**
- **Interferon:** Interferon has the most adverse effects:
  - Flulike symptoms
  - Arthralgia
  - Myalgia
  - Fatigue
  - Thrombocytopenia
  - Depression

Chronic Hepatitis C

Combine **interferon with ribavirin.** The most common adverse effect of ribavirin is **anemia.**

VACCINATION

Vaccination for both **hepatitis A and B** is now done universally in **childhood.**

For **adults,** the strongest indications for vaccination for both **hepatitis A and B** are the following:

- **Chronic liver disease.** Someone with cirrhosis or another cause of liver disease who develops hepatitis A or B is at *much* greater risk of fulminant hepatitis.
- **Household contacts** of those with hepatitis A or B
- **Men who have sex with men**
- **Blood product recipients on a chronic basis**
- **Injection drug users**

Specific indications for vaccines are as follows:

- **Hepatitis A vaccine**
  - Travelers
- **Hepatitis B vaccine**
  - Health care workers
  - Patients on dialysis

A health care worker gets stuck with a needle contaminated with blood from a person with chronic hepatitis B. The health care worker has never been vaccinated. What is the most appropriate action?

Answer: Give hepatitis B immune globulin and hepatitis B vaccine. *The same recommendation would be made for a child born to a mother with chronic hepatitis B. If the person had already been vaccinated, then you would check for levels of protective surface antibody. If hepatitis B surface antibody were already present, then no further treatment would be necessary.*

> There is *no* postexposure prophylaxis for **hepatitis C** and *no* vaccine.

CIRRHOSIS

No matter what the cause of the cirrhosis, it will have a number of features:

- **Edema from low oncotic pressure:** Treat with spironolactone and diuretics
- **Gynecomastia**
- **Palmar erythema**
- **Splenomegaly**

- **Thrombocytopenia from splenic sequestration**
- **Encephalopathy:** Treat with lactulose
- **Ascites:** Treat with spironolactone
- **Esophageal varices:** Propranolol will prevent bleeding. Perform banding of the varices if they bleed.

ASCITES

Perform a **paracentesis** for all patients with ascites if any of the following are present:

- **New ascites**
- **Pain, fever, or tenderness**

Diagnostic Testing

- If the SAAG is < 1.1, then portal hypertension is *not* present.
- If the SAAG is > 1.1, then portal hypertension *is* present.

Perform an ascitic fluid **albumin level.** If the ascites fluid albumin level is low, the gradient or difference between the ascites and the serum level of albumin will be very great. This is a **serum-to-ascites albumin gradient (SAAG).** If the **SAAG is > 1.1, portal hypertension from cirrhosis** or **congestive failure** is present.

Spontaneous bacterial peritonitis (SBP) is diagnosed with a **cell count > 250 neutrophils.** Treat with **cefotaxime.**

CHRONIC LIVER DISEASE (CAUSES OF CIRRHOSIS)

Alcoholic Cirrhosis

This is a **diagnosis of exclusion.** Exclude all the other causes of cirrhosis and look for a history of **longstanding alcohol abuse.**

Treat **as described above for cirrhosis.**

Primary Biliary Cirrhosis (PBC)

PBC presents with a **middle-aged woman** complaining of **itching. Xanthalasmas** (cholesterol deposits) may be found on examination. Also look for a history of **other autoimmune disorders.**

Diagnostic testing is as follows:

- Best initial test: **Elevated alkaline phosphatase with a normal bilirubin level.** IgM level is elevated.
- Most accurate tests: **Antimitochondrial antibody (AMA), liver biopsy**

Treatment is with **ursodeoxycholic acid.**

Primary Sclerosis Cholangitis (PSC)

Inflammatory bowel disease (IBD) accounts for 80 percent of PSC. PSC also presents with **itching** but is much more likely to give an **elevated bilirubin level.** The **alkaline phosphatase level is elevated.**

Diagnostic testing is as follows:

- **Most accurate tests:**
  - **ERCP** shows "beading" of the biliary system
  - **Antismooth muscle antibody (ASMA)**
  - **ANCA** is positive

Treatment is with **ursodeoxycholic acid.**

Wilson's Disease

Wilson's disease involves cirrhosis and liver disease in a person with a **choreiform movement disorder** and **neuropsychiatric abnormalities.** This condition also presents with **hemolysis.**

Diagnostic testing is as follows:

- **Best initial test:** Slit lamp looking for **Kayser Fleischer rings** is more sensitive and specific than a **low ceruloplasmin level.** On CCS, order *both.*
- **Most accurate test:** Liver biopsy is more accurate than a urinary copper level.

Treatment is with **penicillamine.**

Hemochromatosis

Most often, hemochromatosis is from a **genetic disorder** resulting in the over-absorption of iron. The iron deposits throughout the body, most commonly in the liver. Other manifestations include the following:

> The most common cause of death from hemochromatosis is **cirrhosis.** Cardiac disease occurs in only 15 percent of cases.

- **Restrictive cardiomyopathy**
- **Skin darkening**
- **Joint pain** from pseudogout or calcium pyrophosphate deposition disease
- **Damage to the pancreas** leading to diabetes, referred to as **"bronze diabetes"**
- **Pituitary accumulation** with panhypopituitarism
- **Infertility**
- **Hepatoma**

Diagnostic testing is as follows:

- Best initial test: **Elevated serum iron and ferritin levels with a low iron-binding capacity.** The iron saturation is enormously elevated (> 45 percent).

- Most accurate test: **Liver biopsy.** However, an **MRI** of the liver and the specific genetic test, the **HFe gene mutation,** in combination are suffiently diagnostic to spare the patient a liver biopsy.

Treatment is with phlebotomy.

Autoimmune Hepatitis

Look for a **young woman with other autoimmune diseases,** such as Coomb's positive hemolytic anemia, thyroiditis, and ITP.

Diagnostic testing is as follows:

- Best initial tests: **ANA and antismooth muscle antibody test. Serum protein electrophoresis (SPEP)** shows hypergammaglobulinemia. The patient may also have positive ANA and liver/kidney microsomal antibody.
- Most accurate test: **Liver biopsy**

Treatment is with **prednisone.** One may also need to use other immunosuppressive agents, such as azathioprine, if attempting to wean the patient off steroids.

Nonalcoholic Steatohepatitis (NASH)

NASH is strongly associated with **obesity, diabetes, and hyperlipidemia. Hepatomegaly** is often present.

Diagnostic testing is as follows:

- Best initial test: **ALT > AST**
- Most accurate test: **Liver biopsy showing fatty infiltration.** The liver biopsy looks just like alcoholic liver disease.

No specific therapy exists to reverse NASH. **Control the underlying causes** with weight loss, diabetes control, and managment of the hyperlipidemia.

NEUROLOGY

9

STROKE AND TRANSIENT ISCHEMIC ATTACK (TIA)

Strokes and TIAs present with the **sudden onset of weakness on one side of the body. Weakness of half of the face and aphasia are common as well.** Cases may state that there is a **partial or total loss of vision,** which may be transient. The cause is decreased or altered cerebral blood flow.

STROKE

Strokes are discriminated from TIA based on time. **Strokes occur for ≥ 24 hours.** There will be **permanent residual neurologic deficits,** caused by **ischemia** or **hemorrhage:** 80 percent are ischemic in nature, and 20 percent are hemorrhagic. Ischemic strokes can be either from emboli or from a thrombosis. Emboli present with more sudden symptoms.

TRANSIENT ISCHEMIC ATTACK (TIA)

TIAs present exactly the same as a stroke, except that the **symptoms last < 24 hours and resolve completely.** Cases may present only with **transient loss of vision in one eye,** known as **amaurosis fugax.** This happens during a transient ischemic attack because the first branch of the carotid artery is the ophthalmic artery. TIAs are always caused by **emboli** or **thrombosis.** TIAs are *never* due to hemorrhage; hemorrhages do not resolve in 24 hours.

A 67-year-old man with a history of hypertension and diabetes comes to the emergency department with a sudden onset of weakness in the right arm and leg over the last hour. On exam, he cannot lift the bottom half of the right side of his face. What is the best initial step?

a. Head CT with contrast
b. Head CT without contrast
c. Aspirin
d. Thrombolytics
e. MRI

*Answer: The correct answer is **B**. Prior to administering thrombolytics or any anticoagulation, you need to **rule out hemorrhagic stroke**, which is a contraindication to thrombolytics. You cannot even give aspirin without doing a head CT first. Thrombolytics are indicated within the first 3 hours of the onset of the symptoms of a stroke. Remember, 20 percent of strokes are hemorrhagic. You do not need contrast to visualize blood; contrast is used to detect cancer or infection, such as an abscess.*

ARTERIES AND SYMPTOMS

Identifying or localizing a lesion based on characteristic symptoms likely will be important during the exam.

Cerebral Artery	Symptoms
Anterior cerebral artery	• Profound lower extremity weakness (contralateral in the case of unilateral arterial occlusion) • Mild upper extremity weakness (contralateral in the case of unilateral arterial occlusion) • Personality changes • Urinary incontinence
Middle cerebral artery	• Profound upper extremity weakness (contralateral in the case of unilateral arterial occlusion) • Aphasia • Apraxia/neglect • The eyes deviate *towards* the side of the lesion.
Posterior cerebral artery	• Contralateral homonyous hemianopia, with macular sparing • Prosopagnosia (inability to recognize faces)
Vertebrobasilar artery	• Vertigo • Nausea and vomiting • May be described as a "drop attack" • Vertical nystagmus • Dysarthria and dystonia • Sensory changes in face and scalp • Ataxia • Labile blood pressure
Lacunar infarct	• There must be an *absence* of cortical deficits. • Ataxia • Parkinsonian signs • Sensory deficits • Hemiparesis (most notable in the face) • Possible bulbar signs
Opthalmic artery	• Amaurosis fugax

DIAGNOSTIC TESTING

The best initial diagnostic test for either stroke or TIA is a **CT scan of the head** *without* **contrast.** Within the first several days, all **nonhemorrhagic strokes** should be associated with a **normal head CT scan.** MRI is *not* done, because the CT is more widely available, less expensive, and more sensitive for blood.

- **Head CT:** Extremely sensitive for blood. Needs 3–5 days to achieve > 95 percent sensitivity in the detection of nonhemorrhagic stroke.
- **MRI:** Achieves 95 percent sensitivity for a nonhemorrhagic stroke within 24 hours.

TREATMENT

- **Thrombolytics:** These should be administered within **3 hours** of the onset of the symptoms of a stroke. Make sure you *always* get a head CT without contrast *first* to rule out a hemorrhagic stroke before anticoagulating. You must know the contraindications to thrombolytic therapy as well. Following are the **absolute contraindications to thrombolytic therapy:**
  - History of hemorrhagic stroke
  - Presence of intracranial neoplasm/mass
  - Active bleeding or surgery within 6 weeks
  - Presence of bleeding disorder
  - CPR within 3 weeks that was traumatic (e.g., chest compressions)
  - Suspicion of aortic dissection
  - Stroke within 1 year
  - Cerebral trauma or brain surgery within 6 months
- **Aspirin:** Best initial therapy for **those coming too late for thrombolytics.** Also indicated *after* the use of thrombolytics.
- **Dipyridamole:** If the patient is *already* on aspirin when a new stroke or TIA occurs, the best initial therapy is dipyridamole for **those presenting too late to receive thrombolytics.**
- **Clopidogrel:** This is an **alternative to dipyridamole** as an alternative to aspirin for those developing a new stroke on aspirin.
- **Heparin:** There is no clear evidence of heparin's benefit for stroke.
- Ticlopidine is always a *wrong* answer. It has *no* added benefit to the use of clopidogrel and has more adverse effects, such as TTP and neutropenia.

> Less than 20 percent of patients with a stroke come in time to get thrombolytics (< 3 hours).

FURTHER MANAGEMENT

Stroke

When you have done the head CT and given thrombolytics or aspirin, you should move the clock forward on CCS. On subsequent screens, the most important issue is to **determine the origin** of the stroke to prevent another one.

The following are indicated in all patients with stroke or TIA:

- **Echocardiogram:** Warfarin for clots, possible **surgery** for valve vegetations
- **Carotid dopplers/duplex: Endarterectomy** for stenosis > 70 percent, but *not* if it is 100 percent
- **EKG and a Holter monitor** if the EKG is normal: **Warfarin** for atrial fibrillation

Young patients (< 50) with no past medical history (diabetes, hypertension) should also have the following tests:

- **Sedimentation rate**
- **VDRL or RPR**
- **ANA, double-stranded DNA**
- **Protein C, Protein S, factor V Leiden mutation, antiphospholipid syndromes**

Don't forget to control **hypertension, diabetes, and hyperlipidemia** in a patient who has had a stroke. Hypertensive urgency is a relative contraindication to thrombolytic therapy.

> The younger the patient, the more likely the cause of the stroke is a vasculitis or hypercoaguable state.

Condition	Goal
Hypertension	< 130/80 madiabetic
Diabetes	Same tight glycemic control as general population
Hyperlipidemia	LDL < 100 madiabetic

TIA

The management of a TIA is the **same as for a stroke,** except that thrombolytics are not indicated. The object of administering a thrombolytic is to achieve resolution of symptoms. If the symptoms have already resolved, then there is no point in giving thrombolytics.

SEIZURES

Only the management of status epilepticus is clear in seizure disorders. Status epilepticus therapy is as follows:

1. Benzodiazepines, such as Ativan® (lorazepam).

2. If the seizure persists after moving the clock forward 10–20 minutes, then add fosphenytoin.

3. If the seizure persists after moving the clock forward 10–20 minutes, then add phenobarbital.

4. If the seizure persists after moving the clock forward 10–20 minutes, then add general anesthesia, such as pentobarbital.

DIAGNOSTIC TESTING

Testing of a Patient Having a Seizure

- Sodium, calcium, glucose, oxygen, creatinine, and magnesium levels
- Head CT urgently; MRI later if the initial testing shows nothing
- Urine toxicology screening

> Potassium disorders do *not* result in seizures.

Further Management

If the initial set of diagnostic tests does *not* reveal the etiology of the seizure, then an **electroencephalogram (EEG)** should be performed. The EEG should *not* be done first.

Neurology consultation should be ordered in any patient in with a seizure. Consultations will always ask for your reason for the consultation in ten words or less.

On CCS, consultants *never* say anything. CCS is testing your ability to know when you are expected to need help.

LONG-TERM TREATMENT OF FIRST-TIME SEIZURES

Chronic antiepileptic drug therapy is generally not indicated after a single seizure. There are several exceptions, however. Treat chronically after the first seizure in the following circumstances:

- Strong family history of seizures
- Abnormal EEG
- Status epilepticus that required benzodiazepines to stop the seizure

CHRONIC ANTIEPILEPTIC THERAPY

No clear single agent is the best initial therapy for the long-term management of seizures.

- First-line therapies: **Valproic acid, carbamazepine, phenytoin, and levetiracetam (Kepra®)** are all equal in efficacy. **Lamotrigine (Lamictal®)** has efficacy equal to those agents but is associated with the development of **Stevens-Johnson syndrome** and severe skin reactions.
- Second-line therapies: **Gabapentin and phenobarbital** are considered second-line agents for long-term management.
- **Ethosuxamide** is best for **absence or petit mal seizures.**

PARKINSON'S DISEASE (PD)

Parkinson's disease presents with a **tremulous patient with a slow, abnormal "festinating" gait.** PD is predominantly a gait disorder. It is often characterized by **orthostasis.**

PHYSICAL FINDINGS

- **"Cogwheel" rigidity**
- **Resting tremor** (resolves when patient moves or reaches for something)
- **Hypomimia** (a masklike, underreactive face)
- **Micrographia** (small writing)
- **Orthostasis**
- **Intact cognition and memory**

There are *no* specific diagnostic tests to prove that someone has Parkinson's disease.

TREATMENT

Mild Symptoms

- **Under age 60: Anticholinergic agent,** such as benztropine or hydroxyzine
- **Over age 60: Amantadine** (Older patients develop far more adverse effects from anticholinergic agents, including constipation, glaucoma, and urinary retention.)

Severe Symptoms

Severe symptoms are defined as the inability to perform activities of daily living, such as cooking, cleaning, personal grooming, and shopping.

	Levodopa/Carbidopa	Dopamine Agonists (pramipexole, ropinerole, cabergoline)
Advantages	Greatest efficacy	Fewer adverse effects
Disadvantages	"On-off" phenomena with uneven long-term effects and more adverse effects	Less efficacy

If these medications cannot control the patient's symptoms, then use the following:

- **COMT inhibitors:** Tolcapone, entacapone. These medications **block the metabolism of dopamine** and extend the effect of dopamine-based medications. They are not effective by themselves.
- **MAO inhibitors:** Selegilene, rasegilene

TREMOR

Type of Tremor	Resting Tremor	Tremor with Intention (Action) Only	Tremor Both at Rest and with Intention
Diagnosis	Parkinson's disease	Cerebellar disorders	Essential tremor
Treatment	Amantadine	Treat etiology	Propranolol

MULTIPLE SCLEROSIS (MS)

Presents with **abnormalities of *any* part of the central nervous system;** these improve only to have **another defect develop several months to years later.** The most common abnormality to develop is **optic neuritis.** Other abnormalities are **motor and sensory problems and defects of the bladder,** such as an atonic bladder.

Other common features of MS are the following:

- **Fatigue**
- **Hyperreflexia**
- **Spasticity**
- **Depression**

DIAGNOSTIC TESTING

- Best initial diagnostic test: **MRI**
- Most accurate diagnostic test: **MRI**
- There is *no* reason to order a CT scan of the head. The CT is far less sensitive than an MRI.

- **CSF (lumbar tap):** Presence of **oligoclonal bands** is only useful if the MRI is nondiagnostic.
- Visual and auditory evoked potential are *always* wrong answers.

TREATMENT

- Best initial therapy: **Steroids** are the best initial therapy for acute exacerbations to help speed resolution.
- Disease-modifying therapy:
  - **Beta interferon**
  - **Glatiramer**
- These two medications have been associated with a decreased rate of progression of disease.
- Additional medications for other symptoms:
  - **Fatigue: Amantadine**
  - **Spasticity: Baclofen** or **tizanadine**

DEMENTIA

ALZHEIMER'S DISEASE (AD)

Alzheimer's presents with **slowly progressive loss of memory exclusively in older patients** (> 65). Although there are no focal deficits, such as motor or sensory problems, these patients develop apathy and, after several years, imprecise speech.

Diagnostic Testing

For all patients with **memory loss,** you *must* order the following tests:

- **Head CT**
- **B12 level**
- **Thyroid function testing (T4/TSH)**
- **RPR or VDRL**

Alzheimer's disease is a diagnosis of exclusion. The only abnormal test will be the **CT scan** of the head showing **diffuse, symmetrical atrophy.**

Treatment

Anticholinesterase medications (donepezil, rivastigmine, and galantamine) are the standard of care. **Memantine** is a medication from another class with modest benefit. Combinations are *not* effective.

FRONTOTEMPORAL DEMENTIA (PICK DISEASE)

Personality and behavior become abnormal first. Then memory is lost afterwards. There is *no* movement disorder.

Head CT or MRI shows **focal atrophy of the frontal and temporal lobes.** Treat **the same as Alzheimer's** with less response.

CREUTZFELD-JAKOB DISEASE (CJD)

CJD is caused by prions, transmissible protein particles. It manifests as **rapidly progressive dementia and presence of myoclonus.** The patient is younger than in Alzheimer's.

Although the **EEG is abnormal,** the *most* accurate diagnostic test is a **brain biopsy.** On CCS cases, an **MRI** should be performed as well, although there is nothing on MRI to suggest CJD. **CSF shows a 14-3-3 protein.** The presence of the 14-3-3 protein spares the patient the need for brain biopsy.

"LEWY BODY" DEMENTIA

Lewy Body dementia is **Parkinson's disease plus dementia.** Remember: Parkinson's disease is primarily a gait disorder.

NORMAL PRESSURE HYDROCEPHALUS (NPH)

This condition generally presents in older males, but it can affect women as well. Symptoms can be remembered as **WWW: wet, weird, wobbly:**

- Wet: Urinary incontinence
- Weird: Dementia
- Wobbly: Wide-based gait/ataxia

Diagnose by **head CT.** A **lumbar puncture (LP)** will show normal pressure, and this should be done on CCS. Treat with **placement of a shunt.**

HUNTINGTON'S DISEASE/CHOREA

Huntington's presents in a **young patient** (30s) *far* below the age for Alzheimer's disease. The question likely will mention family history. Symptoms are the following:

- **Dementia**
- **Psychiatric disturbance with personality changes**
- **Chorea/movement disorder**

Diagnose with **specific genetic testing.** Inheritance is autosomal dominant. *No* treatment is available.

DEMENTIA SYNDROMES

All patients have memory loss and should have a **head CT/MRI, VDRL, B12, and T4.**

How do the conditions vary?

- **Alzheimer's:** No focal deficits. Treatment is with anticholinesterases and memantine.
- **Picks/Frontotemporal:** Personality and behavior are affected first.
- **Lewy Body:** Parkinsonian symptoms accompany dementia.
- **Huntington's:** Presents with movement (chorea) and personality disorders.
- **Normal pressure hydrocephalus:** Remember WWW: Wet, weird, wobbly.

HEADACHE

MIGRAINE

Of migraines, 60 percent are unilateral, and 40 percent are bilateral.

Triggers include the following:

- Cheese
- Caffeine
- Menstruation
- Oral contraceptive

The following symptoms may precede the headache:

- Aura of bright flashing lights
- Scotomata
- Abnormal smells

Diagnostic Testing

Head CT or **MRI** should be done when the headache has any of the following characteristics:

- Sudden and/or severe
- Onset after age 40
- Associated with focal neurological findings

Treatment

- Best initial (abortive) therapy: **Sumatriptan** or **ergotamine** is the best abortive therapy.
- Prophylactic therapy: It takes **several weeks** for prophylactic therapy to be effective.
  - When four or more headaches occur per month, the patient should receive prophylactic therapy with **beta blockers (propranolol).**
  - Alternate prophylactic medications are **calcium channel blockers, tricyclic antidepressants,** or **SSRIs.**

CLUSTER HEADACHE

Cluster headaches are **10 times more frequent in men than in women.** Cluster headaches are **exclusively unilateral** with **redness and tearing of the eye** and **rhinorrhea.**

Treatment

- Best initial (abortive) therapy: **Sumatriptan** is used in the same way as with migraine headache, but 100 percent **oxygen** or **steroids** can also be used. This treatment is *unique* to cluster headaches.
- Prophylactic therapy: There is *no* prophylactic therapy, because, by definition, cluster headaches occur multiple times in a short period and then resolve. The "cluster" would be over by the time prophylactic therapy had taken effect.

Headache Type	Migraine	Cluster
Gender		Much more common in men
Presentation	• Unilateral or bilateral • Aura	• Only unilateral • Tearing and redness of eye; rhinorrhea • No aura
Abortive	• Sumatiptan	• Sumatriptan • Special: 100% oxygen
Prophylactic	• Propranolol	• None

TEMPORAL ARTERITIS

Temporal arteritis presents with the following:

- Tenderness of the temporal area
- Jaw claudication

Diagnostic testing is as follows:

- **Sedimentation rate (ESR)**
- Most accurate test: **Temporal artery biopsy**

Give **steroids first and fast** if these are available. A delay may result in **permanent vision loss.**

PSEUDOTUMOR CEREBRI

Look for an **obese young woman with a headache and double vision.** On exam, there is **papilledema,** but CT/MRI is normal. **Vitamin A use** is suggestive.

The most accurate test is a **lumbar puncture with opening pressure measurement,** which will show a markedly elevated pressure.

Treatment is as follows:

- **Weight loss**
- **Acetazolamide**

DIZZINESS/VERTIGO

All patients with vertigo will have a subjective sensation of the **room spinning** around them. This is often associated with **nausea and vomiting.** All patients with vertigo will have **nystagmus** (horizontal). When a patient thinks the room is spinning, the eyes should naturally dart back and forth to give the feeling of looking at a single point.

Generally *all* patients with vertigo should have an **MRI of the internal auditory canal.**

The following table summarizes the presentation of a number of conditions that cause vertigo.

Disease	Characteristics	Hearing Loss/Tinnitus
Benign positional vertigo	Changes with position	No
Vestibular neuritis	Vertigo occurs without position changes	No
Labyrinthitis	Acute	Yes
Meniere's disease	Chronic	Yes
Acoustic neuroma	Ataxia	Yes
Perilymph fistula	History of trauma	Yes

BENIGN POSITIONAL VERTIGO (BPV)

This presents as vertigo alone with no hearing loss, no tinnitus and no ataxia. The question may describe a positive Dix-Hallpike maneuver. History may describe onset of symptoms when quickly changing positions.

There is no specific diagnostic test. BPV responds modestly to meclizine (Antivert®).

VESTIBULAR NEURITIS

This is an idiopathic inflammation of the vestibular portion of the VIII (8th) cranial nerve. Because only the vestibular portion is involved, there is no hearing loss and no tinnitus. Presumably, this condition is viral. It is entirely characterized by vertigo and dizziness and is not related to changes in position.

There is no specific diagnostic test. Treat with meclizine.

LABYRINTHITIS

Labyrinthitis is inflammation of the cochlear portion of the inner ear. There is hearing loss as well as tinnitus. This condition is acute and self-limited and may be treated with meclizine.

MENIERE'S DISEASE

Same presentation as labyrinthitis (vertigo, hearing loss, tinnitus), but Meniere's is chronic with remitting and relapsing episodes. Treat with salt restriction and diuretics.

ACOUSTIC NEUROMA

This is an VIII (8th) cranial nerve tumor that can be related to neurofibromatosis, or Von Recklinghausen's disease. Acoustic neuroma presents with ataxia in addition to hearing loss, tinnitus, and vertigo.

Diagnose with an MRI of the internal auditory canal. Treat with surgical resection.

PERILYMPH FISTULA

Head trauma or any form of barotrauma to the ear may rupture the tympanic membrane and lead to a perilymph fistula.

WERNICKE-KORSAKOFF SYNDROME

Wernicke-Korsakoff syndrome presents as follows:

- History of chronic heavy alcohol use
- Confusion with confabulation
- Ataxia
- Memory loss
- Gaze palsy/ophthalmoplegia
- Nystagmus

Diagnostic Testing

With memory loss, it is very important to perform the following tests:

- Head CT
- B12 level
- Thyroid function (T4/TSH)
- RPR or VDRL

Treatment

- Treat with thiamine. Acutely, give IV dose; then may switch to oral.
- Also give glucose with thiamine, but administer thiamine first, then glucose.

CENTRAL NERVOUS SYSTEM INFECTIONS

BACTERIAL MENINGITIS

A 45-year-old man comes to the emergency department with fever, headache, photophobia, and a stiff neck. What is the next best step in the management of this patient?

a. Lumbar puncture

b. Head CT scan

c. Ceftriaxone and vancomycin

d. Penicillin

e. Movement of patient to ICU

*Answer: The correct answer is **A**. When you suspect bacterial meningitis, administer antibiotics quickly. Further, do blood cultures stat simultanenously with a lumbar puncture or immediately prior. Penicillin can never be used as empiric therapy for meningitis; it is not sufficiently broad in coverage to be effective empiric therapy. In this case, perform the LP; answer A is the best choice.*

Often when a CNS infection is suspected, a head CT should be performed before a lumbar puncture. Perform a head CT before a lumbar puncture (LP) in the following circumstances:

- A history of central nervous system disease
- Focal neurologic deficit
- Presence of papilledema
- Seizures
- Altered conciousness
- Significant delay in the ability to perform an LP

If these findings are present, get blood cultures and start empiric antibiotic therapy before ordering the head CT.

Cerebrospinal Fluid (CSF)

The most accurate test for bacterial meningitis is a culture, but you cannot wait for the results of culture before starting therapy. Preliminary analysis of the CSF is useful.

- Gram stain shows: The gram stain is only about 50–60 percent sensitive for bacterial meningitis. Therefore, a negative stain excludes nothing. On the other hand, a positive gram stain is extremely useful and specific. In other words, the gram stain has poor sensitivity but good specificity.
  - Gram-positive diplococcic: Pneumococcus
  - Gram-negative diplococci: Neisseria
  - Gram-negative pleomorphic, coccobacillary organisms: Hemophilus
  - Gram-positive bacilli: Listeria

- Protein: An elevated protein level in the CSF is of marginal diagnostic benefit. Protein elevation is nonspecific; any form of CNS infection can elevate the CSF protein. A normal CSF protein level essentially excludes bacterial meningitis.
- Glucose: Glucose levels below 60 percent of serum levels are consistent with bacterial meningitis.
- CSF cell count: The best initial test for the diagnosis of meningitis is a cell count.
  - Although not as specific as a culture, it is available much sooner.
  - Cell count with a differential is much more specific than an elevated CSF protein level.
  - If thousands of neutrophils are present in the CSF, start IV ceftriaxone, vancomycin, and steroids. Steroids have been associated with a decrease in mortality in bacterial meningitis.

> CSF cell count is the most important criterion to determine the need to treat a patient. Thousands of polys (neutrophils) indicates bacterial meningitis until proven otherwise.

CRYPTOCOCCUS

Look for an HIV-positive patient with < 100 CD4 cells. This infection is slower than bacterial meningitis and may not give severe meningeal signs, such as neck stiffness, photophobia, and high fever, all at the same time.

Diagnostic Testing

- Best initial test: India ink
- Most accurate test: Cryptococcal antigen

Treatment

- Best initial therapy: Amphotericin
- Amphotericin is followed with oral fluconazole.
  - If the patient's CD4 cells do not rise, fluconazole must be continued indefinitely.
  - If the CD4 count rises above 100, the fluconazole can be stopped.

LYME DISEASE

Look for a patient who has recently been on a camping or hiking trip. Tick exposure is remembered only by 20 percent of patients.

There are no characteristic CSF findings to confirm a diagnosis of CNS Lyme. Specific serologic or western blot testing on the CSF is the most accurate test. Look for a patient with a history of joint pain, VII (7th) cranial nerve palsy, or a rash with central clearing (target lesion). Treat with IV ceftriaxone or penicillin

ROCKY MOUNTAIN SPOTTED FEVER

Look for a camper or hiker with a rash that starts on the wrists and ankles and moves centripetally towards the center. Fever, headache, and malaise precede the rash. Only 60 percent at most will remember a tick bite.

Diagnose with specific serology. Doxycycline is the most effective therapy.

TB MENINGITIS

This is an extremely difficult diagnosis to be precise about. Look for an immigrant with a history of lung tuberculosis. The presentation is very slow over weeks to months; if the case describes fever, headache, and neck stiffness over hours then it is not TB.

Diagnostic Testing

TB meningitis has a very high CSF protein level. Acid fast (mycobacterial) stain of the CSF is positive in 10 percent or less of patients. For acid-fast culture, you need three high-volume taps that are centrifuged.

Treatment

Treat with rifampin, isonizaid, pyrizinamide, and ethambutol (RIPE) as you would for pulmonary TB. The only difference is that you should add steroids and extend the length of therapy for meningitis when compared with pulmonary disease.

VIRAL MENINGITIS

Viral meningitis is, in general, a diagnosis of exclusion. There is a lymphocytic pleocytosis in the CSF, and none of the other findings is present. There is no specific therapy for viral meningitis.

An elderly man comes to the emergency department with fever, headache, a stiff neck, and photophobia. He is HIV positive with < 50 CD4 cells and a history of pneumocystis pneumonia. His head CT is normal. CSF shows 2,500 white cells that are all neutrophils; gram stain is normal. What is the best initial therapy?

a. Ceftriaxone and metronidazole

b. Cefoxitin and mefloquine

c. Ceftriaxone, ampicillin, and vancomycin

d. Fluconazole

e. Amphotericin

*Answer: The correct answer is **C**. Listeria monocytogenes is a cause of meningitis that is not adequately treated by any form of cephalosporin. Ampicillin is added to the usual regimen of ceftriaxone and vancomycin to cover Listeria. This cannot be fungal meningitis, because the CSF is characterized exclusively by a high number of neutrophils; neutrophils are not consistent with fungal meningitis.*

A 17-year-old male is brought to the emergency department with fever, headache, stiff neck, and photophobia. He has a petechial rash. CSF shows 2,499 neutrophils. Ceftriaxone and vancomycin are started. What should be done next?

a. Test for HIV

b. Wait for results of culture

c. Add ampicillin

d. Enforce respiratory isolation

e. Enforce respiratory isolation and prescribe rifampin for close contacts

*Answer: The correct answer is **E**. When an adolescent presents with a petechial rash and increased neutrophils on CSF, it is suggestive of Neisseria meningitides. These patients should be placed on respiratory isolation, and close contacts should receive prophylaxis.*

LISTERIA

Look for elderly, neonatal, and HIV-positive patients and those with who have no spleen, are on steroids, or are immunocompromised with leukemia or lymphoma.

There will be elevated neutrophils in the CSF. Add ampicillin to therapy.

NEISSERIA MENINGITIDES

Look for patients who are adolescent, in the military, or asplenic or who have terminal complement deficiency.

> The nurse or medical student taking care of a patient with Neisseria does not need prophylaxis. Those with kissing and other saliva-type contact do need prophylaxis.

Treat as follows:

- Patient: Begin respiratory isolation.
- Close contacts: Start prophylaxis with rifampin or ciprofloxacin for close contacts, such as household members and those who share utensils, cups, or kisses.
- Routine contacts: Routine school and work contacts do not need to receive prophylaxis.

ENCEPHALITIS

Look for a patient with fever and altered mental status over a few hours. If the patient also has photophobia and a stiff neck, you will not be able to diagnose encephalitis. Almost all encephalitis in the United States is from herpes. The patient does not have to recall a herpes infection in the past for the condition to be herpes encephalitis.

> - **Fever + confusion = Encephalitis**

Diagnostic Testing
- Best initial test: Head CT scan
- Most accurate test: PCR of the CSF

The most common wrong answer on questions dealing with the diagnosis of encephalistic is "brain biopsy." A brain biopsy is not necessary. Do a PCR instead.

Treatment
- Best initial therapy: Acyclovir
- For acyclovir-resistant patients: Foscarnet

BRAIN ABSCESS

A brain abscess presents with fever, headache, and focal neurological deficits. A CT scan finds a "ring," or contrast-enhancing, lesion. Contrast ("ring") enhancement basically means either cancer or infection.

Brain Abscess

Consider HIV status in the context of a brain abscess as follows:

- HIV-negative: Brain biopsy is the next best step.
- HIV-positive: Treat for toxoplasmosis with pyrimethamine and sulfadiazine for two weeks and repeat the head CT.

PROGRESSIVE MULTIFOCAL LEUKOENCEPHALOPATHY (PML)

These brain lesions in HIV-positive patients are not associated with ring enhancement or mass effect.

There is no specific therapy. Treat the HIV and raise the CD4. When the HIV is improved, the lesions will disappear.

NEUROCYSTICERCOSIS

Look for a patient from Mexico with a seizure.

Head CT shows multiple 1 cm cystic lesions. Over time, the lesions calcify. Confirm diagnosis with serology.

When still active and uncalcified, the lesions are treated with albendazole. Use steroids to prevent a reaction to dying parasites.

HEAD TRAUMA AND INTRACRANIAL HEMORRHAGE

Any head trauma resulting in a loss of consciousness (LOC) or altered mental status should lead to a CT scan of the head without contrast.

> Do not use skull X-rays in head trauma. If the head trauma is severe, then diagnosis requires a CT scan.

> Loss of consciousness ‡ CT scan

> The following table shows possible outcomes of head trauma that can result in a loss of consciousness and how they vary from one another:

	Concussion	Contusion	Subdural Hematoma	Epidural Hematoma
Focal deficits	Never	Rarely	Yes or no	Yes or no
Head CT	Normal	Ecchymosis	Crescent-shaped collection	Lens-shaped collection

Cortical contusion
> 1cm in diameter

Subdural Hematoma

Epidural Hematoma

TREATMENT

Treatments for various head traumas are as follows:

- Concussion: None
- Contusion: Admit, but vast majority get no treatment.
- Subdural and epidural: Large ones are drained; small ones are left alone to reabsorb on their own.
- Large intracranial hemorrhage with mass effect:
  - Intubation/hyperventilation to decrease intracranial pressure. Decrease pCO2 to 25–30, which will constrict cerebral blood vessels.
  - Administer mannitol as an osmotic diuretic to decrease intracranial pressure.
  - Perform surgical evacuation.

> Steroids do not help intracranial hemorrhage.

Stress Ulcer Prophylaxis

Patients with any of the following conditions should receive proton pump inhibitors as prophylaxis against stress ulcer:

- Head trauma
- Burns
- Endotracheal intubation with mechanical ventilation

SUBARRHACHNOID HEMORRHAGE (SAH)

Look for the following symptoms:

- Sudden, severe headache
- Stiff neck
- Photophobia
- Loss of consciousness (LOC) in 50 percent of patients
- Focal neurological deficits in 30 percent of patients

SAH is like the sudden onset of meningitis with a LOC but without fever.

DIAGNOSTIC TESTING

- Best initial test: A head CT without contrast is 95 percent sensitive. If this is conclusive for an SAH, you do not need to do a lumbar puncture.
- Most accurate diagnostic test: Lumbar puncture. This is not necessary If the head CT scan shows blood.

To tell if an increased number of white cells in CSF is from an infection or just from blood, look for the ratio. A normal number of white cells is 1 for every 500 red cells. An infection is considered to be present only if the number of white cells is greater than the ratio of 1 to 500.

> • Normal white cell count = 1 WBC:500 RBC

TREATMENT

Treatment proceeds as follows:

1. Perform angiography to determine the site of bleeding.
2. Surgically clip or embolize the site of the bleeding.
3. Insert a ventriculoperotoneal shunt if hydrocephalus develops.
4. Prescribe nimodipine orally; this is a calcium channel blocker that prevents stroke.

When SAH occurs, an intense vasospasm can lead to a nonhemorrhagic stroke.

You must clip or embolize the source of bleeding in a SAH before it can rebleed. If it rebleeds, the chances are 50 percent that the patient will die.

SPINE DISORDERS

The following table summarizes some spine disorders and their symptoms:

Lumbosacral Strain	Cord Compression	Epidural Abscess	Spinal Stenosis
Nontender	Tender	Tender and fever	Pain on walking downhill

SYRINGOMYELIA

This is a defective fluid cavity in the center of the cord from trauma, tumors, or a congenital problem. It presents with loss of sensation of pain and temperature in the upper extremities bilaterally in a capelike distribution over the neck, shoulders, and down both arms.

Diagnose with an MRI. Treat surgically.

Syringomyelia

CORD COMPRESSION

Metastatic cancer presses on the cord, resulting in pain and tenderness of the spine. Lumbosacral strain does not give tenderness of the spine itself.

Scan with an MRI. Biopsy is the most accurate test if the diagnosis is not clear from the history.

The most effective therapy depends on the cause. The most urgent step in cases of cord compression is to give steroids to decrease swelling.

SPINAL EPIDURAL ABSCESS

A spinal epidural abscess presents with back pain with tenderness and fever.

Scan the spine with MRI. Give antibiotics against staphylococcus, such as oxacillin or nafcillin. Large accumulations require surgical decompression.

SPINAL STENOSIS

This condition presents with leg pain on walking and can look like peripheral arterial disease. The pulses will be intact, and the pain is worse upon walking downhill, when the patient is leaning backwards, but improved when walking uphill.

Diagnose with an MRI. Treat with surgical decompression.

ANTERIOR SPINAL ARTERY INFARCTION

All sensation is lost except position and vibratory sense, which travel down the posterior column. No specific therapy.

BROWN-SEQUARD SYNDROME

This results from traumatic injury to the spine, such as that from a knife wound. The patient loses ipsilateral position, vibratory sense, contralateral pain, and temperature.

A 58-year-old woman with metastatic breast cancer comes in with back pain. The spine is tender. She has hyperreflexia of the legs. What is the most urgent step?

a. X-ray
b. CT
c. MRI
d. Biopsy
e. Steroids
f. Chemotherapy
g. Radiation

*Answer: The correct answer is **E**. The most urgent step in the management of cord compression is to administer steroids as soon as possible and to relieve pressure on the cord. Imaging studies are done after steroids are given, if the diagnosis of cord compression is clear (as it is in this case with pain, tenderness, and signs of hyperreflexia in the legs).*

AMYOTROPHIC LATERAL SCLEROSIS

This is an idiopathic disorder of both upper and lower motor neurons. It is treated with riluzole, a unique agent that blocks the accumulation of glutamate.

Upper Motor Neuron Signs	Lower Motor Neuron Signs
• Hyperreflexia	• Wasting
• Upgoing toes on plantar reflex	• Fasciculations
• Spasticity	• Weakness
• Weakness	

PERIPHERAL NEUROPATHIES

DIABETES

The most common cause of peripheral neuropathy by far is diabetes. A specific test, such as an electromyogram or nerve conduction study, is not necessary in the majority of cases.

Treat with gabapenin or pregablin. Tricyclic antidepressants are less effective and have more adverse effects.

CARPAL TUNNEL SYNDROME

Look for pain and weakness of the first three digits of the hand. Symptoms may worsen with repetitive use.

Initial management is a splint. In CSS, inject steroids when you move the clock forward if symptoms persist or worsen.

RADIAL NERVE PALSY

Also known as "Saturday night palsy," this results from falling asleep or passing out with pressure on the arms underneath the body or outstretched, perhaps draped over the back of a chair. Radial nerve palsy results in a wrist drop.

PERONEAL NERVE PALSY

This results from high boots pressing at the back of the knee. It results in foot drop and the inability to evert the foot. May see "high boots" in the case.

There is no therapy. Peroneal nerve palsy resolves on its own.

VII (7TH) CRANIAL NERVE (BELL'S PALSY)

Bell's palsy results in hemifacial paralysis of both the upper and lower halves of the face. There is also loss of taste on the anterior two thirds of the tongue, hyperaccusis, and the inability to close the eye at night. Hyperaccusis results in the inability to control the stapedius muscle of the middle ear, which acts as a kind of "shock absorber" for sounds. Bell's palsy is believed to result from a viral infection.

Treat with steroids and acyclovir. It is not clear that acyclovir works, but valacycolvir is often prescribed on a trial basis.

REFLEX SYMPATHETIC DYSTROPHY (CHRONIC REGIONAL PAIN SYNDROME)

This happens in a patient with previous injury to the extremity. Light touch, such as from a sheet touching the foot, results in extreme pain that is "burning" in quality.

Treat with NSAIDs, gabapentin, and occasionally nerve block. Surgical sympathectomy may be necessary.

RESTLESS LEG SYNDROME

This often comes to the health care provider's attention when the bed partner comes in complaining of pain and bruises in the legs. The patient experiences an uncomfortable feeling in the legs, which is relieved by movement.

Treat with pramipexole or ropinerole.

A man comes to the emergency department with weakness in his legs that has been getting markedly worse over the last few days. He has weakness and loss of deep tendon reflexes in the legs. He recalls an upper respiratory illness about 2–4 weeks prior that resolved. What is the most urgent step?

a. Steroids
b. Intravenous immunoglobulins
c. Peak inspiratory pressure
d. Intubation
e. Lumbar puncture

*Answer: The correct answer is **C**. This case is Guillain-Barre. Ascending weakness with loss of deep tendon reflexes is characteristic. Peak inspiratory pressure is the correct answer. The peak inspiratory pressure diminishes as the diaphragm is weakened. Peak inspiratory pressure predicts who will have respiratory failure before it happens. It is more important than to start therapy with either intravenous immunoglobulins (IVIG) or plasmapheresis. Combinations of these medications are not effective. Steroids are not effective. Lumbar puncture will show an elevated protein level with no cells.*

MYASTHENIA GRAVIS

Myasthenia gravis presents with weakness of the muscles of mastication, making it hard to finish meals. Blurry vision from diplopia results from the inability to focus the eyes on a single target. The case may classically report drooping of the eyelids as the day progresses.

Diagnostic Testing

- Best initial test: Anti-acetylcholine receptor antibodies (ACHR)
- Most accurate test: Clinical presentation and ACHR are more sensitive and specific than an edrophonium or "tensilon" stimulation test.

Treatment

- Best initial therapy: Pyridostigmine or neostigmine
- Thymectomy: If pyridostigmine or neostigmine do not work, patients < 60 should undergo thymectomy.
- Prednisone: If thymectomy does not work, or if there simply is no response to pyridostigmine or neostigmine, then prednisone should be started.
- Azathioprine and cyclosporine are used to try to keep the patient off of long-term steroids.

NEPHROLOGY

10

ACUTE RENAL FAILURE

The first step is to **evaluate whether the renal failure is prerenal (perfusion), renal (parenchymal), or postrenal (drainage).**

- Clues to the renal failure being of **short duration** are the following:
  - Normal kidney size
  - Normal hematocrit
  - Normal calcium level

- **Chronic renal failure** will have the following effects:
  - It makes the kidneys smaller.
  - With renal failure of more than two weeks, the hematocrit will drop from loss of erythropoietin production.
  - Calcium levels drop from the loss of vitamin D hydroxylation (i.e., activation).

PRERENAL AZOTEMIA

Any cause of **hypoperfusion** will lead to renal failure:

- **Hypotension,** generally with a systolic pressure < 90 mmHg
- **Hypovolemia** from dehydration or blood loss
- **Low oncotic pressure** (low albumin)
- **Congestive heart failure:** You can't perfuse the kidney if the pump doesn't work.
- **Constrictive pericarditis:** You can't perfuse the kidney if the heart cannot fill.
- **Renal artery stenosis:** Although the systemic pressure may be high, the kidney thinks the body is hypotensive because of the blockage.

Diagnostic Testing

Prerenal azotemia will have the following characteristics:

- **BUN to creatinine ratio of > 15:1 and often > 20:1**
- **Urinary sodium is low** (< 20)
- **Fractional excretion of sodium < 1 percent:** This is largely the same thing as a low urine sodium. Do not spend your time learning to do the calculation.
- **Urine osmolality > 500**
- May have hyaline casts on urinalysis.

Treatment

Treatment of prerenal azotemia is *entirely* based on the underlying cause.

On CCS, all renal cases should have the following tests performed:

- Urinalysis
- Chemistries
- Renal ultrasound

POSTRENAL AZOTEMIA (OBSTRUCTIVE UROPATHY)

Any cause of obstruction of the kidney will lead to renal failure:

- **Stone in the bladder or ureters**
- **Strictures**
- **Cancer of the bladder, prostate, or cervix**
- **Neurogenic bladder** (atonic or noncontracting, such as from multiple sclerosis or diabetes)

Obstuctive uropathy will give an **elevated BUN-to-creatinine ratio of > 15:1**, similar to that seen in prerenal azotemia.

Clues to obstructive uropathy are the following:

- **Distended bladder** on exam
- **Large volume diuresis** after passing a urinary catheter
- **Bilateral hydronephrosis on ultrasound**

Remember: The obstruction *must* be bilateral to cause renal failure. Unilateral obstruction cannot cause renal failure.

INTRARENAL CAUSES OF RENAL FAILURE

Intrarenal causes of renal failure result in the following:

- **BUN-to-creatinine ratio closer to 10:1**
- **Urinary sodium > 40**
- **Urine osmolality < 350**

Acute tubular necrosis (ATN) can be from either **hypoperfusion** to the point of death of the tubular cells or from various **toxic injuries to the kidney.** It is often from a combination of both of these.

Toxin-Induced Renal Insufficiency

In these cases, there is *no* single test to prove that a particular toxin caused the renal failure. Common causes are these:

- **Aminoglycosides,** such as gentamicin, tobramycin, or amikacin: Hypomagnesemia is suggestive of aminoglycoside-induced renal failure, but it is *not* conclusive.
- **Amphotericin**
- **Contrast agents:** In a CCS case, order a **magnesium level** when evaluating possible contrast-induced renal failure.
- **Chemotherapy,** such as cisplatin

The urinalysis may show **"muddy brown" or granular casts.** There is *no* specific therapy to reverse toxin-induced renal failure.

A man is admitted for pneumonia from a nursing home. He is placed on piperacillin-tazobactam, and he becomes afebrile. Two days later, his BUN and creatinine start to rise. He develops a new fever and a rash. What is the most likely diagnosis, and what is the most accurate diagnostic test?

Answer: **Allergic interstitial nephritis** *is a hypersensitivity reaction to medications such as penicillin or sulfa drugs. Other common culprits are phenytoin, allopurinol, cyclosporine, quinidine, quinolones, or rifampin. The clue to the diagnosis is the* **fever and rash.** *The best initial test is a* **urinalysis (UA) that shows white cells.** *However, the UA is not capable of distinguishing between neutrophils and eosinophils. The most accurate test is a* **Wright stain** *or* **Hansel's stain of the urine** *that will show eosinophils. This is more sensitive than either the blood eosinophil level or an elevated IgE level. There is no specific therapy generally given for allergic interstitial nephritis; it resolves on its own.*

Avoid this frequent wrong answer: Cyclophosphamide causes hemorhagic cystitis, *not* renal failure.

Rhabdomyolysis

In cases of rhabdomyolysis, large-volume **muscular necrosis** is associated with renal failure from the direct **toxic effect of myoglobin on the kidney tubule.** Look for the following in presentation:

- Crush injury
- Seizure
- Prolonged immobility in an intoxicated patient
- Hypokalemia resulting in muscle necrosis
- A patient recently started on a "statin" medication for hyperlipidemia

Diagnostic testing is as follows:

- Best initial test: **Urinalysis** showing dipstick positive for large amounts of blood with no cells seen on the microscopic examination
- **CPK level:** Will be elevated.
- Most accurate test: **Urine myoglobin** is probably the single most accurate test.
- On a CCS, also order the following:
  - **Potassium level (hyperkalemia):** Potassium goes up from any cellular destruction, such as from a tumor lysis, hemolysis, or rhabdomyolysis.
  - **Calcium level (hypocalcemia):** Why the calcium level is decreased in rhabdomyolysis is not clear. Damaged muscle may bind increased amounts of calcium. Hyperphosphatemia may lead to binding of calcium with the phosphate.
  - **Chemistries especially for detecting a decreased serum bicarbonate**

Treatment is as follows:

- **Bolus of normal saline**
- **Mannitol and diuresis** to decrease the contact time of myoglobin with the tubule
- **Alkalinization of the urine** may decrease precipitation of myoglobin at the tubule

A patient is brought to the emergency department after a seizure leading to prolonged immobility on a sidewalk. He has dark urine and myalgias. What is the most urgent step in the management of this patient?

a. Urinalysis

b. Urine myoglobin level

c. EKG

d. CPK level

e. Phosphate level

f. Creatinine

*Answer: The correct answer is **C**. EKG is the most urgent step in an acute case of rhabdomyolysis. This case tests your knowledge of how people die with rhabdomyolysis. Severe muscle necrosis leads to **hyperkalemia**, which leads to **arrhythmia.** If this is a CCS case, then all of the tests should be done simultaneously. A specific diagnosis with urinalysis or urine myoglobin is not as important as detecting and treating potentially life-threatening conditions, such as hyperkalemia with peaked T waves. This condition would be treated with immediate intravenous calcium gluconate, insulin, and glucose.*

Crystal-Induced Renal Failure

This condition can result from oxalate crystals or uric acid crystals.

- Oxalate crystals: Look for **suicide from antifreeze ingestion** (ethylene glycol). The patient will be intoxicated with metabolic acidosis with an elevated anion gap.
  - The best initial test is **urinalysis** showing **envelope-shaped oxalate crystals.**
  - The best initial treatment is **ethanol** or **fomepazole** with **immediate dialysis.**

oxalate crystals

- **Uric acid crystals:** Look for **tumor lysis syndrome,** most often after chemotherapy for lymphoma.
  - Treat with hydration and allopurinol.

Prevention of Contrast-Induced Renal Failure

To test your knowledge of this situation, the case will describe a patient who *must* have a radiologic procedure with contrast *and* common reasons for renal insufficiency, such as an elderly patient with hypertension and diabetes. There will be no attempt to hide the etiology. Mild renal insufficiency with a creatinine just above the normal range at 1.5 to 2.5 will be shown.

What is the best method to prevent contrast induced renal failure?

*Answer: Give hydration with **normal saline** and possibly **bicarbonate, N-acetyl cysteine,** or **both.***

Step 3 wants you to know that even a *very slight* elevation in creatinine means the loss of 60–70 percent of renal function at a minimum. Preserve what is left!

NSAIDs AND THE KIDNEY

NSAIDS can cause the following:

- **Direct toxicity and ATN**
- **Allergic interstitial nephritis** with eosinophils in the urine
- **Nephrotic syndrome**
- **Afferent arteriolar vasoconstriction and decreased perfusion of the glomerulus,** worsening renal function

GLOMERULONEPHRITIS

All forms of glomerulonephritis (GN) can have the following characteristics:

- **Red blood cells** in the urine
- **Red cell casts** in the urine
- Mild degrees of **proteinuria** (< 2 grams per 24 hours)
- **Edema**
- May lead to **nephrotic syndrome**
- Are most accurately diagnosed with **kidney biopsy,** although this is not always necessary

Think: What are the few extra words we need to know about each disease to answer the diagnostic and treatment questions? (Step 3 does *not* generally emphasize the "most likely diagnosis" question.)

GOODPASTURE'S SYNDROME

Cough, hemoptysis, shortness of breath, and lung findings will be present in the case.

Diagnostic Testing
- Best initial test: **Anti–basement membrane antibodies**
- Most accurate test: **Renal biopsy showing "linear deposits"**

Treatment
Treatment is with **plasmapheresis.**

Churg-Strauss Syndrome
Asthma, cough, and eosinophilia are present in addition to the **renal abnormalities.**

Diagnostic Testing

- Best initial test: **CBC for eosinophil count**
- Most accurate test: **Biopsy**

Treatment

- Best initial therapy: **Glucocorticoids** (e.g., prednisone)
- If there is no response to prednisone, add **cyclophosphamide.**

WEGENER'S GRANULOMATOSIS

Upper respiratory problems such as **sinusitis and otitis** are the key to diagnosis. **Lung problems** (cough, hemoptysis, abnormal chest X-ray) are present as well.

Wegener's is a **systemic vasculitis,** so joint, skin, eye, brain, and GI problems are also present, but the key is both upper and lower respiratory involvement *in addition* to renal involvement. Often the case will be misdiagnosed as pneumonia.

Diagnostic Testing

- Best initial test: **c-ANCA** (antineutrophil cytoplasmic antibodies)
- Most accurate test: **Biopsy of kidney**

Treatment

The best initial therapy is **cyclophosphamide and steroids.**

POLYARTERITIS NODOSA (PAN)

Polyarteritis nodosa is **systemic vasculitis** with involvement of every organ *except* the lung.

Presentations include the following:

- Renal
- Myalgias
- GI bleeding and abdominal pain
- Purpuric skin lesion
- Stroke
- Uveitis
- Neuropathy

The very nonspecific findings of fever, weight loss, and fatigue will also be present. **Multiple motor and sensory neuropathy with pain** are key to diagnosis.

Diagnostic Testing

- Best initial test: **ESR and markers of inflammation**
- Most accurate test: **Biopsy of sural nerve or the kidney**
- Test for **hepatitis B and C,** which can be associated with PAN.
- **Angiography showing "beading"** can spare the need for biopsy.

Treatment

The best initial therapy is **cyclophosphamide and steroids.**

IGA NEPHROPATHY (BERGER'S DISEASE)

This condition presents with **painless recurrent hematuria,** particularly in an **Asian patient** after a very **recent viral respiratory tract infection.** Proteinuria and red cells and red cell casts can be present in all forms of glomerular disease. There is *no* specific physical finding that clearly defines the disease.

Diagnostic Testing

- Best initial test: There is *no* specific blood test. IgA levels are sometimes elevated.
- Most accurate test: **Renal biopsy is essential,** because there is no blood test or specific physical findings to use in diagnosis. Complement levels are normal.

Treatment

There is *no* proven effective therapy to reverse IgA nephropathy.

- **Steroids** are used in boluses when there is a sudden worsening of proteinuria.
- **ACE inhibitors** are used as they are for all patients with proteinuria.
- **Fish oil** *may* have some effect in delaying progression.

HENOCH-SCHONLEIN PURPURA

This presents in an **adolescent or child** with the following symptoms:

- **Raised, nontender, purpuric skin lesions,** particularly on the buttocks
- **Abdominal pain**
- Possible **bleeding**
- **Joint pain**
- **Renal involvement**

Diagnostic Testing

- Best initial test: The presentation of GI, joint, skin, and renal involvement is the best indicator of Henoch-Schonlein purpura.
- Most accurate test: Although a biopsy is the most accurate test, showing deposition of IgA, it is *not* necessary.

Treatment

No specific therapy is necessary because Henoch-Schonlein purpura **resolves spontaneously** over time.

POST-STREPTOCOCCAL GLOMERULONEPHRITIS (PSGN)

PSGN results in dark urine, described as "tea colored" or "cola colored." **Periorbital edema** and **hypertension** also occur. Many other infections can lead to glomerulonephritis; both throat and skin infections can lead to PSGN.

Diagnostic Testing

- **Best initial test:** Antistreptolysin O (ASLO), anti-DNAse, antihyaluronidase in blood Complement levels are low.
- **Most accurate test:** Although **biopsy** is the most accurate test, it should *not* be done routinely, because the blood tests are most often sufficient. Biopsy shows subepithelial deposits of IgG and C3.

Treatment

- **Penicillin and other antibiotics** for the infection should be given, although they do *not* clearly reverse the disease.
- Control the hypertension and fluid overload with **diuretics.**

CRYOGLOBULINEMIA

This presents in a patient with a history of **hepatitis C with renal involvement.** The patient may have **joint pain and purpuric skin lesions.**

Diagnostic Testing

- Best initial test: **Serum cryoglobulin component levels** (immunoglobulins and light chains, IgM). Complement levels (especially C4) are low.
- Most accurate test: **Biopsy**

Treatment

Treat the hepatitis C with **interferon and ribavirin.**

LUPUS (SLE) NEPHRITIS

The patient presents with a history of SLE. Note that drug-induced lupus spares the kidney and brain.

Diagnostic Testing

- Best initial test: **ANA and anti-double-stranded DNA**

- Most accurate test: **Renal biopsy.** The biopsy in the case of lupus nephritis is very important. It is not to diagnose the presence of renal involvement but to **determine the extent of disease to guide therapy.**

Treatment

- **Sclerosis only:** *No* treatment. This is a "scar" of the kidney.
- **Mild disease, early stage, nonproliferative: Steroids**
- **Severe disease, advanced, proliferative: Mycophenolate mofetil and steroids.** Mycophenolate is superior to cyclophosphamide.

ALPORT'S SYNDROME

Alport's syndrome is a congenital problem with **eye and ear problems,** such as **deafness.**

There is *no* specific therapy.

THROMBOTIC THROMBOCYTOPENIC PURPURA (TTP) AND HEMOLYTIC UREMIC SYNDROME (HUS)

Look for a history of *E. coli* **0157:H7 for HUS.** There is no specific diagnostic test for these conditions.

HUS is a triad:

- **Intravascular hemolysis** (fragmented cells on smear)
- **Elevated creatinine**
- **Thrombocytopenia**

TTP has the same three findings *plus* the following:

- **Fever**
- **Neurological abnormalities**

Treatment is with plasmapheresis in severe cases.

Do *not* give platelets for hemolytic uremic syndrome or thrombotic thrombocytopenic purpura. They can make HUS and TTP worse. Also, do *not* give antibiotics for the infection; doing so may worsen the disease.

NEPHROTIC SYNDROME

Any of the glomerular diseases just described can lead to nephrotic syndrome if they are severe. Nephrotic syndrome is often a term of **severity of renal disease.**

- When the damage becomes severe enough, this leads to the **loss of more than 3.5 grams per day of protein in the urine.** When this happens, **albumin levels in the blood fall,** and there is also **edema.**

- **Hyperlipidemia** is a part of nephrotic syndrome. LDL and VLDL are removed from serum by lipoprotein signals. If the lipoprotein is lost in the urine with nephrotic syndrome, then the lipid levels in the blood rise.
- **Thrombosis** can occur because of the loss of antithrombin, protein C, and protein S in the urine.

Nephrotic syndrome is defined as follows:

- **Hyp*erproteinuria***
- **Hyp*oproteinemia***
- **Hyperlipidemia**
- **Edema**

DIAGNOSTIC TESTING

- Best initial test: **Urinalysis showing a markedly elevated protein level**
- The next best test is one of these:
  - **Spot urine for a protein-to-creatinine ratio > 3.5:1.** The spot urine protein creatinine level is equal in accuracy to a 24-hour urine collection.
  - **24-hour urine protein collection showing > 3.5 grams of protein**
- Most accurate test: **Renal biopsy**

OTHER PRIMARY RENAL DISORDERS

In addition to the glomerular diseases previously described with systemic manifestations and specific blood tests, there are several primary renal disorders with *no* specific physical findings to make a precise diagnosis. There are features in the history that are suggestive. The following table summarizes specific types of nephrotic syndromes and their associations.

Children	Adults, Cancer Such as Lymphoma	Hepatitis C	HIV, Heroin Use	Unclear
Minimal change disease	Membranous	Membranoproliferative	Focal segmental	Mesangial

DIAGNOSTIC TESTING

In all of these cases, testing is as follows:

- Best initial tests: **Urinalysis,** followed by **spot protein-to-creatinine ratio** or **24-hour urine**
- Most accurate test: Renal biopsy

TREATMENT

Treatment for all of these cases is as follows:

- Best initial therapy: **Steroids**
- If there is no response, such as a decrease in urine protein excretion after 12 weeks, **cyclophosphamide** is used.

PROTEINURIA

At any given time, from 2–10 percent of the population has mild proteinuria. The first step when this presents is always to **repeat the urinalysis.** Very often, the proteinuria disappears on repeat testing. These patients need no further follow up.

If proteinuria persists, you should see if the patient has a reason for transient mild proteinuria, such as the following:

- **CHF**
- **Fever**
- **Exercise**
- **Infection**

If these reasons are not present, the next possibility is **orthostatic proteinuria.** Look for a history of **a job in which people must stand all day,** such as waiters, teachers, security, and so on.

DIAGNOSTIC TESTING

1. The first step to confirm orthostatic proteinuria is to **split the urine.** Do a morning urine for protein and then one in the afternoon. If protein is present in the afternoon and not in the morning, then the patient likely has orthostatic proteinuria. Orthostatic proteinuria does *not* need to be treated.
2. If proteinuria is persistent and not orthostatic, a **24-hour urine** or **spot protein/creatinine ratio** is necessary.
3. If this is elevated, a renal biopsy should be performed.

Steps for proteinuria evaluation:

1. Repeat the UA.
2. Evaluate for orthostatic proteinuria.
3. Get a protein/creatinine ratio.
4. Perform a renal biopsy.

END-STAGE RENAL DISEASE

When is dialysis indicated?

Dialysis is essential with renal failure in the following circumstances:
- *Hyperkalemia*
- *Metabolic acidosis*
- *Uremia with encephalopathy*
- *Fluid overload*
- *Uremia with pericarditis*
- *No renal failure, but patient has toxicity with dialysable drug, such as lithium, ethylene glycol, or aspirin.*

The following table summarizes other manifestations of uremia and their treatment.

Hyperphosphatemia	Calcium acetate, calcium carbonate phosphate binders
Hypermagnesemia	Dietary magnesium restriction
Anemia	Erythropoietin replacement
Hypocalcemia	Vitamin D replacement

HYPERNATREMIA

Elevated serum sodium always implies a free water deficit. Dehydration is treated with **normal saline replacement** at first. Step 3 does *not* require knowledge of specific dosing. However, fluids should be first ordered as a bolus, then given continuously.

Besides **simple dehydration,** which can occur from poor oral intake, fever, pneumonia, or other types of increased insensible losses, the other main cause is **diabetes insipidus (DI).** Diabetes insipidus can be either from

- **failure to produce antidiuretic hormone (ADH) in the brain (central);** or
- **insensitivity of the kidney (nephrogenic).** Nephrogenic DI can be from hypokalemia or hypercalcemia or lithium toxicity.

Hypernatremia leads to **neurological abnormalities,** such as confusion, disorientation, or seizures. Sodium disorders do not cause cardiac rhythm disturbance. The worst manifestation is a **coma.**

DIAGNOSTIC TESTING

Both central and nephrogenic DI give the following results:

- **Low urine osmolality**
- **Low urine sodium**

- **Increased urine volume**
- *No* change in urine osmolality with water deprivation

The following table summarizes specific diagnostic tests and treatment for central DI and nephrogenic DI.

Central DI	Nephrogenic DI
Prompt **decrease** in urine volume with administration of vasopressin (DDAVP)	**No change** in urine volume with DDAVP
Prompt **increase** in urine osmolality with DDAVP	**No change** in urine osmolality with DDAVP
Treat with **DDAVP** or **vasopressin**	**Correct underlying cause**, such as hypokalemia or hypercalcemia. **Thiazide diuretics** are used in other cases.

HYPONATREMIA

Hyponatremia presents with **neurological abnormalities, such as confusion, disorientation, seizures, or coma.** There will be *neither* edema *nor* signs of dehydration.

The first step in the management of hyponatremia is to **assess volume status** to determine the cause and, therefore, the treatment.

HYPERVOLEMIC HYPONATREMIA

Hypervolemic causes of hyponatremia are the following:

- **Congestive heart failure (CHF)**
- **Nephrotic syndrome**
- **Cirrhosis**

These are managed by correcting/managing the underlying cause.

HYPOVOLEMIC HYPONATREMIA

Hypovolemic causes of hyponatremia are the following:

- **Diuretics**
- **GI loss of fluids (vomiting, diarrhea)**
- **Skin loss of fluids (burns, sweating)**

The diuretic, sweating, or other cause makes the patient lose water and a little salt, but the patient replaces free water only. Over time the sodium level drops.

Correct the underlying cause and replace with normal (isotonic) saline.
Remember to check serum sodium frequently.

Addison's Disease

Addison's disease also causes hyponatremia from **insufficient aldosterone production.** The key to this diagnosis is the presence of hyponatremia with **hyperkalemia and mild metabolic acidosis.** Treat with **aldosterone replacement, such as fludrocortisone.**

EUVOLEMIC (NORMAL) VOLUME STATUS

This can be caused by the following:

- **Inappropriate ADH release (SIADH)**
- **Hypothyroidism**
- **Psychogenic polydipsia**

SIADH

SIADH can be caused by the following:

- Any **CNS**
- Any **lung disease**
- Medications such as **sulfonylureas or SSRIs**
- **Cancer**

SIADH is associated with the following:

- Inappropriately **high urine sodium** (> 20 meq/L)
- Inappropiately **high urine osmolality** (> 100 mOsm/L)
- **Low serum osmolality** (< 290 mOsm/kg)
- **Low serum uric acid**
- Normal BUN, creatinine, and bicarbonate

TREATMENT

Mild Hyponatremia (no symptoms)
Treat by restricting fluids.

Moderate to Severe Hyponatremia (confused, seizures)
Treat as follows:

- **Saline infusion** with loop diuretics
- **Hypertonic (3 percent) saline**
- **Check serum sodium frequently**

Do not correct serum sodium more than 10–12 meq/L in the first 24 hours or more than 18 meq/L in the first 48 hours. Otherwise, you run the risk of **central pontine myelinosis.**

Chronic SIADH (as from malignancy)
Demeclocycline blocks the effect of ADH at the kidney.

HYPERKALEMIA

Hyperkalemia is predominantly caused by **increased potassium release from tissues, such as muscles, or red blood cells, such as in rhabdomyolysis or hemolysis.** Increased dietary potassium can *only* cause hyperkalemia if it is associated with renal insufficiency. If kidney function is normal, it is almost impossible to ingest potassium faster than the kidney can excrete it. Also, the GI tract is not able to absorb potassium faster than the kidney can excrete it. Aldosterone normally functions to excrete potassium from the body. If there is a **deficiency or blockade of aldosterone,** potassium levels will rise.

Other causes of hyperkalemia are the following:

- **Metabolic acidosis** from transcellular shift out of the cells
- **Adrenal aldosterone deficiency,** such as from Addison's disease
- **Beta blockers**
- **Digoxin toxicity**
- **Insulin deficiency,** such as from diabetic ketoacidosis (DKA)
- **Diuretics,** such as spironolactone
- **ACE inhibitors and angiotensin receptor blockers** by their effect on inhibiting aldosterone
- **Prolonged immobility, seizures, rhabdomyolysis, or crush injury**
- **Type IV renal tubular acidosis,** resulting from decreased aldosterone effect
- **Renal failure,** preventing potassium excretion

> **Pseudohyperkalemia** is an artifact caused by the hemolysis of red cells in the laboratory or prolonged tourniquet placement during phlebotomy. Pseudohyperkalemia does not need therapy; you need only repeat the test.

> Remember: First you get peaked T-waves, then you lose the p-wave, and then comes the widened QRS complex.

Hyperkalemia can lead to **cardiac arrhythmia.** Potassium disorders are not associated with seizures or neurological disorders.

Hyperkalemia Peaked T-Waves

TREATMENT

Severe Hyperkalemia (EKG abnormalities, such as peaked T-waves)

Treat as follows:

- Administer **calcium gluconate intravenously** to protect the heart.
- Follow with **insulin and glucose intravenously.**

Moderate Hyperkalemia (No EKG Abnormalities)

Treat as follows:

- Administer **insulin and glucose intravenously.**
- Use **bicarbonate** to shift potassium into the cell when acidosis is the cause of the hyperkalemia or there is rhabdomyolysis, hemolysis, or another reason to alkalinize the urine.
- **Kayexelate** (potassium-binding resin) is administered **orally** to remove potassium from the body. This takes several hours.

HYPOKALEMIA

Dietary insufficiency can lead to hypokalemia. Other causes are the following:

- Increased urinary loss from **diuretics**
- **High-aldosterone states, such as Conn's syndrome**
- **Vomiting** leads to metabolic alkalosis, which shifts potassium intracellularly, and volume depletion, which leads to increased aldosterone.
- **Proximal and distal renal tubular acidosis (RTA)**
- **Amphotericin** from the RTA it causes
- **Bartter's syndrome** is the inability of the loop of Henle to absorb sodium and chloride. It causes secondary hyperaldosteronism and renal potassium wasting.

Hypokalemia leads to **cardiac rhythm disturbance.** The EKG will show **"U-waves,"** which have an extra wave after the T-wave indicative of Purkinje fiber repolarization. Hypokalemia can also cause muscular weakness from its ability to inhibit contraction; this effect can be so severe that rhabdomyolysis occurs.

mm/mV   1 square = 0.04 sec/0.1mV

EKG-Normal Intervals

TREATMENT

Therapy is to **replace potassium.** There is no maximum rate on oral potassium replacement; the bowel will regulate the rate of absorption.

Avoid glucose-containing fluids in cases of hypokalemia. They will increase insulin release and worsen the hypokalemia.

> In hypokalemia cases, IV potassium replacement must be *slow* so as not to cause an arrhythmia with overly rapid administration.

MAGNESIUM DISORDERS

HYPERMAGNESEMIA

Hypermagnesemia is caused by the **overuse of magnesium-containing laxatives** or from **iatrogenic administration,** such as during premature labor when it is administered as a tocalytic. It is rare to have hypermagnesemia without renal insufficiency. Hypermagnesemia leads to **muscular weakness and loss of deep tendon reflexes.**

Treat hypermagnesemia as follows:

- **Restricting intake**
- **Saline administration** to provoke diuresis
- Occasionally **dialysis**

HYPOMAGNESEMIA

Hypomagnesemia is caused by the following:

- **Loop diuretics**
- **Alcohol withdrawal**
- **Gentamicin**
- **Cis-platin**

Hypomagnesemia presents with **hypocalcemia and cardiac arrhythmias.**

Magnesium is required for parathyroid hormone release. This is particularly important in the management of torsades de pointes.

METABOLIC ACIDOSIS

METABOLIC ACIDOSIS WITH AN INCREASED ANION GAP

This condition is caused by the following:

Lactic Acidosis

This is from any form of **hypoperfusion,** such as hypotension, resulting in **anaerobic metabolism.** Anerobic metabolism leads to glycolysis, which results in the accumulation of lactic acid.

Treat the underlying cause of hypotension.

Aspirin Overdose

Aspirin overdose originally gives **respiratory alkalosis from hyperventilation.** Over a short period, **metabolic acidosis** develops from poisoning of mitochondria and the loss of aerobic metabolism. This gives lactic acidosis.

Treat with **bicarbonate,** which corrects the acidosis and increases urinary excretion of aspirin.

Methanol Intoxication

This toxic alcohol leads to **formic acid and formaldehyde production.** Look for an **intoxicated patient with visual disturbance.**

After **getting a methanol level,** order **fomepizole** or **ethanol** administration. These substances block the production of formic acid and allow time for **dialysis** to remove the methanol.

Uremia

Renal failure prevents the excretion of the 1 meq per kg of organic acid that is formed each day.

This is an indication for dialysis.

Diabetic Ketoacidosis

Acetone, acetoacetate, and beta hydroxybutyric acid lead to an increased anion gap.

A **low serum bicarbonate** is the fastest single test to tell if a patient's hyperglycemia is life threatening. Treat with normal **saline hydration and insulin.** Place the patient in the **ICU.**

Isoniazid Toxicity

Just **stop the medication** and move the clock forward on CCS.

Ethylene Glycol

Look for an **intoxicated patient with a renal abnormality,** such as oxalate crystals in the urine. There is also renal failure and hypocalcemia, because the oxalate binds with calcium to form crystals. **Suicide attempt with ethylene glycol is key.**

Treat the same as methanol intoxication with **fomepizole** or **ethanol,** which blocks the production of oxalic acid and allows time for dialysis to remove the ethylene glycol.

METABOLIC ACIDOSIS WITH A NORMAL ANION GAP

This results from either **diarrhea** or **renal tubular acidosis (RTA).**

Diarrhea

Diarrhea causes metabolic acidosis via **increased bicarbonate loss from the colon.** The colon secretes both bicarbonate and potassium, so the potassium level will be low **(hypokalemia)** as well. Because there is increased chloride reabsorption, there is **hyperchloremia,** and that is why there is a normal anion gap.

Renal Tubular Acidosis (RTA)

- **Distal RTA (Type I):** There is an **inability to excrete acid of hydrogen ions in the distal tubule**. This results in the accumulation of acid in the body. The urine pH rises because the body cannot excrete acid. In an alkaline environment stones will form. **Serum potassium is low** (body excretes +-ions in the form of K since it can't excrete H+) and **serum bicarbonate is low**.

  - Test by **intravenously administering acid** (ammonium chloride—which should lower urine pH secondary to increased H+ formation). In Distal RTA the person cannot excrete the acid, and the urine pH stays abnormally basic.

  - Treat by administering **bicarbonate**. The proximal tubule is still working therefore the patient will still absorb the bicarbonate.

- **Proximal RTA (Type II):** There is an **inability to reabsorb bicarbonate in the proximal renal tubule**. Initially there is an elevated urine pH, but when the body loses substantial amounts of bicarbonate, the **urine pH drops**. Because urine pH is often low, kidney stones do *not* develop. A low serum bicarbonate leeches calcium out of the bones, and there is also **osteomalacia**.
  - Test by giving **bicarbonate**. A normal person with metabolic acisosis will absorb all of the bicarbonate, and there should still be a low urine pH in a normal patient. In proximal RTA, the patient cannot absorb the bicarbonate and the urine pH rises from the bicarbonate malabsorption.
  - Treat by giving a **thiazide diuretic**, which results in a volume contraction. The contracted blood volume raises the concentration of serum bicarbonate. Large quantities of serum bicarbonate are also given (Bicarbonate is generally ineffective and that is why they must be used in such high amounts).

- **Hyporeninemic hypoaldosteronism (Type IV):** There is **decreased aldosterone production or effect**. Look for a **diabetic patient with a normal anion gap metabolic acidosis**. This is the *only* RTA with an **elevated potassium level**.
  - Treat with **aldosterone** administration in the form of **fludrocortisone**, which is the steroid with the highest mineralocorticoid content.

The following table compares Types I, II, and IV RTA.

	Type I Distal RTA	Type II Proximal RTA	Type IV (Diabetes)
Urine pH	High	Low	Low
Serum Potassium	Low	Low	High
Stones	Yes	No	No
Test	Give Acid	Give Bicarbonate	Urine sodium loss
Treatment	Bicarbonate	Thiazide diuretic **High dose** bicarbonate	Fludrocortisone

Urine Anion Gap (UAG)

The UAG is the way to **distinguish between diarrhea and RTA** as the cause of the normal anion gap metabolic acidosis.

- UAG = Urine Na^+ – Urine Cl^-

When acid is excreted from the kidney, it goes out as NH_4Cl. Acid excretion from the kidney goes out with chloride.

If you *can* excrete acid from the kidney, the urine chloride goes up. If the urine chloride is up, then the number (UAG) is negative. **Diarrhea causes a negative UAG**, because the kidney can excrete acid and the net UAG is negative. In metabolic acidosis, a **negative UAG means the kidney works.**

If you *cannot* excrete acid from the kidney, the urine chloride goes down. This gives a positive number (UAG). **In RTA, you cannot excrete acid from the kidney.** The urine chloride will be low, and the **UAG will be positive.**

METABOLIC ALKALOSIS

VOLUME CONTRACTION

Volume contraction leads to metabolic alkalosis because there is a **secondary hyperaldosteronism,** which causes increased urinary loss of acid.

Treat the underlying cause.

CONN'S SYNDROME OR CUSHING'S SYNDROME

Hyperaldosteronism from primary hyperaldosteronism (Conn's syndrome) or Cushing's syndrome causes urinary acid loss.

Surgically remove the adenoma. Also look for **hypokalemia,** which often accompanies the increased urinary acid loss.

HYPOKALEMIA

Hypokalemia causes metabolic alkalosis, because **potassium ions shift out of the cell** to correct the hypokalemia. This shifts hydrogen ions into the cell in exchange for the potassium ions leaving.

MILK-ALKALI SYNDROME

Metabolic alkalosis occurs from the administration of **too much liquid antacid.**

VOMITING

Vomiting causes a **loss of acid from the stomach.** In addition, the loss of fluids leads to **volume contraction** and secondary hyperaldosteronism.

CYSTIC DISEASE

Cystic disease presents with **recurrent hematuria, stones, and infections.** There are **cysts throughout the body,** such as in the liver, ovaries, and circle of Willis; **mitral valve prolapse; and diverticulosis.** The most common site of extrarenal cysts is the **liver.** The most common cause of death is **end-stage renal disease.**

There is *no* specific therapy.

Subarrhachnoid hemorrhage is *not* the most common cause of death in cystic disease.

INCONTINENCE

The following table summarizes the presentation, diagnosis, and treatment of incontinence.

	Urge Incontinence	**Stress Incontinence**
Presentation	Pain followed by urge to urinate	No pain
	No relationship to coughing, laughing, or straining	Brought on by coughing and laughing
Testing	Urodynamic pressure monitoring	Observe leakage with coughing

Treatment	• Behavior modification
	• Anticholinergic medications
	  - Tolterodine
	  - Trospium
	  - Darifenacin
	  - Solifenacin
	  - Oxybutynin
		• Kegel exercises
		• Estrogen cream

HYPERTENSION

A man comes to the office for a routine visit. He is found to have a blood pressure of 145/95. What is the next best step in management?

Answer: Repeat the blood pressure measurement in 1–2 weeks.

The first step when a case of hypertension presents is to **repeat the blood pressure measurement.** It may take from 3 to 6 measurements to get an accurate assessment of blood pressure.

Routine tests for hypertension cases on CCS are the following:

- **Urinalysis**
- **EKG**
- **Eye exam** for retinopathy
- **Cardiac exam** for murmur and S4 gallop

TREATMENT

If the blood pressure is repeatedly abnormal, initiate lifestyle modifications such as these:

- **Sodium restriction**
- **Weight loss**
- **Dietary modification**
- **Exercise**
- **Relaxation techniques**

What is the most effective lifestyle modification for hypertension?

*Answer: **Weight loss***

If lifestyle modifications have no effect over 3–6 months, initiate medical therapy:

- Use a **thiazide diuretic,** such as **hydrochlorothiazide** or **chlorthalidone.**
- In **diabetics,** however, use **ACE/ARB** as the first-line therapy.

About 70 percent of patients will be controlled with a diuretic alone. If pressure control is not achieved with a diuretic alone, add a second drug:

- **Beta blocker** (atenolol, metoprolol)
- **ACE inhibitor**
- **Angiotensin receptor blocker (ARB)**
- **Calcium channel blocker (CCB)**

From 90–95 percent of patients should achieve control with the use of two medications. If two drugs do not work, **add a third drug and investigate for causes of secondary hypertension.**

Compelling Indications for Specific Medications

If any of the conditions in the following table are present, do not start with a diuretic. Go straight to the specific medication.

Condition	Medication
Coronary artery disease	Beta blocker
Congestive heart failure	Beta blocker, ACE, or ARB
Migraine	Beta blocker, CCB
Hyperthyroidism	Beta blocker
Osteoporosis	Thiazide
Depression	*No* beta blockers
Asthma	*No* beta blockers
Pregnancy	Alpha methyldopa
BPH	Alpha blockers
Diabetes	ACE/ARB

SECONDARY HYPERTENSION

Investigate for secondary hypertension if you see the following:

- Young (< 30) or old (> 60) patient
- Failure to control pressure with two medications

• Specific findings in the history or physical (see table below)

Specific Findings in the History or Physical

Condition	Medication
Closure of renal artery (stenosis)	Bruit
Pheochromocytoma	Episodic hypertension
Conn's syndrome	Hypokalemia
Cushing's syndrome	Buffalo hump, truncal obesity, striae
Coarctation of the aorta	Upper extremity > lower extremity pressure
Congenital adrenal hyperplasia	Hirsuitism

RENAL ARTERY STENOSIS

Look for an **abnormal sound (bruit)** auscultated in the flanks or abdomen. **Hypokalemia** may be present.

Diagnostic Testing

• Best initial test: **Renal ultrasound with Dopplers**

• If a **small kidney** is seen, any of the following tests can be done next:

   - **Magnetic resonance angiography (MRA)**

   - **Duplex ultrasonogram**

   - **Nuclear renogram**

• Most accurate test: **Renal angiogram**

Treatment

Best initial therapy: **Renal artery angioplasty angioplasty and stenting**

Oncology

11

For Step 3 in oncology, the most important thing to know *by far* is the **screening tests.**

Which of the following screening tests lowers mortality the most?

a. Mammography above age 50
b. Mammography above age 40
c. Colonoscopy
d. Pap smear
e. Prostate-specific antigen (PSA)

*Answer: The correct answer is **A.** Mammography above age 50 lowers mortality the most. Although **screening should start at the age of 40**, the mortality benefit is greatest above the age of 50, because the number of cases of cancer detected will be greater above the age of 50.*

BREAST CANCER

Screening mammography should be done as follows:

- Age 40: Begins
- Ages 40–50: Every 1–2 years
- Ages 50+: Every year

When a mammogram shows an abnormality, it should be followed up by a **biopsy.** The biopsy will both show the cancer, if present, and allow testing for the presence of **estrogen and progesterone receptors.**

SENTINEL NODE BIOPSY

This is the *first* node detected in the operative field. A dye or tracer is placed into the operative field. The first node it goes to is biopsied. This is the "sentinel node."

- If this node is free of cancer, then an axillary node dissection is *not* necessary.
- If the node *does* have cancer, then an axillary lymph node dissection is performed.

BEST INITIAL THERAPY FOR BREAST CANCER

Lumpectomy with radiation treatment of the site at the breast is equal to modified radical mastectomy.

A 42-year-old woman has a 2 cm breast cancer removed by lumpectomy, and the breast is irradiated. The cancer is negative for estrogen receptors and positive for progesterone receptors. Three of 14 nodes removed from the axilla are positive for cancer. What is the next best step in management?

a. Adjuvant chemotherapy and radiation of the axilla
b. Tamoxifen for 5 years
c. Anastrazole (aromatase inhibitor) for 5 years
d. Tamoxifen, adjuvant chemotherapy, and radiation of the axilla
e. Oophorectomy and chemotherapy

*Answer: The correct answer is **D**. Tamoxifen is used whenever there are either estrogen receptors or progesterone receptors positive. If both receptors are positive, tamoxifen will be of greater benefit. Adjuvant chemotherapy is used whenever the axillary nodes are positive or the cancer is > 1 cm in size.*

HORMONAL INHIBITION THERAPY

Tamoxifen or **raloxifene** is used if *either* the estrogen or progesterone receptors are positive. The response is greater if both are positive. Following are the adverse effects of tamoxifen:

- **Deep venous thrombosis (DVT)**
- **Hot flashes**
- **Endometrial cancer**

Aromatase inhibitors are pure estrogen antagonists. They do *not* have the selective estrogen receptor agonist (stimulatory) activity that Tamoxifen does. Aromatase inhibitors (anastrazole, letrozole, exemestane) do *not* lead to DVT, but they can lead to **osteoporosis,** because they are antagonistic to estrogen receptors in the bone.

ADJUVANT CHEMOTHERAPY

Adjuvant chemotherapy is appropriate under the following circumstances:

- Cancer is in the **axilla.**
- Cancer is **larger than 1 cm.**
- It is *more* efficacious when the **patient is still menstruating.** Breast cancer in menstruating women will not likely be controlled with estrogen antagonists, such as tamoxifen or aromatase inhibitors.

TRASTUZUMAB

- A monoclonal antibody against the breast cancer antigen **HER-2/NEU**
- Useful in metastatic disease
- Modest efficacy with few adverse effects

PRIMARY PREVENTIVE THERAPY

Tamoxifen should be used in any patient with **multiple first-degree relatives** (mother, sister) with breast cancer.

BCRA

BRCA genetic testing is *not* a routine screening test. All we can say for sure about BRCA is the following:

- BRCA is associated with an **increased risk of familial breast cancer.**
- BRCA is associated with an **increased risk of ovarian cancer.**

COLON CANCER

The most important knowledge to have is the **screening** schedule and indicators. Colon cancer is treated with **surgical resection of the colon** and **chemotherapy** centered around a **5-fluorouracil** regimen.

The table below shows the recommended screening for colon cancer.

Routine	Single Family Member with Colon Cancer	Three Family Members, Two Generations, One Premature (< 50)	Familial Adenomatous Polyposis	Juvenile Polyposis, Peutz-Jeghers, Turcot's Syndrome, Gardner's Syndrome
• Colonoscopy starting at age 50, then every 10 years • Sigmoidoscopy every 3–5 years • Occult blood testing starting at age 50, then yearly • Double contrast barium enema at age 50, then every 3–5 years	Colonoscopy at age 40, then every 10 years; or first colonscopy 10 years earlier than the earliest age at which a family member was diagnosed with colon cancer, whichever is earlier	Colonoscopy at age 25, then every 10 years	Screening sigmoidscopy at age 12, then every 1–2 years	No additional screening

There is *no* screening test for lung cancer. Routine chest X-rays yearly and CT scanning have *not* been shown to be beneficial (to lower mortality); those answers are wrong.

LUNG CANCER

A 52-year-old smoker has a 1.5 cm calcified nodule found on chest X-ray done for other reasons. He has no symptoms. What should you do?

Answer: **Excisional biopsy** *should be done on solitary lung nodules in patients who are smokers with nodules > 1 cm in size. Age > 50 lends additional urgency to the need for biopsy. Even though calcification goes against malignancy, the age of the patient, size of the nodule, and history of smoking are more important.*

LUNG CANCER THERAPY

The most important issue in the treatment of lung cancer is whether the **disease is localized enough to be surgically resectable.** Surgery *cannot* be performed if any of the following are present:

- Bilateral disease
- Metastases
- Malignant pleural effusion
- Involvement of the aorta, vena cava, or heart
- Lesions within 1–2 cm of the carina

Small-cell cancer is nonresectable because one of these features is present in > 95 percent of cases.

The size of the lesion alone is *not* the reason a cancer may be unresectable. If the lesion is large but is peripheral, without metastases, it can be resected.

CERVICAL CANCER

Follow up abnormal Pap smears as follows:

1. Abnormal Pap smears with low-grade or high-grade dysplasia should be followed by colposcopy and biopsy.
2a. If the Pap smear shows atypical squamous cells of undetermined significance (ASCUS), the patient should undergo HPV testing.
2b. If the patient is HPV-positive, then proceed to colopscopy; otherwise, repeat the Pap smear in 6 months.
2c. Return to routine screening if the repeat Pap smear is normal.

Pap smears lower mortality in screen populations but not as much as mammography, because the incidence of cervical cancer is much less than that of breast cancer.

> - Start Pap smears at age 21 or 3 years after the onset of sexual activity.
> - Frequency should be every 3 years until age 65. Stop at age 65, unless there has been no previous screening.
> - Administer HPV quadrivalent vaccine (Gardasil®) to all women ages 13–26.

PROSTATE CANCER

Prostate-specific antigen (PSA) and digital rectal exam are not proven to lower mortality from prostate cancer. The area of prostate cancer screening is controversial.

> There is *no* proven screening method that lowers mortality for prostate cancer.

A 65-year-old man comes to you requesting screening for prostate cancer. What should you do?

*Answer: Patients requesting screening for prostate cancer should undergo **PSA and digital rectal exam**. Though seemingly self-contradictory, the recommendation is that the physician should not "routinely offer" screening but, if requested, should perform it.*

DIAGNOSTIC TESTING

Besides the **spread of the disease,** the most important prognostic factor for prostate cancer is the **Gleason score.** The Gleason score is a measure of the level of differentiation of the histology. The higher the score, the more aggressive the cancer is.

TREATMENT

- **Localized prostate cancer: Surgery** and either **external radiation** or **implanted radioactive pellets** are nearly *equal* in efficacy.
- **Metastatic prostate cancer: Androgen blockade** is the standard of care: use **flutamide (testosterone receptor blocker) and leuprolide** *or* **goserelin (gonadotropin-releasing hormone [GNRH] agonists).** There is no particularly good chemotherapy for metastatic prostate cancer. The treatments are hormonal in nature.

Do *not* confuse therapies for prostate cancer with the 5 alpha-reductase inhibitor finasteride. Finasteride treats benign prostatic hypertrophy and male pattern hair loss—not prostate cancer.

What is the fastest way to lower androgen/testosterone levels?

Answer: **Orchiectomy.** *We did* not *say to do it, but this is the fastest way.*

A man with prostate cancer presents with severe, sudden back pain. His MRI shows cord compression, and he is started on steroids. What is the next best step in management?

a. Flutamide

b. Flutamide and leuprolide simultaneously

c. Leuprolide followed by flutamide

d. Ketoconazole

Answer: The correct answer is **A.** *Flutamide should be started first to block the temporary flare up in androgen levels that accompanies GNRH agonist treatments. When cord compression is described, GNRH agonists, if used too soon, can worsen the compression. Ketoconazole, at a high dose, blocks the production of androgens, but it is not as effective as the other therapies.*

Ovarian Cancer

Look for a woman > 50 with **increasing abdominal girth** at the same time as **weight loss.**

DIAGNOSTIC TESTING

There is *no* routine screening test for ovarian cancer. **CA125** is a marker of progression and response to therapy for ovarian cancer, *not* a diagnostic test.

TREATMENT

Treatment is **surgical debulking** followed by **chemotherapy,** even in cases of extensive local metastatic disease. Ovarian cancer is unique in that surgical resection is beneficial even when **there is a large volume of tumor spread through the pelvis and abdomen.** Removing all visible tumor still helps.

TESTICULAR CANCER

Presents with a painless **scrotal lump** in a man under 35.

DIAGNOSTIC TESTING

Do *not* do a needle biopsy of the testicle. Simply perform **inguinal orchiectomy** of the affected testicle.

Of all testicular cancers, 95 percent are **germ cell tumors (seminoma** and **nonseminoma).** Alpha fetoprotein (AFP) is secreted *only* by nonseminomas. Measure **AFP, LDH, and** β**HGC.** Stage with a **CT scan of the abdomen and pelvis.**

TREATMENT

- **Local disease: Radiation**
- **Widespread disease: Chemotherapy.** Chemotherapy can cure even metastatic disease.

> Testicular cancer is **extremely curable** with a 90–95 percent 5-year survival rate. It is *not* diagnosed by biopsy of the testicle: this is the wrong answer.

SECTION 2
PREVENTIVE MEDICINE

CANCER PREVENTION

The single most important oncology question on Step 3 is about prevention. While what you need to know in terms of volume is extremely small, it is very highly tested.

BREAST CANCER SCREENING

The cancer screening test that lowers mortality the most is the **mammogram.** The mortality benefit is greatest in patients > 50 years old, but the test should be started in all women > 40.

Routine breast self-examination has *no* proven benefit.

CERVICAL CANCER SCREENING

Cervical cancer screening with Pap smear also lowers mortality. The Pap smear should start at **age 21 or within three years of the onset of sexual activity,** whichever comes first. Pap smears should be done at least **every 3 years** until age 65, when they can be stopped.

COLON CANCER SCREENING

Colon cancer screening is started with a **colonoscopy at age 50** and is performed **every 10 years.**

Other forms of colon cancer screening, such as sigmoidoscopy, barium enema, or stool for fecal occult blood testing, are not as effective in detecting cancer. Virtual colonoscopy with CT scanning is not as accurate.

If a **close family member has had the disease** then screening should begin at 40 or 10 years earlier than the family member was diagnosed, whichever is earlier. **Hereditary nonpolyposis colon cancer syndrome (HNPCC),** known formerly as Lynch syndrome, is defined as colon cancer in 3 family members in 2 generations having the disease with 1 having it prematurely (defined as occurring before the age of 50). In this case, screening should begin at age 25 and be done every 1–2 years.

PROSTATE CANCER SCREENING

There is *no* recommendation to screen patients routinely for prostate cancer with either a prostate-specific antigen (PSA) or a digital rectal examination. There is specific evidence to recommend *against* the PSA for men > 75 on the basis that they will accrue the disadvantages of treatment, such as erectile dysfunction or incontinence, without any benefit.

Summary of Cancer Screening Guidelines	
Breast cancer	Mammography at age 40, then every 1–2 years
Colon cancer	Colonoscopy at age 50, then every 10 years
Cervical cancer	Pap smear at age 21 or within 3 years of first sexual activity, whichever is first, then every 3 years; stop at age 65 unless no previous screening

VACCINATIONS

INFLUENZA AND PNEUMOCOCCAL VACCINE

The indications for influenza vaccination and pneumococcal pneumonia vaccination have a lot of overlap:

- Patients with chronic lung, heart, liver, kidney, and cancer conditions
- HIV-positive patients
- Patients on steroids
- Patients with diabetes

Influenza vaccine is *different* from pneumococcal vaccine in that it is indicated in the following persons:

- Everyone > 50
- Yearly
- Pregnant women
- Health care workers

Pneumococcal vaccine is *different* from influenza vaccine in that it is indicated in the following persons:

- Single injection in all patients > 65

MENINGOCOCCAL VACCINATION

Meningococcal vaccination is now routine at **age 11.** Children at especially high risk who should be vaccinated even earlier are those with **functional or anatomic asplenia** or those with **terminal complement deficiency.**

HPV VACCINATION

Vaccine is a quadrivalent vaccine that should be administered to **all females between 13 and 26.** Studies are looking at the benefits of administering the vaccine to women outside this age range, but currently the guideline is ages 13–26.

SMOKING CESSATION

All patients should be screened for tobacco use and advised against it. The most effective method of achieving smoking cessation is the use of **oral medication, such as bupropion and varenicline.** Less effective therapies that can be tried first are **nicotine patches and gums.**

OSTEOPOROSIS

All women should be screened with bone densitometry at age 65.

ABDOMINAL AORTIC ANEURYSM

All men about **age 65** who were **ever smokers** should be screened once with an ultrasound.

DIABETES

There is *no* recommendation to screen patients routinely for diabetes.

HYPERTENSION

All patients should have their blood pressure checked at every office visit.

HYPERLIPIDEMIA

Men > 35 and women > 45 should be screened for hyperlipidemia.

BULLOUS AND BLISTERING DISEASES

PEMPHIGUS VULGARIS

This is an **autoimmune disease** of unclear etiology in which the body becomes, essentially, allergic to its own skin. Antibodies are produced against antigens **in the intercellular spaces of the epidermal cells.** Its causes are as follows:

- Idiopathic
- ACE inhibitors
- Penicillamine

Pemphigus vulgaris acts like a burn, because the bullae occur from destruction *within* the epidermis and so are **relatively thin and fragile.**

Nikolsky's sign is present: Nikolsky's sign is the easy removal of skin by just a little pressure, with the examiner's finger pulling it off like a sheet. Note that Nikolsky's sign is present in pemphigus vulgaris, staphylococcal scalded skin syndrome, and toxic epidermal necrolysis.

The lesions of pemphigus vulgaris are **painful,** not pruritic.

Diagnostic Testing

The most accurate diagnostic test is a biopsy of the skin.

Treatment

Treatment is as follows:

- Use **glucocorticoids,** such as prednisone.
- When steroids are ineffective, use the following:
  - **Azathiaprine**

- **Mycophenolate**
- **Cyclophosphamide**

BULLOUS PEMPHIGOID

Pemphigoid can be drug induced by sulfa drugs and others.

The fracture of the skin causing the blisters is **relatively deep,** and the **bullae are thicker walled and much less likely to rupture** than the bullae of pemphigus vulgaris. Oral lesions are rare. Because the bullae are tense and intact, the skin is better protected. There is no dressing for skin as good as the skin. Hence, there is much less fluid loss and infection is much less likely as compared with pemphigus vulgaris. Mortality is much less likely in bullous pemphigoid.

Diagnostic Testing

Test for bullous pemphigoid by performing a **biopsy with immunofluorescent antibodies.**

Treatment

Treatment is as follows:

- Use **systemic steroids,** such as prednisone.
- Alternatives to steroids:
  - **Tetracycline**
  - **Erythromycin with nicotinamide**

The following table compares pemphigus vulgaris and bullous pemphigoid.

	Pemphigus Vulgaris	**Bullous Pemphigoid**
Age range	30s and 40s	70s and 80s
Severity	Life-threatening	Resolves
Bullae	Thin and fragile	Thick and intact
Mouth involved	Yes	No
Other features	Nikolsky's sign	

PEMPHIGUS FOLIACEUS

This blistering disease is associated with **other autoimmune diseases,** or it can be **drug induced from ACE inhibitors or NSAIDs.** Foliaceus is much more superficial than pemphigus vulgaris and bullous pemphigoid, and intact bullae are not seen because they break so easily. There are no oral lesions.

Foliaceus is **diagnosed by biopsy** and **treated with steroids** in the same fashion as pemphigus vulgaris.

PORPHYRIA CUTANEA TARDA (PCT)

This is a disorder of porphyrin metabolism resulting in a **photosensitivity reaction** to an **abnormally high accumulation of porphyrins.**

The following are associated with PCT:

- Alcoholism
- Liver disease
- Chronic hepatitis C
- Oral contraceptives
- Liver disease, such as chronic hepatitis or hemochromatosis PCT, is associated with increased liver iron stores.
- Diabetes is found in 25 percent of patients.

PCT presents with the following:

- **Nonhealing blisters on the sun-exposed parts of the body,** such as the backs of the hands and the face
- **Hyperpigmentation of the skin**
- **Hypertrichosis of the face**

Diagnostic Testing

Test for **urinary uroporhyrins.** Uroporphyrins are elevated 2–5 times above the coproporphyrins in this disease.

Treatment

Manage this disease as follows:

- **Stop drinking alcohol.**
- **Stop all estrogen use.**
- **Use barrier sun protection.**
- **Use phlebotomy** to remove iron. **Deferoxamine** is used to remove iron if phlebotomy is not possible.
- **Chloroquine** increases the excretion of porphyrins.

DRUG ERUPTIONS/HYPERSENSITIVITY

Urticaria

Acute urticaria is a **hypersensitivity reaction,** most often **mediated by IgE and mast cell activation,** which results in **evanescent wheals and hives.** It is a type of localized, cutaneous anaphylaxis but without hypotension and hemodynamic instability. The onset of the wheals and hives is usually within 30 minutes and lasts for < 24 hours. **Itching** is prominent.

The most common causes are the following:

- **Medications** (aspirin, NSAIDs, morphine, codeine, penicillins, phenytoin, and quinolones)
- **Insect bites**
- **Foods** (peanuts, shellfish, tomatoes, and strawberries)
- **Emotions** (occasionally)
- **Contact with latex** (in any form)

Chronic urticaria is associated with the following:

- **Pressure on the skin:** Pressure on the skin resulting in localized urticaria is also known as **dermatographism.**
- **Cold**
- **Vibration**

Treat urticaria with the following:

- **H1 antihistamines:** Severe, acute urticaria is treated with older medications, such as **diphenhydramine** (benadryl), **hydroxyzine** (atarax), or **cyproheptadine.**
- For **life-threatening** reactions, add **systemic steroids.**
- **Chronic therapy:** Treat with newer, nonsedating antihistamines, such as **loratadine, desloratadine, fexofenadine,** or **cetirizine.**
- **Desensitization** is the answer when the **trigger cannot be avoided.** An example of this is a bee sting in a person who is a farmer. Beta blocker medications *must* be stopped prior to desensitization, because they inhibit the epinephrine that may be used if there is an anaphylactic *re*action.

Morbilliform Rashes

Morbilliform rash is a milder version of a hypersensitivity reaction than urticaria. This is the **"typical" type of drug reaction** and is usually secondary to medications to which the patient is allergic, such as penicillin, sulfa, allopurinol, or phenytoin. The rash **resembles measles; it is a generalized maculopapular eruption that blanches with pressure.** The reaction can appear a few days after the exposure and may begin even after the medication has been stopped.

Morbilliform rash is lymphocyte mediated and is treated with **antihistamines.** Steroids are rarely necessary.

Erythema Multiforme (EM)

Erythema multiforme is caused by the following:

- **Penicillins**
- **Phenytoin**
- **NSAIDs**
- **Sulfa drugs**
- **Infection with *Herpes simplex* or *Mycoplasma***

This condition presents with **targetlike lesions** that especially occur on the **palms and soles.** These lesions can also be described as "irislike." Bullae are not uniformly found. EM of this type usually does not involve mucous membranes.

Treatment is with **antihistamines** and **treatment of the underlying infection.**

Stevens-Johnson Syndrome (SJS)

It is sometimes difficult to distinguish SJS from toxic epidermal necrolysis (TEN), and, in fact, the two diseases may be considered as being on a spectrum of severity of the same disorder.

Disorders along this spectrum may arise as a **hypersensitivity response** to the same set of medications, such as **penicillins, sulfa drugs, NSAIDs, phenytoin, and phenobarbital.** SJS usually involves < 10–15 percent of the total body surface area, and the overall mortality is < 5–10 percent. There is **mucous membrane involvement,** most often of the oral cavity and the conjunctivae, although there may be extensive involvement of the respiratory tract. **Respiratory tract involvement may be so severe as to require mechanical ventilation.** These patients should be managed **in a burn unit.** Death occurs from a combination of infection, dehydration, and malnutrition.

Steroids have *no* proven benefit. Other therapies of unclear value are intravenous immunoglobulins, cyclophosphamide, cyclosporine, and thalidomide.

Toxic Epidermal Necrolysis (TEN)

TEN is the **most serious version** of cutaneous hypersensitivity reaction.

- Much more of the body surface area (BSA) is involved, up to 30–100 percent.
- Mortality may be as high as 40–50 percent.

Nikolsky's sign is present, and the **skin easily sloughs off.** TEN has certain similar features to staphylococcal scalded skin syndrome. However, TEN is drug induced as opposed to being caused by a toxin coming from an organism. Sepsis is the most common cause of death, but prophylactic systemic antibiotics are *not* indicated.

Diagnosis is with a **skin biopsy.** Systemic steroids are *not* an effective treatment and may, in fact, decrease chances of survival.

Fixed Drug Reaction

This is a **localized allergic drug reaction** that recurs at precisely the same anatomic site on the skin with repeated drug exposure. Fixed drug reactions are generally **round, sharply demarcated lesions that leave a hyperpigmented spot at the site** after they resolve.

Fixed drug reactions can be treated with **topical steroids.**

Erythema Nodosum

This condition presents as follows:

- Painful, red, raised nodules appear on the anterior surface of the lower extremities.
- Nodules are tender to palpation.
- Nodules do not ulcerate.
- Nodules last about 6 weeks.

Erythema nodosum is **secondary to recent infections or inflammatory conditions,** including the following:

- **Pregnancy**
- **Recent streptococcal infection**
- **Coccidioidomycoses**
- **Histoplasmosis**
- **Sarcoidosis**
- **Inflammatory bowel disease**
- **Syphilis**
- **Hepatitis**
- **Enteric infections,** such as *Yersinia*

Treatment is with **analgesics and NSAIDs** and by **treating the underlying disease.**

INFECTIONS

FUNGAL INFECTIONS

These are the following:

- **Tinea pedis**
- **Tinea cruris**
- **Tinea corporis**
- **Tinea versicolor**
- **Tinea capitis**
- **Onychomycosis**

Diagnostic Testing

- First, perform a **potassium hydroxide (KOH) test of the skin.** The leading edge of the lesion on the skin or nails is scraped with a scalpel to remove some of the epithelial cells or some of the nail and hair. KOH has the ability to dissolve the epithelial cells and collagen of the nail but does not have the ability to melt away the fungus.
- Most accurate test: The most accurate test is to **culture the fungus.** Molds that grow on the skin (dermatophytes) take up to 6 weeks to grow, even on specialized fungal media. A specific species usually does not need to be isolated in most cases, unless the infection is of the hair or nails.

Treatment

For onychomycosis (nail infection) or **hair infection** (tinea capitus), the medications with the greatest efficacy are **oral terbinafine or itraconazole.** These medications are used for 6 weeks for fingernails and 12 weeks for toes.

- **Terbinafine is potentially hepatotoxic,** and it is important to check liver function tests periodically.
- Griseofulvan must be used for 6–12 months and has much less antifungal efficacy than terbinafine.

All of the other fungal infections of the skin that don't involve the hair or nails may be treated with any of the following topical medications:

- **Ketoconazole**
- **Clotrimazole**
- **Econazole**
- **Terbinafine**
- **Miconazole**
- **Sertaconazole**
- **Sulconazole**
- **Tolnaftate**
- **Naftifine**

There is no clear difference in efficacy or adverse effects among them when they are used topically.

- When used systemically, **ketoconazole** has the following adverse effects: **hepatotoxicity and gynecomastia.** This is why ketoconazole is not a good choice for onychomycosis.
- There is no topical form of fluconazole. Fluconazole also has less efficacy for dermatophytes of the nails when used systemically.

BACTERIAL INFECTIONS

These include the following:

- **Impetigo**
- **Erysipelas**
- **Cellulitis**
- **Folliculitis**
- **Furuncles**
- **Carbuncles**
- **Necrotizing fasciitis**
- **Paronychia**

Treatment of Bacterial Skin Infections in General (Impetigo, Erysipelas, Cellulitis, Folliculitis, Furuncles, Carbuncles)

- **Dicloxacillin, cephalexin (Keflex), or cefadroxyl (Duricef)**
- The intravenous equivalent of dicloxacillin is **oxacillin or nafcillin.** The intravenous equivalent of cefadroxyl is **cefazolin.**
- If a patient is allergic to penicillin but the reaction is **only a rash,** then **cephalosporins** can be safely used. There is far less than 1 percent cross-reaction between penicillins and cephalosporins. (The cross-reactivity is actually estimated to be 0.1 percent).
- If the penicillin reaction is **anaphylaxis,** cephalosporins *cannot* be used. The alternative antibiotics that will treat the skin are **macrolides,** such as **erythromycin, azithromycin, and clarithromycin,** or the **newer fluoroquinolones levofloxacin, gatifloxacin,** or **moxifloxicin.**
  - Ciprofloxacin will *not* adequately cover the skin.
  - Vancomycin is *only* for intravenous use for skin infections. Oral vancomycin is not absorbed and is used only for *Clostridium difficile* intestinal infection.
- Consider using **IV vancomycin** if you suspect methicillin-resistant *Staphylococcus aureus* (MRSA), such as in a nursing home patient or a patient who has been in the hospital for a long time. The oral alternative would be **linezolid or bactrim.**

Impetigo

This is a **superficial bacterial infection** of the skin limited largely to the epidermis and not spreading below the dermal-epidermal junction. The infection is described as **"weeping," "oozing," "honey-colored," or "draining."** It occurs more often in **warm, humid conditions,** particularly when there is poverty and crowding of children. It is both contagious and autoinnocuable. Impetigo can cause glomerulonephritis, but it will not cause rheumatic fever.

Impetigo is more often caused by *Staphylococcus* but is sometimes caused by *Streptococcus pyogenes,* also known as group A *Streptococcus.*

Impetigo is treated as follows:

- Apply **topical antibiotics,** such as **mupirocin.**
- If topical antibiotics are not effective, then **antistaphylococcal oral antibiotics** should be used.

Erysipelas

Erysipelas involves both the dermis and epidermis and is most commonly caused by **group A *Streptococcus (pyogenes).*** Erysipelas is more likely than other bacteria infections to result in the following:

- Fever, chills, and bacteremia
- Bright red, angry, swollen appearance to the face

Treatment is as follows:

- **Use the systemic oral or intravenous antibiotics previously described.**
- If there is culture confirmation of the organism as *Streptococcus,* then **penicillin G** or ampicillin can be used.

Cellulitis

This is a bacterial infection of the dermis and subcutaneous tissues with *Staph* and *Strep.*

Cellulitis is treated with **the antibiotics previously described,** based on the severity of the disease. If there is **fever, hypotension, or signs of sepsis** or if **oral therapy has not been effective,** then the patient should receive intravenous therapy. **Oxacillin, nafcillin,** or **cefazolin** is the best therapy. Treatment is generally empiric, because injecting and aspirating sterile saline for a specific microbiological diagnosis has only a 20 percent sensitivity.

Folliculitis, Furuncles, and Carbuncles

These three disorders represent three different degrees of severity of **staphylococcal infection occurring around a hair follicle.** Occasionally, folliculitis can occur from *Pseudomonas* in those who contract it in a **whirlpool or hot tub.** As folliculitis worsens from a simple infection superficially around the hair follicle, it becomes a small collection of infected material known as a **furuncle.** When several furuncles become confluent into a single lesion, it becomes known as a **carbuncle,** essentially a localized skin abscess that must be drained. Folliculitis is rarely tender, while furuncles and carbuncles are often extremely tender.

Treatment is as follows:

- Folliculitis can be treated with **topical mupirocin.**
- Furuncles and carbuncles must be treated with **systemic antistaphylococcal antibiotics,** such as **dicloxacillin** or **cefadroxyl.**

Necrotizing Fasciitis

This is an **extremely severe, life-threatening infection** of the skin. It starts as a **cellulitis that dissects into the fascial planes of the skin.** *Streptococcus* and *Clostridia* are the most common organisms involved, because they are able to produce a toxin that further worsens the damage to the fascia. **Diabetes** increases the risk of developing fasciitis.

Necrotizing fasciitis presents as follows:

- **Very high fever**
- **Portal of entry into the skin**
- **Pain out of proportion to the superficial appearance**
- **Bullae**
- **Palpable crepitus**

The following diagnostic tests can be used:

- Elevated CPK
- X-ray, CT scan, or MRI that show air in the tissue or necrosis

All of these laboratory methods of establishing a diagnosis *lack both sensitivity and specificity.* **Surgical debridement** is both the best way to confirm the diagnosis, as well as being the mainstay of therapy. If presented with an obvious clinical case with **crepitus,** pain, high fever, and a portal of entry, you should answer surgery, *not* a test, such as X-ray, as the best initial step.

Treat with **beta lactam/beta lactamase combination medications:**

- **Ampicillin/sulbactam (Unasyn)**
- **Ticarcillin/clavulanate (Timentin)**
- **Piperacillin/tazobactam (Zosyn)**

If there is a definite diagnosis of **group A** *Streptococcus (pyogenes),* then the treatment is with **clindamycin and penicillin.**

Without adequate therapy, necrotizing fasciitis has an **80 percent mortality.**

Paronychia

This is an infection **loculated under the skin surrounding a nail.**

It is generally treated with a **small incision** to allow drainage and **antistaphylococcal antibiotics** as previously described.

VIRAL INFECTIONS

Herpes simplex

Herpes simplex infections of the **genitals** are characterized by **multiple, painful vesicles.** They are usually obvious by examination, and you should proceed directly to therapy with **acyclovir, famciclovir,** or **valacyclovir.**

Diagnostic testing, if needed, is as follows:

- Best initial test: In the event that the diagnosis is not clear or the lesions have become confluent into an ulcer, then the best initial test is a **Tzanck smear.** The Tzanck smear is somewhat nonspecific in that it will only determine that the infection is in the *Herpes* virus family. Tzanck smears detect multinucleated giant cells and are similar in technique to a Pap smear. A scraping of the lesion is immediately placed on a slide and sprayed with fixative.
- Most accurate test: **Viral culture.** This grows in 24–48 hours.
- The most common wrong answer is serology; serology is *not* a useful test for diagnosing acute *Herpes* infections.

Treat with the following:

- **Oral acyclovir, famciclovir, or valganciclovir**
- Topical acyclovir has extremely little efficacy.
- Topical penciclovir has some utility for oral herpetic lesions, but it must be used every 2 hours.
- The treatment of acyclovir-resistant *Herpes* is with **foscarnet.**

Herpes zoster/varicella

Chicken pox is primarily a disease of children. It is generally *not* treated with antivirals. *If* the child is immunocompromised or the primary infection occurs in an adult, then **acyclovir, valacyclovir, or famciclovir** should be given.

Complications of varicella are the following:

- **Pneumonia**
- **Hepatitis**
- **Dissemination**

Outbreaks of **shingles,** also known as **dermatomal *Herpes zoster,*** occur more frequently in the elderly and those with defects of the lymphocytic portion of the immune system, such as leukemia, lymphoma, or HIV, or those on steroids.

The vesicles are 2–3 mm in size at all stages of development and are on an erythematous base.

Although Tzanck prep and viral culture are the best initial and most accurate diagnostic tests, they are generally *not* necessary, because little else will produce a band of vesicles in a dermatomal distribution besides *Herpes zoster.*

Treat with the following:

- **Steroid** use is still not clearly beneficial, although the best evidence for its efficacy is in **elderly patients with severe pain.**
- The **rapid administration of acyclovir** still has the best efficacy for decreasing the risk of postherpetic neuralgia.
- Other treatments for managing the pain:
    - **Gabapentin:** The most effective analgesic specifically for postherpetic neuralgia is gabapentin.
    - **Tricyclic antidepressants**
    - **Topical capsaicin**
- **Nonimmune adults exposed to chicken pox** should receive *Varicella zoster immune globulin within 96 hours* of the exposure for it to be effective.

SEXUALLY TRANSMITTED DISEASES (STDs)

HUMAN PAPILLOMAVIRUS (HPV; WARTS) OR CONDYLOMATA ACCUMINATA

These conditions present as heaped up, translucent, white or flesh-colored lesions on mucous surfaces.

Diagnostic Testing

No form of testing is routinely necessary. Biopsy, scraping, smears, and serology are of *no* definite benefit. There is *no* benefit to routine subtyping of the specific strain of papillomavirus.

Treatment

- **Mechanical removal:** This can involve **cryotherapy** with liquid nitrogren, **laser removal,** or **trichloroacetic acid** or **podophyllin** to melt them away.
- **Imiquimod** is a local immunostimulant that takes several weeks to result in sloughing off of the wart. Resolution is slower; however, there is *never* any damage to the surround normal tissue and *no* pain.
- Podophyllin is potentially teratogenic and should be scrupulously avoided in pregnancy.

SYPHILIS

Both primary and secondary syphilis present mainly with **cutaneous disorders.**

Primary Syphilis

The chancre of primary syphilis is an **ulceration with heaped-up indurated edges** that is painless the majority of the time.

The best initial test is a **darkfield examination.** This is because there is a false negative rate of 25 percent for both the VDRL and RPR. In other words, these serologic tests need several weeks to become positive, and they are only 75 percent sensitive in primary syphilis.

Both primary and secondary syphilis are treated with a **single intramuscular dose of penicillin.** In those patients allergic to penicillin, **doxycycline orally for 2 weeks** is the alternative therapy.

Secondary Syphilis

Secondary syphilis presents with a generalized copper-colored, maculopapular rash that is particularly intense on the palms and soles of the feet. The other manifestations of secondary syphilis are predominantly dermatologic as well: the **mucous patch, alopecia areata, and condylomata lata.**

The **VDRL and RPR tests** have nearly 100 percent sensitivity in secondary syphilis.

As above, both primary and secondary syphilis are treated with a **single intramuscular dose of penicillin.** In those patients allergic to penicillin, **doxycycline orally for 2 weeks** is the alternative therapy.

SCABIES, PEDICULOSIS

SCABIES

Scabies involves primarily the **web spaces of the hands and feet,** as well as giving **pruritic lesions around the penis and breast. Itching** can be extreme in both cases. Because *Sarcoptes scabiei* is quite small, all that can be seen with the naked eye are the **burrows and excoriations around small pruritic vesicles.** Scabies often *spares* the head.

Immunocompromised patients, such as those with HIV, are particularly vulnerable to an extremely exuberant form of scabies with severe crusting known as *"Norwegian scabies."*

Diagnosis

Scabies is confirmed by **scraping out the organism after mineral oil is applied to a burrow.**

Treatment

Treatment is with **permethrin.** Lindane has equal efficacy but greater toxicity; thus, it is *not* the best initial therapy. Scabies, particularly Norwegian scabies, can be treated with **ivermectin orally.**

PEDICULOSIS (LICE AND CRABS)

Pediculosis **tends to include the head** and is **easily transmitted** by sharing hats and hairbrushes. Both organisms have an enormously high rate of transmission sexually with 90 percent transmission from a single contact. They are sometimes rust colored from their ingestion of blood.

Diagnosis

Because pediculosis is from a much larger organism, scraping is *not* necessary. The organisms can readily be **seen attached to hair-bearing areas,** particularly with magnification.

Treatment

* Permethrin

As for scabies, treatment is with **permethrin.** Lindane has equal efficacy but greater toxicity; thus, it is *not* the best initial therapy. Pediculosis can be treated with **over-the-counter pyrethins.**

LYME

More than 85 percent of patients who have Lyme disease develop a rash. The **rash must be erythematous with central clearing and be at least 5 centimeters in diameter.** It usually occurs 7–10 days after the tick bite.

This rash is so characteristic of Lyme that it is more important than serological testing in terms of confirming a diagnosis. If the rash is described, then go straight to therapy with **oral doxycycline, amoxicillin,** or **cefuroxime.** Without therapy,

* two-thirds of these patients will develop **joint disease.**
* a smaller number will develop **neurological or cardiac disorders.**

Toxin-Mediated Diseases

TOXIC SHOCK SYNDROME (TSS)

TSS is caused by *Staphylococcus* **attached to a foreign body.** Nasal packing, retained sutures, or any other form of surgical material retained in the body can promote the growth of the type of *Staph* that produces the toxin.

Diagnosis

Because there is no single specific test, cases are matters of definition. The definition of a case of toxic shock syndrome is as follows:

- **Fever > 102°F**
- **Systolic blood pressure < 90**
- **Desquamative rash**
- **Vomiting**
- **Involvement of the mucous membranes of the eye, mouth, and genitals**

In addition, toxic shock is a systemic disease that

- **raises the creatinine, CPK, and liver function tests;**
- **lowers the platelet count;** and
- can cause **central nervous system dysfunction,** such as confusion.

Treatment

Treatment is with the following:

- **Vigorous fluid resuscitation**
- **Pressors,** such as **dopamine**
- **Antistaphylococcal medications,** such as **oxacillin, nafcillin,** or **cefazolin**
- For methicillin- (oxacillin-) resistant strains, **vancomycin** or **linezolid** can be used.

STAPHYLOCOCCAL SCALDED SKIN SYNDROME (SSSS)

SSSS is mediated by a **toxin from *Staphylococcus*.** It presents with **loss of the superficial layers of the epidermis in sheets** and **Nikolsky's sign.** SSSS is different from other conditions in the following ways:

- SSSS is markedly different from toxic shock syndrome in that there is normal blood pressure and no involvement of the liver, kidney, bone marrow, or central nervous system.
- SSSS differs from TEN in that it is from an infection and not from drug toxicity. In addition, SSSS only splits off the superficial granular layer of skin and is not a full thickness split, such as in TEN.

This condition should be managed in a **burn unit.** Give **oxacillin/nafcillin** or other antistaphylococcal antibiotics.

ANTHRAX

Bacillus anthracis is usually a **cutaneous infection** acquired from **contact with infected livestock.** It is an occupational hazard of wool sorters. **Bioterrorism** is also a potential source. A papule appears that later becomes inflamed and develops **central necrosis that is black in color;** hence the name *anthrax,* which is the Greek word for "coal." Of untreated cases, 20 percent are fatal.

The diagnosis is confirmed with **gram stain and culture of the lesion. Ciprofloxacin** or **doxycycline** is the treatment.

MALIGNANT AND PREMALIGNANT DISEASES

BENIGN LESIONS

The predominant method of distinguishing between benign and malignant lesions is by the **shape and color of the lesion. Benign lesions,** such as the junctional or intradermal nevus, have the following characteristics:

- They do not grow in size.
- They have smooth, regular borders.
- Their diameter is usually < 1 cm.
- They are homogenous in color, and the color remains constant.

Biopsy is the most accurate method of making a diagnosis. Benign lesions only need to be removed for cosmetic purposes.

MELANOMA

These **malignant** lesions **grow in size, have irregular borders, are uneven in shape, and have inconsistent coloring.**

Biopsy diagnosis is best performed with a full thickness sample, because **tumor thickness** is by far the most important prognostic factor. Treatment of melanoma is by **excision. Interferon** seems to reduce the recurrence rates of melanoma.

SEBORRHEIC KERATOSIS

This is a **benign** condition with **hyperpigmented lesions occurring in the elderly with a "stuck on" appearance.** They are most common on the face, shoulders, chest, and back.

They are removed with **liquid nitrogen** or **curettage** *only* for cosmetic purposes and have *no* malignant potential. There is *no* relationship to either actinic keratosis or seborrheic dermatitis.

ACTINIC KERATOSIS

These are **precancerous** lesions occurring on **sun-exposed areas of the body in older persons.** They occur more often in those with light skin color. Although they are usually asymptomatic, they can be tender to the touch.

Therapy is universally with **sunscreen** to prevent their progression and recurrence. Lesions should be removed with **cryotherapy, topical 5 fluorouracil (5FU), imiquimod, topical retinoic acid derivatives,** or **even curettage.**

SQUAMOUS CELL CARCINOMA

Of all skin cancers, 10–25 percent are squamous cell. Squamous cell carcinoma develops on **sun-exposed skin surfaces in elderly patients.** It is particularly common on the lip, where the carcinogenic potential of tobacco is multiplicative. **Ulceration** of the lesion is common. Metastases are rare, with only 3–7 percent of patients developing them.

Diagnosis is with a **biopsy,** and the treatment is **surgical removal.**

BASAL CELL CARCINOMA

Of all skin cancers, 65–80 percent are basal cell. Basal cell carcinoma has a shiny or "pearly" appearance. The rate of metastases is < 0.1 percent.

The diagnosis is confirmed by **shave or punch biopsy.** Treatment is with **surgical removal. Moh's microsurgery** has the greatest cure rate. In this technique, instant frozen sections are done to determine when enough tissue has been removed to give a clean margin.

KAPOSI'S SARCOMA

These are **purplish lesions found on the skin predominantly of patients with HIV and CD4 counts < 100.** Human *Herpes* virus 8 is the causative organism.

The best therapy is to **start antiretroviral therapy and raise the CD4 count.** In those in whom this does not occur, the specific chemotherapy for Kaposi's sarcoma is **liposomal adriamycin and vinblastine.**

SCALING DISORDERS (ECZEMA)/ PAPULOSQUAMOUS DERMATITIS

PSORIASIS

Silvery scales develop on the extensor surfaces. Psoriasis can be local or enormously extensive. **Nail pitting** is a common accompaniment. A **Koebner phenomenon** is the development of lesions with epidermal injury.

Treatment

All patients should use **emollients,** such as eucerin, lubriderm, aquaphor, and Vaseline or mineral oil. **Salicylic acid** is used to remove heaped up collections of scaly material so the other therapies can make contact.

- If the disease is relatively localized, **topical steroids** are used.
- Severe disease also needs **coal tar** or **anthralin derivatives.**
- To avoid the long-term use of steroids, which can cause skin atrophy, and to avoid coal tars, which are messy, one can substitute **topical vitamin D and vitamin A derivatives.** The vitamin D derivative most frequently used is **calcipotriene. Tazarotene** is a topical vitamin A.

When > 30 percent of the body surface area is involved, it is difficult to use topical therapy routinely to control disease. These patients can be treated with **ultraviolet light.** This is the most rapid way to control extensive disease.

The most severe, widespread, and progressive forms of the disease can be controlled with **methotrexate.** However, this therapy has the highest toxicity and may cause **liver fibrosis.**

The newest therapies are **immunomodulatory biological agents,** such as **alefacept, efalizumab, etanercept, and infliximab.**

XEROSIS/ASTEATOTIC DERMATITIS

Xerosis and dry skin are managed with **humidifiers and emollients,** such as lubriderm, eucerin, Vaseline, dermasil, mineral oil, or lac-hydrin. In those who are especially inflamed, **topical steroids** can be used briefly.

ATOPIC DERMATITIS

This extraordinarily pruritic disorder presents with the following:

- **High IgE levels**
- **Red, itchy plaques of the flexor surfaces**

Treatment

- **Preventive therapy:** Keep the skin moist with emollients, avoid hot water and drying soaps, and use only cotton clothes, because these patients are extremely sensitive to drying.
- **Active disease** is managed with the following:
  - **Topical steroids**
  - **Antihistamines**
  - **Coal tars**
  - **Phototherapy**
  - **Antistaphylococcal antibiotics,** if there is impetiginization of the skin
  - **Topical immunosuppressants,** such as tacrolimus and pimecrolimus, can be used to decrease dependence on steroid use.
  - **Every effort has to be made to avoid scratching.** The topical tricyclic **doxepin** can be used to help stop pruritus.

SEBORRHEIC DERMATITIS

An **oversecretion of sebaceous material,** as well as a **hypersensitivity reaction to a superficial fungal organism, pityrosporum ovale,** underlies seborrheic dermatitis. These patients present with **"dandruff," which may also occur on the face.** Scaly, greasy, flaky skin is found on a red base on the scalp, around the eyebrows, and in the nasolabial fold.

Treatment

- **Low-potency topical steroids,** such as **hydrocortisone**
- **Topical antifungal,** such as **ketoconazole** or **selenium sulfide**
- **Zinc pyrithione** used as a shampoo

STASIS DERMATITIS

There is *no* way to reverse this problem. It occurs over a long period from **venous incompetence of the lower extremities** leading to the microscopic extravasation of blood in the dermis. It is a **hyperpigmentation** that is built up from hemosiderin in the tissue.

Prevention of progression is with **elevation of the legs and lower-extremity support hose.**

CONTACT DERMATITIS

This is a **hypersensitivity reaction to soaps, detergents, latex, sunscreens, or neomycin** over the area of contact. Jewelry is a frequent cause, as is contact with the metal nickel from belt buckle and wristwatches. It can present as **linear streaked vesicles,** particularly when it is from **poison ivy.**

A definitive diagnosis can be determined with **patch testing.**

Treatment is by properly **identifying the causative agent** and with **antihistamines and topical steroids.**

PITYRIASIS ROSEA

This is a **pruritic eruption** that begins with a **"herald patch"** 70–80 percent of the time. It is **erythematous and salmon colored** and looks like secondary syphilis, except that it spares the palms and soles, has a herald patch, and the VDRL/RPR is negative. The lesions on the back appear in a pattern like a Christmas tree if the observer is especially imaginative.

It is **mild and self-limited** and usually resolves in 8 weeks without scarring. Lesions that are very itchy may be treated with topical steroids.

ACNE

Pustules and cysts occur and rupture, releasing free fatty acids that cause further irritation. The contributing organism is *Propionibacterium acnes.* The discharge, although purulent, is odorless.

Treatment

Mild disease is treated with the following:

- **Topical antibiotics,** such as **clindamycin, erythromycin,** or **sulfacetamide.** In addition, the bacteriostatic agent **benzoyl peroxide** is used.
- **Topical retinoids** are used if these attempts to control the load of bacteria locally are ineffective.

Moderate disease is treated with the following:

- **Benzoyl peroxide,** combined with the retinoids **tazarotene, tretinoin, and adapalene.**

Severe cystic acne is treated with the following:

- **Oral antibiotics, such as minocycline, tetracycline, clindamycin, and isotretinoin:** Oral retinoic acid derivatives are **strong teratogens.** Check urine pregnancy test and make sure patients are on oral contraceptives if they are females of childbearing age.

Section 4
Surgery

Trauma

AIRWAY

Establishing and securing the airway is always the first step in management in any patient with acute trauma or change in mental status. **Altered mental status** is the most common indication for intubation in the trauma patient (unconscious patients can't maintain their airways). The exam will want you to know the *best* step in securing an airway.

- **Orotracheal intubation** is the preferred method of securing an airway.
- If the case describes **trauma with cervical spine injury,** orotracheal intubation can still be performed with manual cervical immobilization. The best answer is **the use of a flexible bronchoscope.**
- If the case describes **extensive facial trauma and bleeding into the airway** (listen for gurgling sounds), **cricothyroidotomy** is the best answer. **Percutaneous tracheostomy** is also acceptable.

BREATHING

Always check the oxygen saturation. If the saturation is < 90 percent, do the following:

- **Increase the oxygen concentration and flow rate.**
- Obtain an **arterial blood gas (ABG).**
- **Determine likely causes of hypoxia** based on the history.

CIRCULATION

Chest Trauma

Circulatory disturbances in the setting of trauma may have one of three major causes. In the exam, you will need to determine quickly the likely cause to institute prompt therapy.

1. **Hypovolemic shock** is the most common type of shock.
   - The case will describe a pale, cold, shivering patient with diaphoresis, hypotension, and tachycardia.
   - Look for a source of bleeding. (The patient may lose a large volume of blood in the abdomen or thigh following diaphyseal fracture of the femur.)
2. **Pericardial tamponade** and **tension pneumothorax** can both result from thoracic trauma.
   - Both result in **distended neck veins,** or a high central venous pressure (CVP).

Pericardial tamponade involves the following:
   - Look for an **enlarged heart** on chest X-ray.
   - Immediately perform **pericardiocentesis tap** or **pericardial window.**
   - Look for **electrical alternans** on EKG.
   - Remember to note presence of **pulsus paradoxus** on vital signs.
3. **Tension pneumothorax:**
   - Look for **respiratory distress, tracheal deviation, absent breath sounds, and hyperresonance to percussion.**
   - Immediately place a **large-bore needle or IV catheter** into the pleural space. *Then* place a **chest tube.**
   - *Never* wait for a chest X-ray for diagnosis.

> Do *not* be distracted by head trauma or dilated pupils in a hypotensive trauma patient. Intracranial bleeds are *never* the cause of hypotensive shock. The first step in management is to identify and control the site of bleeding.

Abdominal Trauma

A 22-year-old male arrives in the ER with multiple gunshot wounds to the abdomen. He is diaphoretic, pale, cold, shivering, anxious, and asking for a blanket and a drink of water. His blood pressure is 60/40 mm Hg, pulse rate 150/min and thready. What is the next step in management?

a. Blood transfusion

b. Direct pressure to the abdomen

c. Foley catheter

d. Intravenous antibiotics

e. Intravenous fluids

*Answer: The correct answer is **E.** Administering large volumes of intravenous fluid is the first step in management. If an identifiable source of bleeding is readily seen (e.g., bleeding extremity), the first step in management is to control the bleeding. In this patient, there are likely multiple sources of bleeding, which will require surgery to correct.*

Spleen injury!

Management of circulatory disturbances in cases of abdominal trauma involves the following:

- The first step in management is *always* to **control the site of bleeding** if known.
  - Apply **direct local pressure** when the site is visible (e.g., extremity).
  - Blind clamping and the use of a tourniquet is *never* the answer.
- The next priority is **fluid resuscitation.**
- Do several things at once in **preparation for immediate exploratory laparotomy:**

  → confirm bleeding c̄ fast or DPL prior to ex lap

  - Set up two large-gauge IV lines
  - Give fluids and blood
  - Type and screen
  - Insert Foley catheter
  - Administer IV antibiotics.
- **If surgery isn't needed** (e.g., blunt trauma), **fluid resuscitation is the first step in management and is also diagnostic.** (If the patient responds promptly, then he's probably no longer bleeding.)

Vasomotor Shock

Vasomotor shock is the cause of hypotension and tachycardia in patients who are **warm and flushed** (rather than pale and cold). Look for a history of **medication use** (e.g., penicillin that may have triggered a penicillin allergy), **spinal anesthesia,** or **exposure to allergen** (e.g., bee sting).

> Intraosseous cannulation in the proximal tibia is used in children (generally < 6 years old). Give an initial bolus of Ringers lactate at 20 ml/kg of body weight.

The first step in management is to administer **vasoconstrictors and fluids.**

TRAUMA TO LOCALIZED SITES

All penetrating wounds with damage to internal organs will need to go to the OR. If the case describes an object embedded in the patient, *never* remove it in the ER or at the scene of the accident.

HEAD TRAUMA

Management Steps for the Exam

A man was hit over the head with a baseball bat during a mugging. He has a scalp laceration and a linear skull fracture on CT scan. He denies loss of consciousness. There are no neurological signs on exam. Is surgery indicated?

*Answer: No surgical intervention is needed for an **asymptomatic head injury with a closed skull fracture** (no overlying wound) alone. The next step in management is to **clean any lacerations.***

A woman was hit over the head with a baseball bat during a mugging. She has a scalp laceration, and a comminuted, depressed fracture is seen on CT scan. She denies loss of consciousness. There are no neurological signs on exam. Is surgery indicated?

Answer: **Surgery** *(repair or craniotomy) is* always *done for* **comminuted** *or* **depressed skull fracture,** *even if the patient is asymptomatic. Send the patient to the OR.*

A man is hit over the head with a baseball bat during a mugging. He reports "being out of it for a few seconds," but then he came to without any symptoms. There are no neurological signs on exam. What is the next step in management? He wants to go home—what will you tell him?

For **head trauma and loss of consciousness,** *the first step in management is to order a* **CT** *of the head* and **neck without contrast.** *If the head CT and neurological exam are normal, he can go home if someone can closely observe him over the next 24 hours (i.e., wake him up frequently and watch for changes in mentation).*

> Give **tetanus toxoid and prophylactic antibiotics** to *all* patients with open skull fractures.

Basal Skull Fracture

Look for ecchymosis around both eyes (**raccoon's eyes**) or behind the ear (**Battle's sign**) or **clear fluid dripping from the ear or nose** (cerebral-spinal fluid [CSF] leak).

Management of this injury involves the following:

- **CT scan of the head** *and* **neck** (which will show a basal skull fracture). X-ray is *not* the correct answer.
- A CSF leak will stop by itself and requires no specific management. Prophylactic antibiotics are *not* indicated.
- **Facial palsy** may occur 2–3 days later due to neuropraxia. **Steroids** will resolve the symptoms.

Epidural Hematoma

A 14-year-old boy is hit over the side of the head with a baseball bat. He loses consciousness for a few minutes, but he recovers promptly and wishes to continue playing. He is brought to the ER; the CT is shown in Image 4.1. The patient has no complaints and has no neurologic dysfunction on exam. What is the next step in management?

a. Admit and observe for 24 hours.
b. Perform emergency craniotomy.
c. Give mannitol.
d. Send the patient home with frequent neurological checks.

*Answer: The correct answer is **B**. The patient is at risk of sudden deterioration. Emergency craniotomy is needed for* all *epidural hematomas.*

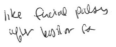
middle meningeal arterial

Epidural hematomas present with **trauma** and **sudden loss of consciousness.** The period when the patient immediately awakes and appears normal is referred to as the "honeymoon period," but then the patient quickly deteriorates. It is important to move quickly.

- **Diagnosis: CT scan** shows a **lens-shaped hematoma** with or without midline deviation.

- **Management:** Perform an **emergency craniotomy.** If the patient is treated, the prognosis is good; if not, epidural hematoma is fatal within hours.

Acute Subdural Hematoma

Bleeding is low pressure from the venous system. Suspect acute subdural hematoma in cases of **head trauma with fluctuating consciousness** (gradual headaches, memory loss, personality changes, dementia, confusion, and drowsiness).

slow bleed = fluctuating consciousness pain from dural rupture

- **Diagnosis: CT scan** shows **semilunar, crescent-shaped hematoma** with or without midline deviation.

- **Management:** Conservative management is usually done with **steroids.** Emergency craniotomy is done only if there are lateralizing signs and midline displacement.

like facial palsy after lesion ca

craniotomy if epidural or midline displacement p subdural.

Subdural Hematoma

Diffuse Axonal Injury

Diffuse axonal injury results from **acceleration-deceleration injuries to the head.** The patient will be deeply unconscious.

- **Prognosis is terrible,** and surgery *cannot* help.
- Therapy is directed at **preventing further injury** from increased intercranial pressure (ICP).

ELEVATED INTRACRANIAL PRESSURE (ICP)

The classic history proceeds as follows:

1. **Briefly depressed consciousness after head trauma**
2. **Improvement**
3. **Progressive drowsiness**

Elevated intracranial pressure is a **medical emergency.**

Diagnosis

- **Gradual dilatation of one pupil and a decreasing responsiveness to light** is an important sign, as it indicates clot expansion on the ipsilateral hemisphere.
- Get a head CT and look for midline shift or dilated ventricles.
- Do *not* think about performing a lumbar tap in anyone *without* first getting a head CT. If you perform a lumbar puncture on a person with increased intracranial pressure, you will herniate the brain, kill the patient, and fail the exam.

Management

- **First-line measures** are the following:
  - **Head elevation** ~reverse trendelenburg~
  - **Hyperventilation** ↓CO2
  - **Avoid fluid overload**
- **Second-line measures** are the following:
  - **Mannitol and furosemide:** Use these *very* cautiously; they can reduce cerebral perfusion.
  - **Sedation and/or hypothermia:** These lower oxygen demand.

Caution! Do *not* overdo the treatment for elevated intracranial pressure. Lowering ICP is *not* the ultimate goal; preserving brain perfusion is. Systemic hypotension or excessive cerebral vasoconstriction may be counterproductive.

> Steroids are good for cerebral edema secondary to tumors and abscesses, but they have *no* role in head trauma patients.

GENERAL SURGERY

ACUTE ABDOMEN

The four main causes of an acute abdomen are these:

1. Perforation
2. Obstruction
3. Inflammatory/infection
4. Ischemia

The most important question to ask yourself when presented a case of an acute abdomen is **when to operate and when to treat medically.**

When is **surgery** the answer?

- **Peritonitis** (excluding primary peritonitis)
- **Abdominal pain/tenderness plus signs of sepsis**
- **Acute intestinal ischemia**
- **Pneumoperitoneum**

In all of the above cases, make sure pancreatitis is first ruled out.

> Primary peritonitis is spontaneous inflammation in children with nephrosis or an adult with ascites and mild abdominal pain (even if there is fever and leukocytosis).

SBP fluid in abdomen that spontaneously gets infected.

Pneumoperitoneum in a child with perforated small bowel

When is **"treat medically"** the answer?

- **Primary peritonitis**
- **Pancreatitis**
- **Cholangitis**

- **Urinary stones:** Look for stones on X-ray.
- Things that can mimic an acute abdomen:
  - **Lower lobe pneumonia:** Look for infiltrate on chest X-ray.
  - **Myocardial ischemia:** Look for EKG changes.
  - **Pulmonary embolism:** Always suspect this in any immobilized patient.
- **Ruptured ovarian cysts**

Nonsurgical causes of an acute abdomen are the following:

- Myocardial infarction, acute pericarditis
- Lower lobe pneumonia, pulmonary infarction
- Hepatitis, GERD
- DKA, adrenal insufficiency
- Pyelonephritis, acute salphingitis
- Sickle cell crisis
- Acute porphyria

PERFORATION

Gastrointestinal Perforation

The question will describe **acute abdominal pain that is sudden, severe, constant, and generalized.** Pain is excruciating with any movement (it may be blunted in elderly patients). The most common causes of gastrointestinal perforation are these:

- **Diverticulitis:** Elderly patient with lower abdominal pain and fever
- **Perforated peptic ulcer:** Epigastric pain that classically awakes patient at night and, possibly, referred pain to the scapula
- **Crohn's disease**

Diagnose with a **supine and erect abdominal X-ray** (free air under diaphragm, or falciform ligament).

Management is as follows:

- Order **nothing per mouth (NPO) and IV fluid hydration.**
- Prescribe **IV antibiotics such as flagyl and gentamicin** or second-generation cephalosporins (**cefotetan** or **cefoxitin**).
- Perform **emergency surgery.**

Esophageal Perforation

The most common cause of esophageal perforation is **iatrogenic.** The case will describe the following:

- Pain in chest or upper abdomen
- Dysphagia or odynophagia
- Subcutaneous emphysema shortly after endoscopy

Esophageal perforation is a **surgical emergency. Gastrograffin contrast esophogram** is the first study of choice (do *not* use barium).

OBSTRUCTION

Suspect obstruction in patients with the following symptoms:

- **Severe colicky pain**
- **Absence of flatus or feces**
- **Nausea and vomiting** in patients with **risk factors:** Risk factors are these:
  - Prior surgery (think adhesions)
  - Elderly patient with weight loss and anemia or melanotic stools (think tumor)
  - History of recurrent lower abdominal pain (think diverticulitis)
  - History of hernia (incarcerated hernia)
  - Sudden abdominal pain in elderly patient (don't forget about volvulus)
- **Constant movement,** as the patient tries to find a position of comfort

Diagnosis

- **CBC and lactate level**
- **Supine and erect abdominal X-ray:** Look for dilated loops of bowel, absence of gas in rectum, bird's beak sign for volvulus.

Management

- **NPO, nasogastric (NG) suction, and IV fluid hydration**
- Consider **gastrograffin contrast study** (until perforation has been ruled out).
- **Volvulus:** Perform **proctosigmoidoscopy** with rigid instrument. Leave the rectal tube in place. Perform **sigmoid resection** for recurrent cases.
- **Abdominal hernias:** Perform **elective repair** for all abdominal hernias, *except* umbilical hernia in patients < 2 years old and esophageal sliding hiatal hernia.
- **All other obstructions:** Perform **emergency surgery.**

In a patient with a hernia, immediate surgery is the answer *if* the case describes fever, leukocytosis, constant pain, and signs of peritoneal irritation (think strangulated obstruction).

INFLAMMATION

Inflammatory causes of acute abdomen include the following:

- **Acute diverticulitis**
- **Acute pancreatitis**
- **Acute appendicitis**

The question will describe the following:

- Gradual onset of constant abdominal pain that slowly builds up over several hours
- Initially ill-defined pain that eventually becomes localized to the site of inflammation
- Note that signs of peritoneal irritation are absent in pancreatitis.

Acute Diverticulitis

Acute diverticulitis is one of the very few inflammatory processes presenting with acute abdominal pain in the **left lower quadrant.** Look for a patient in **middle age or older with fever, leukocytosis, and peritoneal irritation in the left lower quadrant with a palpable tender mass.** In women, think about fallopian tube and ovaries as potential sources.

Diagnose with a **CT**—look for abscess and free air. *Never* order contrast studies or endoscopy in the acute phase.

> When diagnosing acute diverticulitis, don't forget to order a **urine pregnancy test** on *all* women of childbearing age.

Treat as follows:

- **No peritoneal signs:** Manage as outpatient with antibiotics.
- **Localized peritoneal signs and abscess:** Admit the patient. Order NPO, IV fluids, and IV antibiotics.
- **Generalized peritonitis or perforation:** Perform *emergency* surgery.
- **Recurrent attacks of diverticulitis:** Perform *elective* surgery.

Acute Pancreatitis

Suspect this in the **alcoholic** who develops an **acute (over several hours) upper abdominal pain, radiating to the back, with nausea and vomiting.** Acute pancreatitis may be

- **edematous,**
- **hemorrhagic,** or
- **suppurative** (pancreatic abscess).

Late complications include **pancreatic pseudocyst and chronic pancreatitis.**

Diagnose with a **serum or urinary amylase or lipase** (serum from 12 to 48 hours, urinary from 3rd to 6th day). Perform a **CT** if diagnosis is uncertain.

Treat with **NPO, NG suction, and IV fluids.**

Complications can include the following:

- **Abscess:** Often appears 10 days after onset with persistent fevers and WBC count. **Surgical drainage** is the treatment.
- **Pseudocyst:** Appears 5 weeks after initial symptoms, when a collection of pancreatic juice causes anorexia, pain, and a palpable mass.
  - If < 6 cm and present < 6 weeks: **Observe.**
  - If > 6cm or present > 6weeks: **Perform percutaneous drainage** or **endoscopic drainage.**
- **Chronic damage:** Causes diabetes and steatorrhea. Treat with **insulin and pancreatic enzyme supplements.**

> Warning signs for **hemorrhagic pancreatitis** are the following:
> - Lower hematocrit that continues to fall the day after presentation
> - Very high WBC (> 18,000), glucose BUN
> - Very low calcium

Acute Appendicitis

Acute appendicitis presents as follows:

- It classically begins with **anorexia**
- This is followed by vague **periumbilical pain,** which several hours later becomes sharp, severe, constant, and localized to the **right lower quadrant of the abdomen.**
- **Tenderness, guarding, and rebound are found to the right and below the umbilicus** (but not elsewhere in the belly).

Diagnose as follows:

- Look for **fever and leukocytosis in the 10,000–15,000 range,** with neutrophilia and immature forms.
- If diagnosis is unclear by clinical history and exam, get an **ultrasound** or **CT scan.**

Manage as follows:

- Administer an **IV before appendectomy.**
- If appendix is **perforated, continue IV** until fever and WBC count have normalized.

Chronic Ulcerative Colitis (CUC)

CUC is managed medically. *Elective* surgery is the answer under the following conditions:

- Disease has been **present more than 20 years** (high incidence of malignant degeneration).
- There have been **multiple hospitalizations.**
- The patient needs **high-dose steroids** or **immunosuppressant.**
- There is **toxic megacolon** (abdominal pain, fever, leukocytosis, epigastric tenderness, massively distended transverse colon on X-rays with gas within the wall of the colon).

ISCHEMIA

Always consider the following:

- Acute mesenteric ischemia in older patients
- History of arrhythmia (atrial fibrillation)
- Coronary artery disease
- Recent MI

Classically, **pain is out of proportion to the exam.** Diagnosis is clinical but look for acidosis and signs of sepsis. If ischemia is suspected, do *not* wait for lab findings (acidosis, elevated lactate); go straight to **surgery** or **order angiography.**

- If diagnosis is during surgery: **Perform embolectomy and revascularization of resection.**
- If diagnosis is during angiography: **Give vasodilators** or **thrombolysis.**

When you think a patient has an acute abdomen or one that may become acute, make sure to get a *surgical consultation* on the CCS. The consultation will not offer useful information; the test is checking if you know to get surgery involved.

ABSCESS

Intra-Abdominal Abscess

Consider the possibility of an abscess in any patient with a **history of a previous operation, trauma, or intra-abdominal infection/inflammation.** Abscesses can occur anywhere in the abdomen or retroperitoneum.

Diagnose with a **CBC and a contrast CT of the abdomen/pelvis.**

Management of an intra-abdominal abscess is as follows:

- Always **drain an abscess** (either surgically or percutaneously).
- Give **antibiotics** to prevent spread of infection (does not cure abscess).

SURGICAL JAUNDICE

Obstructive Jaundice Caused by Stones

The question will describe an **obese, fecund woman in her 40s** with the following signs:

- **Recurrent episodes of abdominal pain**
- **High alkaline phosphatase**
- **Dilated ducts on sonogram**
- **Nondilated gallbladder full of stones**

Diagnose with the following:

1. Order a **sonogram.**
2. Confirm with **endoscopic retrograde cholangiopancreatography (ERCP).**

Manage the condition as follows:

1. Perform a **sphincterotomy** and remove the common duct stone.
2. **Cholecystectomy** should follow.

Obstructive Jaundice Caused by Tumor

In patients with progressive symptoms in the preceding weeks and weight loss, suspect a **tumor:**

- Adenocarcinoma at the head of the pancreas
- Adenocarcinoma of the ampulla of Vater
- Cholangiocarcinoma arising in the common duct itself

Diagnose with the following:

- Sonogram
- CT scan
  - For lesions seen on CT scan, get a **percutanous biopsy.**
  - If no lesion is seen on CT scan, order an **endoscopic retrograde cholangiopancreatography (ERCP)** (shows ampullary or common bile duct tumors not seen on CT scan).

Management is with **surgical resection.**

gall stone ileus!

GALLSTONES

Biliary Colic

Temporary occlusion of the cystic duct causes **colicky pain in the right upper quadrant, radiating to the right shoulder and back,** often triggered by **fatty food.** Episodes are **brief** (20 minutes), and there are *no* signs of peritoneal irritation or systemic signs.

Diagnosis is with a **sonogram.**

Treatment is with *elective* **cholecystectomy.**

Acute Cholecystitis

Persistent occlusion of the cystic duct from a stone causes **constant pain,** as well as **fever, leukocytosis, and peritoneal irritation in the right upper quadrant.**

Diagnosis is with a **sonogram,** which will show gallstones, a thick-walled gallbladder, and pericholecystic fluid.

Treatment is as follows:

1. **NG suction, NPO, IV fluids, and antibiotics**
2. These are followed by *elective* **cholecystectomy** (after 6–12 weeks).

Emergency cholecystectomy is needed if there is **generalized peritonitis** or **emphysematous cholecystitis** (suggestive of perforation or gangrene).

Acute Ascending Cholangitis

Obstruction of the common duct causes **obstruction and ascending infection.** There is **high fever and very high white blood cell sepsis.** A key finding is **extremely high levels of alkaline phosphatase.**

Treatment is with the following:

- **IV antibiotics**
- **Emergency decompression of the common duct** is lifesaving:
  - Ideally by ERCP
  - Alternatively through the liver by percutaneous transhepatic cholangiogram (PTC)
  - Rarely by surgery.
- Eventually **cholecystectomy** must follow

PREOPERATIVE AND POSTOPERATIVE CARE

PREOPERATIVE ASSESSMENT

The most important aspect of preoperative assessment is being able to **identify comorbidites that preclude surgery.** Other aspects of preoperative assessment include understanding the modifications that may need to be instituted to **prepare patients for surgery.**

A 72-year-old man is scheduled to have an elective sigmoid resection for diverticular disease. His exercise tolerance has remained stable as 3 blocks. On examination, he has Jugular venous distention (JVD) 5 cm above the sternal angle. His medications include aspirin, metoprolol, lasix, and albuterol, which he uses every fortnight. What is the most important next step in management to address his perioperative risk?

a. Order echocardiogram.
b. Start statin preoperatively.
c. Start enalapril preoperatively.
d. Start long acting beta agonist inhaler
e. Perform coronary angiography.

*Answer: The correct answer is **C**. JVD is one of the most important indicators of congestive heart failure—a major preoperative risk. The priority in management is first to ensure that the heart failure is optimized with ACE inhibitors, beta blockers, and diuretics. Further cardiac workup and interventions are indicated only when symptoms have increased or outcomes have worsened in the past 1–2 years.*

A 42-year-old man with hepatitis C presents with severe-onset epigastric pain and altered mental status. Upper GI series reveals a duodenal ulcer. His hemoglobin decreases 2 grams from presentation. Surgical intervention is being considered. His bilirubin is 2.9, his prothrombin time is 22 seconds, and his serum albumin is 2.3. Which of the following is the best next step in management?

a. Proceed to emergency surgery.
b. Proceed with surgery after first giving vitamin K.
c. Proceed with surgery after total parenteral nutrition (TPN).
d. Proceed with surgery after albumin infusion.
e. Do not perform surgery.

*Answer: The correct answer is **E**. Do not do surgery in any patients with derangements in all 4 hepatic risk factors. Any 1 of the hepatic risks alone—bilirubin above 2, albumin below 3, prothrombin above 16, and encephalopathy (as suggested by altered mental status)—predicts a mortality of over 40 percent. If 3 of them are present, the risk is 85 percent, All 4 risks constitute almost 100 percent risk of mortality.*

A 59-year-old male is scheduled for prostatectomy. He has a history of HTN, COPD, and diabetes mellitus. He takes atenolol for blood pressure, tiotropium and albuterol for COPD, and glipizide for diabetes. BP is 145/89 mm Hg, and HgbA1c is 7.1. Recent pulmonary tests document FEV1 1.3. Blood CO2 is 47. Which of the following is this patient most at risk of developing?

a. Intraoperative myocardial infacrtion

b. Pneumothorax

c. Postoperative pneumonia

d. Hypercapneic failure

*Answer: The correct answer is **C**. Severe COPD (FEV1 < 1.5 L) increases surgical risk, mainly because patients have an ineffective cough and cannot clear secretions. They are subsequently at risk for postoperative pneumonia.*

The following table summarizes important principles in preoperative assessment.

Organ System	Risk Factor	Modifications/Interventions
Cardiac risk	Ejection fraction < 35%	Prohibits noncardiac surgery.
	Jugular venous distention (sign of CHF)	Optimize medications with ACE inhibitors, beta blockers, digitalis, and diuretics should precede surgery.
	Recent myocardial infarction	Defer surgery for 6 months after MI.
	Severe progressive angina	Perform cardiac catheterization to evaluate for possible coronary revascularization.
Pulmonary risk	Smoking (compromised ventilation (high PCO2, FEV1 < 1.5)	Order PFTs to evaluate FEV. If FEV1 is abnormal, obtain blood gas. Cessation of smoking for 8 weeks prior to surgery.
Hepatic risk	Bilirubin > 2.0 Prothrombin time > 16 Serum albumin < 3.0 Encephalopathy	~ 40% mortality with any single risk factor. ~ 80–85% mortality is predictable if three or more risk factors are present.
Nutritional Risk	Loss of 20% of body weight over several months Serum albumin < 3.0 Anergy to skin antigens Serum transferrin < 200 mg/dL Diabetic coma	Provide 5–10 days of nutritional supplements (preferably via gut) before surgery. Absolute contraindication to surgery. First stabilize diabetes. Rehydrate and normalize acidosis prior to surgery.

The following table shows the calculation of the cardiac risk index in noncardiac surgery.

Cardiac Risk Index in Noncardiac Surgery		
Criteria	**Finding**	**Points***
Age	> 70	5
Cardiac status	MI within 6 months	10
	Ventricular gallop or jugular venous distention (signs of heart failure)	11
	Significant aortic stenosis	3
	Arrhythmia other than sinus or premature atrial contractions	7
	≥ 5 premature ventricular contractions/minute	7
General medical condition	PO2 < 60 mm Hg, PCO2 > 50 mm Hg, K < 3 mmol/L, HCO3 < 20 mmol/L, BUN > 50 mg/dL, serum creatinine > 3 mg/dL, elevated AST, a chronic liver disorder, or bedbound	3
Type of surgery needed	Emergency surgery	4
	Intraperitoneal, intrathoracic, or aortic surgery	3
*Risk is based on the total number of points: Level I: 0–5 Level II: 6–12 Level III: 13–25 Level IV: > 25		
Adapted from Goldman, L. et al., 1997. "Multifactorial index of cardiac risk in noncardiac surgical procedures." *New England Journal of Medicine* 297:845–850.		

POSTOPERATIVE COMPLICATIONS

In each of the following cases, which diagnostic tests will likely show the cause of the patient's postoperative fever?

A) A patient who had major abdominal surgery is afebrile during the first 2 postoperative days but on Day 3 has a fever to 103°F.

B) A patient who had major abdominal surgery is afebrile during the first 4 postoperative days but on Day 5 has a fever to 103°F.

C) A patient who had major abdominal surgery is afebrile during the first 6 postoperative days but on Day 7 has a fever to 103°F.

a. Chest X-ray

b. CT of the abdomen

c. CT of the chest

d. Doppler of the lower extremities

e. Urinalysis

Answers:

A) **A.** *Chest X-ray*

B) **D.** *Doppler of the lower extremities*

C) **B.** *CT of the abdomen*

Every *potential source of post-op fever must be investigated, but the timing of the first febrile episode gives a clue as to the most likely source. While not a hard and fast rule, the "four Ws" mnemonic gives a clue to the likely cause of the fever:*

- *"Wind" for atelectasis, common post-op Day 1: Order a* **chest X-ray.**
- *"Water" for urinary tract infections, common post-op Day 3: Order* **urinalysis and urine culture.**
- *"Walking" for thrombophlebitis, common post-op Day 5: Order* **Dopplers.**
- *"Wound" for wound infections, common post-op Day 7: Conduct a* **complete physical exam** *and consider* **CT scan** *to evaluate for deep infections.*

A 46-year-old female with past medical history significant for large fibroids and anemia becomes disorientated 18 hours after an uncomplicated hysterectomy. What is the next step in management?

a. Obtain arterial blood gas.

b. Obtain CT scan of the pelvis.

c. Give intravenous fluids.

d. Give ativan.

e. Give blood transfusion.

Answer: The correct answer is **A.** *There are a long list of causes for post-op disorientation; however, the most lethal one if not recognized and treated early is* **hypoxia.** *Unless the vignette clearly identifies other possible metabolic causes of disorientation—uremia, hyponatremia, hypernatremia, ammonium, hyperglycemia, delirium tremens (DTs), or iatrogenic medications—the safest thing is to obtain a blood gas first.*

A 52-year-old woman is found to have brown feculent fluid draining from her wound drain 9 days after a sigmoid resection for colorectal cancer. The patient is afebrile, has stable vital signs, and is without complaints. What is the next step in management?

a. Administer intravenous antibiotics.

b. Order a CT of the abdomen.

c. Flush the drain with normal saline.

d. Perform an urgent laparotomy.

e. Conduct observation only.

Answer: The correct answer is **E.** *Observation is all that is needed. A fecal fistula, if draining to the outside, is not serious. It will close eventually with little or no therapy. If feces were accumulating on the inside, the patient would be febrile and would have other systemic signs. This would require drainage and probably a diverting colostomy.*

The leakage of fecal, gastric, or duodenal contents to the outside postoperatively is *not* an indication for emergency surgery. Observe stable patients. Dehydration and electrolyte derangements must be corrected before surgery.

Nutritional support should always first be given via the gut whenever possible. Total parenteral nutrition is almost *never* the right answer on the exam due to the high risk of infection.

The following table summarizes the features and management of postoperative complications.

Postoperative Complication	Features	Management
Fever		
Malignant hyperthermia exceeding 104°F	Shortly after the onset of the anesthetic (halothane or succinylcholine) Treat with IV dantrolene, 100 percent oxygen, correction of the acidosis, and cooling blankets	Watch for development of myoglobinuria
Bacteremia exceeding 104°F	Within 30–45 minutes of invasive procedures (instrumentation of the urinary tract is a classic example)	Blood cultures times 3 Start empiric antibiotics
Postoperative fever in the usual range (101°–103°F)	Atelectasis (Day 1)	Incentive spirometry
	Pneumonia (Day 3)	CXR: Infiltrate Sputum culture Antibiotics (hospital-acquired pneumonia)
	Urinary tract infection (Day 3)	Urinalysis and urinary culture Antibiotics
	Deep venous thrombophlebitis (Day 5)	Doppler ultrasound of deep veins of legs and pelvis Anticoagulation
	Wound infection (Day 7)	Antibiotics if only cellulitis Incision and drainage if abscess is present
	Deep abscesses (subphrenic, pelvic, or subhepatic) (Days 10–15)	CT scan of the appropriate body cavity is diagnostic Percutaneous radiologically guided drainage is therapeutic
Perioperative myocardial infarction	Precipitated by hypotension when intraoperative Post-op MI seldom presents with chest pain	Thrombolytics are contraindicated, even in post-op setting Mortality rate is higher than for nonsurgery-related MI

Postoperative Complication	Features	Management
Fever		
Pulmonary embolus (PE) (Day 7)		CTA (CT Angiogram) Anticoagulate with heparin IVC filter if recurrent PE
Aspiration		Lavage and remove gastric contents Bronchodilators and respiratory support. Steroids do *not* help
Intraoperative tension pneumothorax	Positive-pressure breathing; patient becomes progressively more difficult to "bag" BP steadily declines, and CVP steadily rises	Insert needle to decompress and place chest tube later
Postoperative confusion	Suspect hypoxia first Consider sepsis	Check blood gases Get blood cultures and CBC
Adult respiratory distress syndrome (ARDS)	Bilateral pulmonary infiltrates and hypoxia, with no evidence of CHF	Positive end-expiratory pressure (PEEP)
Delirium tremens (Days 2–3)	Tachycardia, hyperthermia, hypertension, altered mental status	Give benzodiazepines (barbiturates are second-line agents because of lower therapeutic range); watch for seizures and rhabdomyolysis

PEDIATRIC SURGERY

CONDITIONS THAT NEED SURGERY AT BIRTH

Congenital anomalies constitute the conditions that need surgery at birth. On the Step 3 exam, the most important first step before surgery is to rule out other associated congenital conditions. In any of the following presentations, look for other associated elements of the VACTER (vertebral, anal, cardiac, tracheal, esophageal, renal, and radial) constellation:

- Look at anus for imperforation.
- Check the X-ray for vertebral and radial anomalies.
- Do echocardiogram looking for cardiac anomalies.
- Do sonogram looking for renal anomalies.

Esophageal Atresia

Excessive salivation is noted shortly after birth, or **choking spells** are noticed when first feeding is attempted.

Confirm the diagnosis with an **NG tube,** which becomes coiled in the upper chest on X-ray.

Treat as follows:

- Primary **surgical repair** is indicated.
- If surgery needs to be delayed for further workup, perform **gastrostomy** to protect the lungs from acid reflux.

Imperforated Anus

This is indicated by an **absence of flatus or stool.** The anal canal is absent on exam.

Treat as follows:

- Look for a **fistula nearby** (to vagina or perineum).
  - If **present,** delay repair until further growth (but before toilet training time).
  - If **not present,** a **colostomy** needs to be done for high rectal pouches.

Congenital Diaphragmatic Hernia

Dyspnea is noted at birth, and **loops of bowel in left chest are seen on X-ray.** The primary abnormality is the **hyoplastic lung with fetal-type circulation.**

Treat by performing **endotracheal intubation, low-pressure ventilation, sedation, and NG suction.** Delay repair 3–4 days to allow lung maturation.

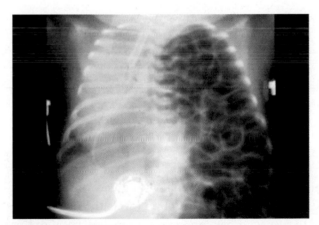

Congenital Diaphragmatic Hernia

Gastroschisis and Omphalocele

- **Gastroschisis:** The umbilical cord is normal (it reaches the baby); the defect is to the right of the cord, where there is no protective membrane and the bowel looks angry and matted.
- **Omphalocele:** The umbilical cord goes to the defect, which has a thin membrane under which one can see normal-looking bowel and a little slice of liver.

Treat as follows:

- **Small defects:** Close small defects primarily.
- **Large defects:** These require a silastic "silo" to protect the bowel and **manual replacement of the bowel daily** until complete closure (in about 1 week). In the meantime, give parenteral nutrition (the bowel will not work in gastroschisis).

Exstrophy of the Urinary Bladder

This is an abdominal wall defect over the pubis.

Transfer the patient to a specialized center that offers surgical repair in first 1–2 days of life. Do *not* delay surgery.

A newborn is vomiting greenish liquid material. A "double-bubble" is seen on X-ray. What is the diagnosis?

a. Annular pancreas
b. Congenital diaphragmatic hernia
c. Gastroschisis
d. Imperforated anus
e. Intestinal atresia

*Answer: The correct answer is **A**. Don't be fooled into thinking that only duodenal atresia presents with double-bubble sign. Annular pancreas and malrotation also present with double-bubble sign. All of these anomalies require surgical correction, but malrotation is the most dangerous because the bowel can twist on itself, cut off its blood supply, and die.*

Intestinal Atresia

Like annular pancreas, this condition also presents with green vomiting. But instead of a double-bubble, there are **multiple air-fluid levels throughout the abdomen.** There is no need to suspect other congenital anomalies, because this condition results from a vascular accident in utero.

SURGICAL CONDITIONS IN THE FIRST TWO MONTHS OF LIFE

Necrotizing Enterocolitis

This shows up as **feeding intolerance in premature infants** when they are first fed. There is **abdominal distention** and a **rapidly dropping platelet count** (in babies, this is a sign of sepsis).

Treatment is as follows:

- **Stop all feedings.**
- Prescribe **broad-spectrum antibiotics.**
- Deliver **IV fluids and nutrition.**
- Do **surgery** if there are signs of necrosis or perforation (abdominal wall erythema, portal vein gas, or gas in the bowel wall).

Meconium Ileus

Symptoms are **feeding intolerance and bilious vomiting** in a baby with **cystic fibrosis** (look for cystic fibrosis in family history).

Diagnose by **X-rays,** which show **multiple dilated loops of small bowel** and a **ground-glass appearance** in the lower abdomen.

Gastrografin enema is both

- **diagnostic** (microcolon and inspissated pellets of meconium in the terminal ileum); and
- **therapeutic** (gastrografin draws fluid in and dissolves the pellets).

Hypertrophic Pyloric Stenosis

This shows up as **nonbilious projectile vomiting after each feeding** at approximately 3 weeks of age. Look for **gastric peristaltic waves** and a **palpable "olive-size" mass** in the right upper quadrant.

Diagnose with a **sonogram.**

Treat as follows:

- **Correct dehydration and associated hypochloremic, hypokalemic metabolic alkalosis.**
- Follow this with **Ramstedt pyloromyotomy.**

Biliary Atresia

This appears in 6- to 8-week-old babies who have **persistent, progressively increasing jaundice** (conjugated fraction).

Diagnose in the following ways:

- Conduct **serologies and sweat test** to rule out other problems.
- Order **HIDA scan** after 1 week of phenobarbital (a powerful choleretic).
- If no bile reaches the duodenum even with phenobarbital stimulation, **surgical exploration** is needed.

Hirschsprung Disease (Aganglionic Megacolon)

The most important clue to diagnosis is **chronic constipation.** A **rectal exam** may lead to explosive expulsion of stool and flatus with relief of abdominal distention.

Diagnose by getting a **full-thickness biopsy of rectal mucosa.**

SURGICAL CONDITIONS LATER IN INFANCY

Intussusception

This presents in 6- to 12-month-old **chubby, healthy-looking kids** with **brief episodes of colicky abdominal pain** that makes them "double up and squat." There is also the following:

- A vague mass on the right side of the abdomen
- An "empty" right lower quadrant
- "Currant jelly" stools

A barium or air enema is both diagnostic and therapeutic. Perform **surgery** if enema fails to achieve reduction.

Intussusception

Meckel Diverticulum

This presents as **lower GI bleeding** in a child of pediatric age.

Diagnosis is with a **radioisotope scan,** which looks for gastric mucosa in the lower abdomen.

ORTHOPEDICS

COMMON ADULT ORTHOPEDIC INJURIES

General Rules about Fractures

- When you suspect a fracture, order **two views at 90° to one another** and *always* include the joints above and below the broken bone.
- *Always* X-ray other sites **"in the line of force"** (e.g., lumbar spine for someone who falls and lands on the feet, hips in a patient who has been in a motor vehicle accident with force of knees against the dashboard).
- **Closed reduction** is the answer for fractures that are not badly displaced or angulated.
- **Open reduction and internal fixation** is the answer when the fracture is severely displaced or angulated or cannot be aligned.
- **Open fractures** (the broken bone sticking out through a wound) require cleaning in the OR and reduction within 6 hours from the time of the injury.
- *Always* perform **cervical spine films** in any patient with **facial injuries.**

> Always worry about **gas gangrene** in any deep-penetrating or dirty wounds. Three days later, the patient will be septic with a tender, swollen injury site with gas crepitus. Treatment is large doses of **IV penicillin and hyperbaric oxygen.**

Fractures Management

A 27-year-old woman with known seizure disorder has a grand mal seizure. She complains of left shoulder pain. PA and lateral X-rays are obtained and fail to reveal fracture or dislocation. She is given ibuprofen for pain. She returns 3 days later with persistent pain with her arm held close to her side. She reports that she is unable to move the left arm. What is the next step in management?

a. Axillary radiograph of the left shoulder
b. Change analgesic to Percocet
c. CT of the left shoulder
d. MRI of the left shoulder
e. Ultrasound of tendon insertion sites

*Answer: The correct answer is **A**. Although **anterior shoulder dislocations** are easily seen on erect posterior-anterior (PA) and lateral films—look for adducted arm and externally rotated forearm with numbness over deltoid (axillary nerve is stretched)—posterior shoulder dislocations are commonly missed on these views. **Posterior shoulder dislocations** should be suspected in a patient with a recent seizure or electrical burn and shoulder injury or pain. Order axillary or scapular views of the affected shoulder.*

- **Hypospadias** (urethral opening on ventral side of penis) is easily seen on routine newborn physical exam.
  - *Never* perform circumcision on this child. The prepuce will be needed for the **plastic reconstruction.**
- A child who has **hematuria from trivial trauma** has an **undiagnosed congenital anomaly** until proven otherwise.
- A child with a **urinary tract infection** has an **undiagnosed congenital anomaly** until proven otherwise (e.g., vesicoureteral reflux).
  - Order a voiding cystogram to look for the reflux.
  - If found, give long-term antibiotics until the child "grows out of the problem."
- Suspect **low implantation of a ureter** in girls who void appropriately but are also found to be constantly wet from **urinating into the vagina.**
- **Ureteropelvic junction (UPJ) obstruction** is only symptomatic when diuresis occurs. UPJ presents classically in a teenager who drinks large volumes of beer and develops **colicky flank pain.**

VASCULAR SURGERY

A 48-year-old laborer complains of coldness and tingling in his left hand as well as pain in the forearm when he does strenuous work. Recently he's complained of dizziness, with blurred vision and trouble keeping steady during these episodes. Which of the following is the most important management?

a. Aspirin

b. Clopidogrel

c. Coumadin

d. Bypass surgery

e. Carotid endarterectomy

*Answer: The correct answer is **D**. Bypass surgery is needed for **subclavian steal syndrome.***

SUBCLAVIAN STEAL SYNDROME

Although this condition is rare in practice, it is a classic board vignette. An arteriosclerotic stenotic plaque at the origin of the subclavian allows enough blood supply to reach the arm for normal activity but not enough to meet the increased demands of an exercised arm, resulting in **blood being "stolen" from the vertebral artery.** Classic symptoms are the following:

- **Posterior neurological signs:** Visual symptoms, equilibrium problems
- **Claudication** in the arm during arm exercises

Don't confuse this condition with thoracic outlet syndrome, which causes vascular symptoms only with *no* neurologic signs.

Diagnose with an **angiography.**

Treatment is with **bypass surgery.**

AORTIC ANEURYSMS

A 66-year-old man has vague, poorly described epigastric and upper-back discomfort. He is found on physical examination to have a pulsatile mass, which is tender to palpation. Ultrasound reveals a 6 cm abdominal aneurysm. What is the next step in management?

Abdominal Aortic Aneurysm with mural thrombus

a. *Emergent surgery*
b. *Urgent surgery*
c). *Elective repair*
d. *Repeat abdominal ultrasound in 6 months*
e. *Order CT angiogram of the chest*

*Answer: The correct answer is **B**. Urgent surgery within the next day is the most appropriate management.*

Size and symptoms are key to management of abdominal aortic aneurysms.

- Aneurysms < 5 cm can be observed with **serial annual imaging.**
- Aneurysms ≥ 5 cm should have **elective repair.**

More urgent surgery is needed in the following cases:

- A **tender abdominal aortic aneurysm** will rupture within a day or two and, thus, requires **urgent repair.**
- **Excruciating back pain in a patient with a large abdominal aortic aneurysm** means that the aneurysm is already leaking, necessitating **emergency surgery.**

A 65-year-old man presents with severe sharp chest and back pain down the spine that started 1 hour ago. His blood pressure is 219/115 mm Hg. Chest X-ray is shown. ECG and cardiac enzymes are nonrevealing. Which of the following is the most important intervention that would have prevented this presentation?

a. Aspirin prophylaxis
b. Blood pressure control
c. Cessation of smoking
d. Low fat diet
e. Serial CT scans

*Answer: The correct answer is **B.** Blood pressure control is the most important strategy to prevent progression of thoracic aortic aneurysms.*

Risk Factors

The following contribute to the *development* of thoracic aortic aneurysms:

- **Chronic hypertension**
- **Hyperlipidemia**
- **Smoking**
- **Marfan syndrome**
- **Untreated tertiary syphilis**

The most important modifiable risk to prevent *worsening* of existing aneurysms is **uncontrolled hypertension.**

- **Asymptomatic lesions: Blood pressure management** is the most important factor in controlling asymptomatic lesions.
- **Symptomatic lesions,** including active dissection (look for chest pain and sudden-onset "tearing" pain in the back): These require **surgical intervention.**

ARTERIOSCLEROTIC OCCLUSIVE DISEASE OF THE LOWER EXTREMITIES

The classic presentation of this condition is **pain in the legs on exercise that is relieved by rest** (intermittent claudication).

If the claudication does *not* interfere significantly with the patient's lifestyle, *no* workup is indicated. The only management indicated is

- cessation of smoking and
- the use of **cilostazol.**

If the pain is more severe, diagnosis is with the following:

- Doppler studies looking for a pressure gradient
- Arteriogram to identify stenosis

If the case describes **disabling symptoms** (affects work or activities of daily living) or if there is **impending ischemia to the extremity,** then **surgery** is indicated. This involves the following:

- Angioplasty and stenting for stenotic segments
- More extensive disease requires bypass grafts or sequential stents.

Pain at rest indicates **end-stage disease** (the patient complains of calf pain at night with disturbed sleep).

ARTERIAL EMBOLIZATION OF THE EXTREMITIES

Look for a history of the following:

- Atrial fibrillation
- Recent MI with sudden-onset painful, pale, cold, pulseless, paresthetic, and paralytic lower extremity.

Get **Doppler studies** to locate the obstruction and consider **thrombolytics** (if early) or **embolectomy** (if later) with **fasciotomy.**

SECTION 5
PEDIATRICS

THE NEWBORN

MANAGEMENT OF THE NEWBORN

At delivery, give the following:

- **1 percent silver nitrate eye drops or 0.5 percent erythromycin ophthalmic ointment**
- **1 mg of vitamin K IM** to prevent hemorrhagic disease

Before discharge, do the following:

- **Perform hearing test** to rule out congenital sensorineural hearing loss (SNHL).
- Order neonatal screening tests. These are more reliable if done after 48 hours. Routine screening tests include the following:
  - **Phenylketonuria**
  - **Galactosemia**
  - **Hypothyroidism**

Apgar Score

The Apgar score is a measure of the need and effectiveness of resuscitation. The Apgar score does *not* predict outcome, but a persistently low Apgar (0–3) is associated with high mortality.

- The **1-minute** score gives an idea of what was going on **during labor and delivery.**
- The **5-minute** score gives an idea of **response to therapy** (resuscitation).

ABNORMALITIES IN THE NEWBORN

The table below lists both the benign findings in the newborn and the disorders that require further management.

Figure	Finding/Description	Diagnosis	Association	Further Management
	Blue/gray macules on presacral back/posterior thighs	Mongolian spots	Usually fade in first few years	Rule out child abuse
	Firm, yellow-white papules/pustules with erythematous base, which peak on second day of life	Erythema toxicum		Self-limited
	Permanent, unilateral vascular malformation on head and neck	Port wine stain (nevus flammeus)	Sturge-Weber syndrome (AV malformation that results in seizures, mental retardation, and glaucoma)	Pulsed laser therapy For Sturge-Weber, evaluate for glaucoma and give anticonvulsives
	Red, sharply demarcated, raised lesions appearing in first 2 months, rapidly expanding, then involuting by age 5–9 years.	Hemangioma	Consider underlying organ involvement with deep hemangiomas. (If it involves the larynx, it can cause obstruction.) May cause high output cardiac failure when large.	Treat with steroids or pulsed laser if large or interferes with organ function.

Figure	Finding/ Description	Diagnosis	Association	Further Management
	Preauricular tags/ pits	Preauricular tags/ pits	Hearing loss Genitourinary abnormalities	Hearing test Ultrasound of kidneys
	Defect in the iris	Coloboma of the iris	Other eye abnormalities CHARGE syndrome (Coloboma, Heart defects, Atresia of the nasal choanae, growth Retardation, Genitourinary abnormalities, and Ear abnormalities)	Screen for CHARGE syndrome
	Absence of the iris	Aniridia	Wilms' tumor	Screen for Wilms' tumor with abdominal ultrasound Q3 months until age 8
	Mass lateral to midline	Branchial cleft cyst	Remnant of embryonic development associated with infections	Surgical removal
	Mass in midline that moves with swallowing	Thyroglossal duct cyst	Associated with infections May have thyroid ectopia	Surgical removal
	GI tract protrusion through the umbilicus with sac	Omphalocele (failure of GI sac to retract at 10–12 weeks gestation)	Malformations, chromosomal disorders	Screen for trisomy 13, trisomy 18, and trisomy 21
	Abdominal defect lateral to midline without sac	Gastroschisis	Intestinal atresia	

Figure	Finding/ Description	Diagnosis	Association	Further Management
	Congenital weakness where vessels of the fetal and infant umbilical cord exited through the rectus abdominus muscle	Umbilical hernia	Congenital hypothyroidism	Screen with TSH May close spontaneously
	Scrotal swelling, transillumination	Hydrocele	Inguinal hernia	Differentiate from inguinal hernia
	Unilateral absence of testes in scrotal sac	Undescended testes	Associated with malignancy if > 1 year of age	Surgical removal
	Urethral opening on ventral surface	Hypospadias	Other GU anomalies may be present (most common is undescended testes and inguinal hernias).	Do *not* circumcise
	Urethral opening on dorsal surface	Epispadias	Urinary incontinence (form of urinary exstrophy)	Surgical evaluation for bladder exstrophy
	Inguinal bulge or reducible scrotal swelling	Inguinal hernia (usually indirect)		Surgery

You are called to see a 9.5-pound newborn infant male who is jittery. The pregnancy was complicated by prolonged delivery with shoulder dystocia. Physical exam reveals a large, plethoric infant who is tremulous. A pan-systolic murmur is heard. Which of the following is the most appropriate diagnostic test?

a. Bilirubin level
b. Blood glucose
c. Galactose level
d. Serum calcium level
e. Serum TSH

*Answer: The correct answer is **B.** Blood glucose is the best initial diagnostic exam to evaluate in infants that present large for gestation, plethora, and jitteriness. This child is most likely born an **infant of a diabetic mother (IODM).***

*Look for **macrosomia** (all organs except the brain are enlarged), **history of birth trauma, and cardiac abnormalities** (cardiomegaly). The case may not give a history of diabetes in the mother. Treat with **glucose and small, frequent meals.***

Infant of a Diabetic Mother (IODM)

Lab abnormalities are the following:

- *Hypoglycemia (after birth)*
- *Hypocalcemia*
- *Hypomagnesemia*
- *Hyperbilirubinemia*
- *Polycythemia*

IODM is associated with the following:

- **Cardiac abnormalities** (ASD, VSD, truncus arteriosus)
- **Small left colon syndrome** (abdominal distension)

IODM is associated with an **increased risk of developing diabetes and childhood obesity.**

RESPIRATORY DISTRESS IN THE NEWBORN (RDS)

Keep the following in mind for *all* cases of respiratory distress in the newborn:

- Best initial therapy: Chest X-ray
- Other diagnostic studies:
  - **ABG**
  - **Blood cultures** (sepsis)
  - **Blood glucose** (hypoglycemia)
  - **CBC** (anemia or polycythemia)
  - **Cranial ultrasound** (intracranial hemorrhage)
- Best initial treatment:
  - **Oxygen:** Keep SaO2 > 95 percent.
  - Give **nasal CPAP** if high O2 requirements to prevent barotrauma and bronchopulmonary dysplasia.
  - Consider **empiric antibiotics** for suspected sepsis.

In cases of newborn respiratory distress, when hypoxia does not improve with oxygen therapy, evaluate the patient for cardiac causes of hypoxia (i.e. congenital heart defects).

Respiratory Distress Syndrome (RDS)

Clinical features are a **premature neonate** with the following:

- Tachypnea
- Nasal grunting
- Intercostals retractions within hours of birth

The hallmark finding is **hypoxemia.** Eventually **hypercarbia and respiratory acidosis develop.**

Diagnostic testing

- Best initial tests:
  - **Chest X-ray:** Ground-glass appearance
  - **Atelectasis**
  - **Air bronchograms**

- Most accurate test: **Lecithin-sphingomyelin (L/S) ratio on amniotic fluid prior to birth**

Pneumonia and RDS look identical on chest X-ray. If in doubt, give antibiotics.

Treatment:

- Best initial treatments: **Oxygen and nasal CPAP**
- Most effective treatment: **Exogenous surfactant administration** (proven to decrease mortality)

Do the following for primary prevention:

- **Antenatal betamethasone:** This is *most* effective if > 24 hours before delivery and < 34 weeks gestation.
- **Avoid prematurity:** Give **tocolytics.**
- Postnatal corticosteroids do *not* help and are *not* indicated.

Possible Complications:

- **Retinopathy of prematurity (ROP)** (hypoxemia)
- **Bronchopulmonary dysplasia** (prolonged high-concentration oxygen): Prevent with CPAP.
- **Intraventricular hemorrhage**

Give corticosteroids *immediately* to any fetus in danger of preterm delivery < 34 weeks.

Transient Tachypnea of the Newborn (TTN)

This presents as tachypnea after a **term birth** of infant delivered by **cesarean section or rapid second stage of labor.**

Perform a **chest X-ray** to look for the following:

- **Air trapping**
- **Fluid in fissures**
- **Perihilar streaking**

The best initial treatment is **oxygen** (minimal requirements needed), which results in rapid improvement within hours to days.

Meconium Aspiration

This presents as **severe respiratory distress and hypoxemia** in a **term neonate** with **hypoxia or fetal distress in utero.** (Meconium passed may be aspirated in utero or with the first postnatal breath.)

Diagnostic Testing: Perform a **chest X-ray** to look for the following:

- **Patchy infiltrates**
- **Increased AP diameter** (barrel chest)
- **Flattening of diaphragm**

Treatment:

- **Positive pressure ventilation**
- **High-frequency ventilation**
- **Nitric oxide therapy**
- **Extracorporeal membrane oxygenation**

Prevent by performing an **endotracheal intubation and airway suction** of depressed infants.

Possible Complications:

- Pulmonary artery hypertension
- Air leak (pneumothorax, pneumomediastinum)
- Aspiration pneumonitis

Diaphragmatic Hernia

This presents as **respiratory distress and scaphoid abdomen** (distress related to pulmonary hypoplasia).

Diagnostic Testing: Perform a **chest X-ray** to **look for loops** of bowel visible in the chest.

Treatment: Perform **immediate intubation** (may require extracorporeal membrane oxygenation), followed by **surgical correction.**

GASTROINTESTINAL AND HEPATOBILIARY DISORDERS

Meconium Plugs (Lower Colon) and Meconium Ileus (Lower Ileum)

This presents initially with an intestinal obstruction.

Associated conditions are the following:

- Plugs:
  - **Small left colon in IODM**
  - **Hirschsprung disease**
  - **Cystic fibrosis**
  - **Maternal drug abuse**
- Ileus: **Cystic fibrosis**

Diagnostic Testing: The best initial diagnostic test is an **abdominal X-ray.**

Treatment: Ileus with **gastografin enema.**

Upper Gastrointestinal Malformation

A newborn is born by normal vaginal delivery without complication. There is no respiratory distress. Upon his first feed, he is noted to have prominent drooling; he gags and develops respiratory distress. Chest X-ray reveals an infiltrate in the lung. Which of the following will confirm the diagnosis?

a. Arterial blood gas
b. Blood cultures
c. CT scan of chest
d. Nasogastric tube placement
e. Gastrograffin enema

*Answer: The correct answer is **D**. This patient has a **tracheoesophageal fistula (TEF)**. Classically, there is choking and gagging with the first feeding and then respiratory distress develops due to aspiration pneumonia. The feeding tube will be coiled in the chest. Don't forget to look for other abnormalities associated with VACTERL syndrome.*

> VACTERL abnormalities are the following:
> • Vertebral defects
> • Anal atresia
> • Cardiac abnormalities
> • Tracheoesophageal fistula with esophageal atresia
> • Radial and Renal anomalies
> • Limb syndrome

A premature infant is born by normal vaginal delivery without complication. There is no respiratory distress. Upon her first feed, she begins vomiting gastric and bilious material. Chest X-ray is shown. What is the most likely diagnosis?

*Answer: The most likely diagnosis is **duodenal atresia**. Half of infants with this condition are born prematurely, and the condition is associated with Down syndrome. Look for **polyhydramnios** in the prenatal exam. Treatment involves **nasogastric decompression and surgical correction**. You must search for other abnormalities (VACTERL association) with X-ray of the spine, abdominal ultrasound, and echocardiogram.*

> Differential diagnosis of double-bubble seen on X-ray includes duodenal atresia, annular pancreas, malrotation, and volvulus.

Necrotizing Enterocolitis (NEC)

NEC presents in a premature infant with **low Apgar scores** and **bloody stools, apnea, and lethargy** when feeding is started. **Abdominal wall erythema and distension are signs of ischemia.** NEC is a true medical/surgical emergency with 50 percent mortality related to ischemia and inflammation of the bowel and ultimately perforation. The greatest risk factor for NEC is premature delivery.

Diagnostic Testing: The best initial diagnostic test is an **abdominal X-ray.** (**Pneumatosis intestinalis** is pathognomonic.)

The best initial therapy is as follows:

- **Stop all feeds**
- **Decompress the gut**
- Begin **broad spectrum antibiotics**
- Evaluate for **surgical resection**

Pneumatosis intestinal is associated with necrotizing enterocolitis.

Failure to Pass Meconium

When the case describes a neonate with failure to pass meconium, proceed as follows:

- The best initial test is to perform a **rectal examination.** A patent rectum with passage of a large voluminous stool after digital exam suggests **Hirschsprung disease.**
- The next step in the workup is to obtain a **barium enema** (megacolon proximal to obstruction).
- The best confirmation test is **rectal biopsy** (absent ganglionic cells). Treatment is **surgical resection.**

An absent anal opening on exam suggests **imperforate anus.** Treatment is **surgical resection.**

JAUNDICE IN THE NEWBORN

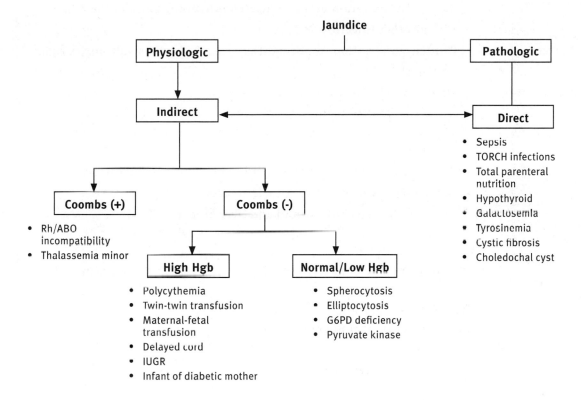

When is hyperbilirubinemia considered pathological?

- It appears on the first day of life.
- Bilirubin rises > 5 mg/dL/day.
- Bilirubin > 12 mg/dL in term infant.
- Direct bilirubin > 2 mg/dL at any time.
- Hyperbilirubinemia is present after the 2nd week of life.

Diagnostic Workup

If jaundice presents in the first 24 hours, workup includes:

- Total and direct bilirubin
- Blood type of infant and mother: Look for ABO or Rh incompatibility.
- Direct Coombs' test
- CBC, reticulocyte count, and blood smear: Assess for hemolysis.
- Urinalysis and urine culture if elevated direct bilirubin: Assess for sepsis.

If prolonged jaundice (> 2 weeks) presents, workup includes:

- If there is **NO elevation of unconjugated bilirubin,** consider the following:
  - **UTI or other infection**
  - **Bilubin conjugation abnormalities** (e.g., Gilbert's syndrome, Crigler-Najjar syndrome)
  - **Hemolysis**
  - **Intrinsic red cell membrane or enzyme defects** (spherocytosis, elliptocytosis, glucose-6-phosphate dehydrogenase deficiency, pyruvate kinase deficiency)
- If there **IS elevation of conjugated bilirubin,** consider **cholestasis:**
  - Initial diagnostic tests: **liver function tests**
  - Most specific tests: **ultrasound and liver biopsy**

Treatment

- **Phototherapy** when bilirubin > 10–12 mg/dL (normally decreases by 2 mg/dL every 4–6 hours)
- **Exchange transfusion** in any infant with suspected bilirubin encephalopathy or failure of phototherapy to reduce total bilirubin

NEONATAL SEPSIS

A 5-week-old infant is brought into the clinic with irritability, weight loss of 3lbs over the past week, and "grunting". Physical examination reveals temperature of 102.5F. There is a bulging anterior fontanel, delayed capillary refill. What is the next step in management?

*Answer: Next step in management includes transferring the patient to the emergency room and initiating a **full sepsis workup**. This includes: 1. CBC with differential 2. blood culture 3. urinalysis/urine culture and 4. chest x-ray BEFORE antibiotics are given).*

In cases of **early-onset sepsis** (within first 24 hours), **pneumonia** is the most common cause. The most common organisms involved are these:

- **Group B** *Streptococcus*
- *E. coli*
- *Haemophilus influenza*
- *Listeria monocytogenes*

In cases of **late-onset sepsis** (after first 24 hours), meningitis and bacteremia are the most common causes. The most common organisms are these:

- *Staphylococcus aureus*
- *E. coli*
- *Klebsiella*
- *Pseudomonas*

The most feared complication of jaundice is due to elevated indirect (*un*conjugated) bilirubin, which can cross the blood brain barrier, deposit in the basal ganglia and brainstem nuclei, and cause **kernicterus.** Watch out for hypotonia, seizures, opisthotonos, delayed motor skills, choreoathetosis, and sensorineural hearing loss. Management is **immediate exchange transfusion.**

A lumbar puncture is *not* part of the standard sepsis workup, *unless* the case describes irritability or lethargy suggestive of meningitis.

Treatment

- If there is *no* evidence of meningitis, prescribe **ampicillin and aminoglycoside** until 48- to 72-hour cultures are negative.
- If meningitis is possible, prescribe **ampicillin and third-generation cephalosporin** (*not* ceftriaxone).

TORCH INFECTIONS SUMMARY

Many of the TORCH infections have similar presentations. The following table highlights the distinguishing features to look for in the exam. (Refer to section 6 on obstetrics for more details.)

Infection	Classic Feature(s)	Diagnostic Workup
General features	Intrauterine growth retardation, hepatosplenomegaly, jaundice, mental retardation	Elevated total cord blood IgM
Toxoplasmosis	Hydrocephalus with generalized intracranial calcifications and chorioretinitis	IgM against toxoplasmosis
Rubella	Cataracts, deafness, and heart defects Blueberry muffin spots (extramedullary hematopoiesis)	Maternal rubella immune status negative or unknown—obtain IgM against rubella
CMV	Microcephaly with periventricular calcifications Petechiae with thrombocytopenia, sensorineural hearing loss	Urine CMV culture—if negative, excludes CMV
Herpes	First week: Pneumonia/shock Second week: Skin vesicles, keratoconjunctivitis Third to fourth week: Acute meningoencephalitis	Best initial test: Tzanck smear/culture (does not exclude disease if negative) Most specific test: PCR
Syphilis	Osteochondritis and periostitis; desquamating skin rash of palms and soles, snuffles (mucopurulent rhinitis)	Best initial test: VDRL screening Most specific test: IgM-FTA-ABS
Varicella	Neonatal: Pneumonia Congenital: Limb hypoplasia, cutaneous scars	Best initial test: IgM serology Most specific test: PCR of amniotic fluid

SEIZURES

In the newborn intensive care unit, an infant is noted to be "jittery" and has repetitive sucking movements, tongue thrusting, and brief apneic spells. Blood counts and chemistries are within normal limits. What is the initial workup of this patient?

*Answer: Seizures classically present with **subtle repetitive movements**, such as chewing, tongue thrusting, apnea, staring, blinking, or desaturations. Classic tonic-clonic movements are uncommon. Look for **ocular deviation and failure of jitteriness to subside with stimulus** (e.g., passive movement of a limb).*

Diagnostic Testing

- **EEG:** May be normal
- **CBC electrolytes, calcium, magnesium, phosphorous, glucose** (Hypoglycemia is a common cause of seizures in infants of diabetic mothers.)
- **Amino acid assay and urine organic acids** to detect inborn errors of metabolism
- To look for infectious causes, perform the following:
  - TORCH infection studies: **Total cord blood IgM** for screening
  - **Blood and urine cultures**
  - **Lumbar puncture** if meningitis is suspected
- **Ultrasound of head in preterms** to look for intraventricular hemorrhage

Treatment

- **Phenobarbital** is the initial drug of choice.
- If seizures persist, use **phenytoin.**

SUBSTANCE ABUSE AND NEONATAL WITHDRAWAL

Neonatal withdrawal presents with the following:

- **Hyperactivity**
- **Irritability**
- **Fever**
- **Diarrhea**
- **Tremors/jitters**
- **High-pitched crying**
- **Sneezing**
- **Restlessness**
- **Vomiting**
- **Nasal stuffiness**
- **Poor feeding**
- **Seizures**
- **Tachypnea**

The timing of withdrawal:

- **Heroin, cocaine, amphetamine, and alcohol withdrawal:** Presents within the first 48 hours of life.
- **Methadone withdrawal:** Presents within the first 96 hours (up to 2 weeks). This drug is associated with a higher risk of seizures.

Complications

Infants of addicted mothers are at higher risk for the following complications:

- **Low birth weight**
- **Intrauterine growth restriction (IUGR)**
- **Congenital anomalies** (alcohol, cocaine)
- **Sudden infant death syndrome (SIDS)**

Also, watch out for complications of the mother's conditions, such as the following:

- **Sexually transmitted diseases**
- **Toxemia**
- **Breech**
- **Abruption**
- **Intraventricular hemorrhage** (cocaine use)

Treatment

The best initial treatment is to prescribe **opioids** (especially if specific prenatal opioid use was known) and **phenobarbital.**

Never give naloxone to an infant born from mother with known narcotics use. It may precipitate sudden withdrawal, including seizures.

TERATOGENESIS AND THE EFFECT OF DRUGS ON THE NEONATE

Drug	Effect	Drug	Effect
Anesthetics	Respiratory, CNS depression	**Isotretinoin**	Facial and ear anomalies, congenital heart disease
Barbiturates	Respiratory, CNS depression	**Phenytoin**	Hypoplastic nails, typical facies, IUGR
Magnesium sulfate	Respiratory depression	**Diethylstilbestrol (DES)**	Vaginal adenocarcinoma
Phenobarbital	Vitamin K deficiency	**Tetracycline**	Enamel hypoplasia, discolored teeth
Sulfonamides	Displaces bilirubin from albumin	**Lithium**	Ebstein's anomaly
NSAIDs	Premature closure of ductus arteriosus	**Warfarin**	Facial dysmorphism and chondrodysplasia
ACE inhibitors	Craniofacial abnormalities	**Valproate/ Carbamezepine**	Mental retardation, neural tube defects

GENETICS/DYSMORPHOLOGY

Condition	Classic Feature(s)	Diagnostic Workup/Disease Associations
Trisomy 21: Down syndrome Risk associated with advanced maternal age (> 35 years)	Upward slanting palpebral fissures; speckling of iris (Brushfield spots); inner epicanthal folds; small stature; late fontanel closure; mental retardation	• Hearing exam • Echocardiogram: Endocardiac cushion defect > VSD > PDA, ASD; MVP (Cardiac abnormalities are a major cause of early mortality.) • Gastrointestinal: TEF, duodenal atresia • TSH: Hypothyroidism • With advancing age, have a low probability of developing acute lymphocytic leukemia and early-onset Alzheimer's disease
Trisomy 18: Edwards syndrome	Low-set, malformed ears; microcephaly; micrognathia; clenched hand—index over third, fifth over fourth; rocker-bottom feet and hammer toe; omphalocele	• Echocardiogram: VSD, ASD, PDA • Renal ultrasound: Polycystic kidneys, ectopic or double ureter • Most patients do not survive first year
Trisomy 13: Patau syndrome	Defect of midface, eye, and forebrain development: Holoprosencephaly, microcephaly, microphthalmia, cleft lip/palate	• Echocardiogram: VSD, PDA, ASD • Renal ultrasound: Polycystic kidneys • Single umbilical artery
Aniridia-Wilms' tumor association (WAGR syndrome)	**W**ilms' **A**niridia **G**U anomalies Mental **R**etardation	• When you see an infant with aniridia, do a complete workup for WAGR syndrome.
Klinefelter syndrome (XXY) 1:500 males	Low IQ, behavioral problems, slim with long limbs, gynecomastia	• Testosterone levels: Hypogonadism and hypogenitalism • Replace testosterone at 11–12 years of age.
Turner syndrome (XO) Sporadic; no association with maternal age	Small-stature female, gonadal dysgenesis, low IQ, congenital lymphedema, webbed posterior neck, broad chest, wide-spaced nipples	• Renal ultrasound: Horseshoe kidney, double renal pelvis • Cardiac: Bicuspid aortic valve, coarctation of the aorta • Thyroid function: Primary hypothyroidism • Can give estrogen, growth hormone, and anabolic steroid replacement
Fragile X syndrome Fragile site on long arm of X Molecular diagnosis—variable number of repeat CGG	Macrocephaly in early childhood, large ears, large testes Most common cause of mental retardation in boys	• Attention deficit hyperactivity syndrome

Condition	Classic Feature(s)	Diagnostic Workup/Disease Associations
Beckwith-Wiedemann syndrome IGF-2 disrupted at 11p15.5	Multiorgan enlargement: Macrosomia, macroglossia, pancreatic beta cell hyperplasia (hypoglycemia), large kidneys, neonatal polycythemia	• Increased risk of abdominal tumors • Obtain ultrasounds and serum AFP every 6 months through 6 years of age to look for Wilms' tumor and hepatoblastoma
Prader-Willi syndrome Deletion at 15q11q13 paternal chromosome responsible	Obesity, mental retardation, binge eating, small genitalia	• Decreased life expectancy related to morbid obesity
Angelman syndrome (happy puppet syndrome) Deletion of 15q11q13 that is maternally derived	Mental retardation, inappropriate laughter, absent speech or < 6 words, ataxia and jerky arm movements resembling a puppet gait, recurrent seizures	• 80 percent develop epilepsy
Robin sequence (Pierre Robin) Associated with fetal alcohol syndrome, Edwards syndrome	Mandibular hypoplasia, cleft palate	• Monitor airway: Obstruction possible over first 4 weeks of life

GROWTH, NUTRITION, AND DEVELOPMENT

EXAM TIPS ON PEDIATRIC GROWTH

- Birth weight normally doubles by 6 months and triples by 1 year.
- Height percentile at 2 years of age normally correlates with final adult height percentile.
- Best indicator for acute malnutrition is weight/height < 5th percentile.
- Best indicator for under- and overweight is BMI.
- Skeletal maturity is related to sexual maturity (less related to chronologic age).
- The most common cause of failure to thrive in all age groups is psychosocial deprivation.
- All cases of underfeeding must be reported to child protective services (CPS).
- You must work up any child who has crossed 2 major growth percentiles.

> Birth weight is normal in patients with *either* genetic short stature or constitutional delay of growth. Patients with both conditions have normal growth velocity, which is below and parallel to the normal growth curve.

Description of Growth Pattern	Differential Diagnosis	Workup
↓ weight gain more than ↓ length/height	• Undernutrition • Inadequate digestion • Malabsorption (infection, celiac disease, cystic fibrosis, disaccharide deficiency, protein-losing enteropathy)	Assess caloric intake Perform stool studies for fat Perform sweat chloride test
Normal weight gain ↓ length/height	• Growth hormone or thyroid hormone deficiency • Excessive cortisol secretion • Skeletal dysplasias	Growth Hormone (GH) deficiency: • Insulin-like growth factor 1 (IGF-1) and IGF-binding protein 3 (IGF-BP3) Thyroid hormone: • TSH, free T4, free T3 Cushings: • 24-hour urinary cortisol or free cortisol Bone age (X-ray of hand and wrist): • Skeletal dysplasia: no delay in bone age and disproportionate bone length on exam
↓ weight gain equals ↓ length/height	Systemic illness: • Heart failure • Inflammation (e.g., inflammatory bowel disease or arthritis) • Renal insufficiency • Hepatic insufficiency Genetic short stature Constitutional delay in growth and development	Inflammatory markers: • CRP, ESR, CBC with dif Organ dysfunction: • LFT, creatinine, BUN • Electrolytes Bone age: • Genetic short stature: The bone age is close to the chronological age; puberty occurs at the normal time. • Constitutional delay of growth: The bone age is delayed, and puberty occurs later than in most children.

BREASTFEEDING

The advantages of breastfeeding:

- **Passive transfer of T-cell immunity:** Decreased risk of allergies and gastrointestinal and respiratory infections
- **Psychological/emotional:** Maternal-infant bonding

Following are the contraindications to breastfeeding:

- **HIV**
- **CMV**
- **HSV** *if* lesions on breast
- **HBV** *until* neonate has received HBV vaccine
- **Acute maternal disease if absent in infant** (e.g., tuberculosis, sepsis)
- **Breast cancer**
- **Substance abuse**
- **Drugs,** as shown on the following table:

Breast feeding is *not* contraindicated in mastitis.

Absolute Contraindications	Relative Contraindications
Antineoplastics	Neuroleptics
Iodide/mercurials	Sedatives
Lithium	Metronidazole
Chloramphenicol	Tetracycline
Nicotine	Sulfonamides
Alcohol	Steroids

HIGH-YIELD DEVELOPMENTAL MILESTONES

The absence of milestone behavior or persistence of it beyond a given time frame signifies **CNS dysfunction.** Exam questions typically describe an infant's/child's skills and ask for the corresponding age.

Age	Milestone
Newborn reflexes	Moro, grasp, rooting, tonic neck, and placing reflexes: Appear at birth and disappear at 4–6 months Parachute reflex (extension of arms when fall simulated): Present at 6–8 months and persists
9 months	Has pincer grasp, creeps and crawls, knows own name
12 months	Cruises, says one or more words, plays ball
15 months	Builds 3-cube tower, walks alone, makes lines and scribbles
18 months	Builds 4-cube tower, walks down stairs, says 10 words, feeds self
24 months	Builds 7-cube tower, runs well, goes up and down stairs, jumps with 2 feet, threads shoelaces, handles spoon, says 2–3 sentences
36 months	Walks downstairs alternating feet, rides tricycle, knows age and sex, understands taking turns
48 months	Hops on one foot, throws ball overhead, tells stories, participates in group play

BEHAVIORAL DISORDERS

A 4-year-old boy has problems with bedwetting. The mother says that during the day, he has no problems but is usually wet 6 of 7 mornings. He does not report dysuria or frequency and has not had increased thirst. The mother also says that he is a deep sleeper. Which of the following is the most appropriate next step in management?

a. Give anticholinergics.

b. Give desmopressin.

c. Give prophylactic antibiotics.

d. Perform renal ultrasound.

e. Reassure mother that bedwetting is normal.

*Answer: The correct answer is **E**. Bedwetting before age 5 (before bladder control is anticipated) is normal.*

ENURESIS

Enurese is the **involuntary voiding of urine, occurring at least twice a week for at least 3 months in children over 5 years** (when bladder control is anticipated). **Nocturnal enuresis** (nighttime wetting) is more common in boys, whereas **diurnal enuresis** (daytime wetting) is more common in girls and is associated with a higher rate of urinary tract infections (UTIs).

Diagnostic Testing

- Best initial test: **Urinalysis** in all patients
- If signs of infection are present: **Urine culture**
- If recurrent UTIs: **Bladder/renal ultrasound** (postvoid residual, anatomical abnormalities) or **voiding cystourethrogram**

Treatment

- Best initial treatment: Behavior and motivational therapy (Never punish the child.)
- If behavioral therapy fails: **tricyclic drugs, imipramine, and desmopressin** (to decrease the volume of urine produced)

Of patients with enuresis, 15 percent spontaneously resolve each year.

ENCOPRESIS

Encopresis is the **intentional or involuntary passage of feces in inappropriate settings,** such as into clothing or onto the floor, **in children > 4 years** (the age by which most children control bowel movements).

Diagnostic Testing

- Best initial test: **Abdominal X-ray.** This distinguishes between retentive (most common; associated with constipation and overflow incontinence) and nonretentive (associated with abuse).
- Do *not* miss uncommon causes: Hirschprung's disease, anal fissure, ulcerative colitis, or spinal cord abnormalities.

Treatment

- Best initial therapies:
  - **Retentive** encopresis: **Disimpaction, stool softeners, and behavior intervention**
  - **Nonretentive** encopresis: **Behavior modification alone**

IMMUNIZATIONS

EXAM TIPS

- Premature infants or low-birth-weight babies:
  - Do *not* delay immunizations—immunize at chronological age.
  - Do *not* dose-adjust immunizations.
- Do *not* give live vaccines to immunocompromized patients.

- The following are *not* contraindications to immunization:
  - A reaction to a previous DPT of temperature < 105°F, redness, soreness, and swelling
  - A mild, acute illness in an otherwise well child
  - Concurrent antimicrobial therapy
  - A family history of seizures or sudden infant death syndrome
- **MMR:** Documented egg allergy is *not* a contraindication.
- **Influenza vaccine** and **yellow fever** vaccines: Egg allergy *does* contraindicate.
- MMR does *not* cause autism or inflammatory bowel disease.
- Hepatitis B vaccine does *not* cause demyelinating neurologic disorders.
- Meningococcal vaccination is *not* related to development of Guillain-Barré.

Recommended Immunization Schedule for Persons Aged 0–6 Years—UNITED STATES • 2008
For those who fall behind or start late, see the catch-up schedule

Vaccine ▼ Age ▶	Birth	1 month	2 months	4 months	6 months	12 months	15 months	18 months	19–23 months	2–3 years	4–6 years
Hepatitis B[1]	HepB	HepB		see footnote 1		HepB					
Rotavirus[2]			Rota	Rota	Rota						
Diphtheria, Tetanus, Pertussis[3]			DTaP	DTaP	DTaP	see footnote 3	DTaP				DTaP
Haemophilus influenzae type b[4]			Hib	Hib	Hib[4]	Hib					
Pneumococcal[5]			PCV	PCV	PCV	PCV				PPV	
Inactivated Poliovirus			IPV	IPV		IPV					IPV
Influenza[6]						Influenza (Yearly)					
Measles, Mumps, Rubella[7]						MMR					MMR
Varicella[8]						Varicella					Varicella
Hepatitis A[9]						HepA (2 doses)				HepA Series	
Meningococcal[10]										MCV4	

Range of recommended ages
Certain high-risk groups

Recommended Immunization Schedule for Persons Aged 7–18 Years—UNITED STATES • 2008
For those who fall behind or start late, see the green bars and the catch-up schedule

Vaccine ▼ Age ▶	7–10 years	11–12 years	13–18 years
Diphtheria, Tetanus, Pertussis[1]	see footnote 1	Tdap	Tdap
Human Papillomavirus[2]	see footnote 2	HPV (3 doses)	HPV Series
Meningococcal[3]	MCV4	MCV4	MCV4
Pneumococcal[4]	PPV		
Influenza[5]	Influenza (Yearly)		
Hepatitis A[6]	HepA Series		
Hepatitis B[7]	HepB Series		
Inactivated Poliovirus[8]	IPV Series		
Measles, Mumps, Rubella[9]	MMR Series		
Varicella[10]	Varicella Series		

Range of recommended ages
Catch-up immunization
Certain high-risk groups

www.cdc.gov/vaccines/recs/schedules/child-schedule.htm

ACTIVE IMMUNIZATIONS AFTER EXPOSURE

Measles	0–6 months: Ig
	6–12 months: Ig plus vaccine
	> 12 months: Vaccine only within 72 hours of exposure
	Pregnant or immunocompromised: Ig only
Varicella	Susceptible children and household contacts: VZIG and vaccine
	Susceptible pregnant women, newborns whose mothers had chicken pox within 5 days before delivery to 48 hours after delivery: VZIG
Hepatitis	Hepatitis B: Ig plus vaccine; repeat vaccine at 1 and 6 months
	Hepatitis A: > 2 years only, Ig plus vaccine
Mumps and Rubella	No postexposure protection available

SPECIFIC ROUTINE VACCINATIONS

Hepatitis B	If mother is HBsAg negative:
	• First dose at birth. A total of 3 doses by **18 months**.
	If mother is HBsAg positive:
	• First dose of hepatitis B virus (HBV) plus hepatitis B Ig at 2 different sites within 12 hours of birth. A total of 3 doses by **6 months**.
DTaP	Total of 5 doses is recommended before school entry (last dose age 4–6 years).
	Pertussis booster vaccine *also* given during adolescence, regardless of immunization.
	Td is given at 11–12 years, then every 10 years.
HiB conjugated vaccine	Does not cover nontypeable *Haemophilus*.
	Not given after age of 5.
	Invasive disease does not confirm immunity; patients still require vaccines if < 5.
Varicella	Has been associated with the development of herpes zoster after immunization.
Meningococcal conjugate vaccine	Given at age 11–12 or at age 15.
	Indicated for all college freshmen living in dormitories.
	Menomune® (MPSV4) indicated in children aged **2–10**.

CHILD ABUSE

Workup

- Laboratory studies: **PT, PTT, platelets, bleeding time**
- **Skeletal survey**
- If **severe injuries** (even with no neurological signs), perform the following:
  - **Head CT scan ± MRI**
  - **Ophthalmologic examination**
- If **abdominal trauma,** perform the following:
  - **Urine and stool for blood**
  - **Liver and pancreatic enzymes**
  - **Abdominal CT scan**

Treatment

1. The first step is *always* is to **address medical and/or surgical issues.**
2. Then report any child suspected of being abused or neglected to **child protective services (CPS).** Initial action includes a phone report; in most states, a written report is then required within 48 hours.

The following are indications for hospitalization:

- **Medical condition requires it.**
- **Diagnosis is unclear.**
- **There is no alternative safe place.**

If parents refuse hospitalization or treatment, the physician must get an **emergency court order.**

You *must* explain to the parent why an inflicted injury is suspected abuse, that you are legally obligated to report it, that you have made a referral to protect the child, and that a CPS worker and law enforcement officer will be involved.

RESPIRATORY DISEASES

Condition	Classic Presentation	Diagnosis	Steps in Management	Complication(s)/ Prognosis
Croup *Parainfluenza 1 or 3, Influenza A or B*	Child age 3 months to 5 years with URT symptoms: Rhinorrhea, sore throat, hoarseness and deep barking cough, inspiratory stridor, tachypnea. Symptoms are worse at night.	Neck X-ray (*not* needed for diagnosis)	1. Humidified oxygen 2. Nebulized epinephrine and corticosteroids Antitussives, decongestants, sedatives, or antibiotics are *not* used in the management of croup.	Spontaneous resolution in 1 week Always suspect diagnosis of epiglottitis.
Epiglottitis *H. influenza type B* (now less common) *S. pyogenes, S. pneumoniae, S. aureus, Mycoplasma*	Sudden onset muffled voice, drooling, dysphagia, high fever, and inspiratory stridor Patient prefers sitting in the tripod position. Patient has a toxic appearance.	This is a medical emergency. Go straight to management based on clinical diagnosis. Perform diagnostic workup *after* stabilization: • Neck X-ray (thumb-print sign) • Blood cultures • Nasopharyngoscopy in the OR • Epiglottic swab culture	1. Transfer to hospital/OR 2. Consult ENT and anesthesia 3. Intubate 4. Give antibiotics (ceftriaxone) and steroids 5. Give rifampin prophylaxis to household contacts if *H. influenza* positive	Airway obstruction and death
Bacterial tracheitis *S. aureus*	Brassy cough, high fever, respiratory distress, but *no* drooling or dysphagia; child < 3 years; usually occurs after viral URTI	Clinical plus laryngoscopy: • Chest X-ray shows subglottic narrowing plus ragged tracheal air column • Blood cultures • Throat cultures	Antistaphylococcal antibiotics May require intubation if severe.	Airway obstruction

Differentiate epiglottitis from croup by the *absence* of a barking cough.

Following are clues to less-common disorders:

- **Diphtheritic croup** (extremely rare in North America): Presents with a gray-white pharyngeal membrane; may cover soft palate; bleeds easily. Don't forget that diphtheria is a notifiable disease!

- **Foreign body aspiration:** Look for sudden choking/coughing without warning.

- **Retropharyngeal abscess:** Patient has drooling and difficulty swallowing.

- **Extrinsic compression** (vascular ring) or **intraluminal obstruction** (masses): Patient has continued symptoms and does not improve with treatment.

- **Angioedema:** This is due to a sudden allergic reaction. (Trigger is given in the case.) Manage with steroids and epinephrine. If severe, intubate for airway protection.

- **Pertussis:** Severe cough develops after 1–2 weeks with characteristic whoop and spells of cough (paroxysms). Look for child with incomplete immunization history.

The most common sites of foreign body aspiration are the following:
- In children > 1 year: Larynx
- In children < 1 year: Trachea or right mainstem bronchus

A toddler presents to the emergency center with sudden onset respiratory distress. The mother reports that the child was without symptoms, playing with LEGOS in the living room with her siblings. On physical examination, the patient is drooling and in moderate respiratory distress. There are decreased breath sounds on the right with intercostal retractions. Which of the following is the most appropriate next step in management?

a. Antibiotics

b. Bronchoscopy

c. Chest X-ray

d. Cricothyroidotomy

e. Throat cultures

*Answer: The correct answer is **B**. Bronchoscopy is indicated both to visualize a suspected foreign body and for foreign body retrieval. If there is significant respiratory distress and hypoxemia, emergency cricothyroidotomy may be indicated. Foreign bodies are found most commonly in children < 4 years.*

Recurrent infections in a young child should always raise the suspicion of previously undiagnosed aspiration. Get a chest X-ray to look for postobstruction atelectasis or visualization of the foreign body.

INFLAMMATION OF THE SMALL AIRWAYS

Bronchiolitis

A 6-month-old infant presents to the physician with a 3-day history of upper respiratory tract infection, wheezy cough, and dyspnea. On physical examination, the patient has a temperature of 39°C (102°F), respirations of 60 breaths/minute, nasal flaring, and accessory muscle usage. The patient appears to be air hungry, and the oxygen saturation is 92 percent.

The pathophysiology of bronchiolitis is as follows:

- Respiratory syncytial virus (RSV) (50 percent)
- Parainfluenza
- Adenovirus
- Other viruses

Bronchiolitis results in **inflammation,** which results in **ball-valve obstruction,** which results in **air trapping and overinflation.**

The classic presentation is in a **child < 2 years of age** (most severe in children 1–2 months old) with the following symptoms:

- **Mild URI**
- **Fever**
- **Paroxysmal wheezy cough**
- **Dyspnea**
- **Tachypnea**
- **Apnea** (in young infants)
- On exam, there is **wheezing and prolonged expirations.**

Diagnosis

Is **clinical.** Following are diagnostic tests to perform:

- Best initial test: **Chest X-ray** shows hyperinflation with patchy atelectasis (May look like early pneumonia.)
- Most specific test: **Immunofluorescence of nasopharyngeal swab**

Treatment

Is **supportive only:**

- Hospitalize *if* severe tachypnea (> 60/minute), pyrexia, and intercostals retractions are present. Give trial of beta-agonists nebulizers.
- Steroids are *not* indicated.

Prevention

In high-risk patients *only,* is by giving hyperimmune RSV IVIG or monoclonal antibody to RSV F protein (palivizumab).

Pneumonia

Classic presentations:

- **Viral:** Most common cause in children < 5 years. Most commonly RSV.
  - **URI symptoms**
  - **Low-grade fever**
  - **Tachypnea** (most consistent finding)
- **Bacterial:** Most common cause in children > 5 years. Most commonly *S. pneumoniae, M. pneumoniae,* or *C. pneumoniae* (*not* trachomatis).
  - **Acute-onset, sudden, shaking chills**
  - **High fever**
  - **Prominent cough**
  - **Pleuritic chest pain**
  - **Markedly diminished breath sounds**
  - **Dullness to percussion**
- *Chlamydia trachomatis:* Infants 1–3 months of age with insidious onset.
  - *No* fever or wheezing (distinguishes from RSV) +/– conjunctivitis at birth
  - Classic findings are **staccato cough** and **peripheral eosinophilia.**

Diagnostic testing:

- **Chest X-ray:**
  - **Viral:** Hyperinflation with bilateral interstitial infiltrates and peribronchial cuffing
  - **Pneumococcal:** Confluent lobar consolidation
  - *Mycoplasma/Chlamydia:* Unilateral lower-lobe interstitial pneumonia; looks worse than presentation
- **CBC with differential:**
  - Viral usually < 20,000
  - Bacterial 15,000–40,000
- **Viral antigens:** IgM titers for mycoplasma
- **Blood cultures**

In cases of pneumonia, do *not* order sputum cultures. They are of no help in the management of pneumonia in children.

Treatment:

- **Outpatient (mild cases): Amoxicillin** is the best choice. (Alternatives are cefuroxime and amoxicillin/clavulanic acid.)
- **Hospitalized: IV cefuroxime.** (If *S. aureus,* add **vancomycin.**)

- If viral origin suspected, may withhold antibiotics. However, give antibiotics if the child deteriorates. (Up to 30 percent may have coexisting bacterial pathogens.)
- *Chlamydia or Mycoplasma:* **Erythromycin** or other macrolide

CYSTIC FIBROSIS (CF)

A 3-year-old white female presents with rectal prolapse. She is noted to be in the less-than-5th percentile for weight and height. The parents also note that she has a foul-smelling bulky stool each day that "floats." They also state that the child has developed a repetitive cough over the last few months. What is the first step in workup in this patient?

a. Genetic testing

b. Pulmonary function tests

c. Rectal biopsy

d. Sweat chloride

e. Stool studies

*Answer: The answer is **D**. Sweat chloride is the best initial test to diagnose cystic fibrosis.*

Clinical Presentation

The most common initial presentation of cystic fibrosis is **meconium ileus.** Other signs and symptoms that warrant workup for CF are the following:

- **Failure to thrive** from malabsorption (steatorrhea due to pancreatic exocrine insufficiency, vitamin ADEK deficiency)
- **Rectal prolapse:** Most often in infants with steatorrhea, malnutrition, and cough
- **Persistent cough** in first year of life with copious purulent mucus production

Other associated conditions are **infertility and allergic bronchopulmonary aspergillosis.**

Diagnostic Testing

- Best initial and most specific test: **Two elevated sweat chloride concentrations (> 60 mEq/L) obtained on separate days.**
- **Genetic testing** is highly accurate but does not detect all chromosome-7 mutations. It is done to detect carrier status and for prenatal diagnosis.
- **Newborn screening:** Determine immunoreactive trypsinogen in **blood spots** and then confirm with **sweat** or **DNA testing.**
- **Chest X-ray** is useful in monitoring course of disease and acute exacerbations.
- **Pulmonary function testing** is not done until age 5 or 6 to evaluate disease progression (obstructive → restrictive).

Treatment

Supportive care consists of the following:

- Aerosol treatment
- Albuterol/saline
- Chest physical therapy with postural drainage
- Pancrelipase: Aids digestion in patients with pancreatic dysfunction.

The following treatment has shown to improve survival:

- **Ibuprofen** is used to reduce inflammatory lung response and slows the patient's decline.
- **Azithromycin** has also been shown to slow rate of decline in FEV1 in patients < 13 years.
- **Antibiotics** during exacerbations delay progression of lung disease.

Other important management considerations are these:

- Give all routine vaccinations *plus* pneumococcal and yearly influenza vaccine.
- *Never* delay antibiotic therapy (even if fever and tachypnea are absent).
- Steroids improve PFTs in the short term, but there's no persistent benefit when steroids are stopped.
- Expectorants (guaiphenesin or iodides) are *not* effective in the removal of respiratory secretions.

Use antibiotics to treat CF as follows:

- **Mild disease:** Give macrolide, trimethoprim-sulfamethoxazole (TMP-SMX), or ciprofloxacin.
- **Documented infection with *Pseudomonas* or *S. aureus:*** Treat aggressively with piperacillin plus tobramycin or ceftazidime.
- **Resistant pathogens:** Use inhaled tobramycin.

> When is a murmur on the exam innocent?
> - When the question includes fever, infection, or anxiety
> - When it is *only* systolic (never diastolic)
> - When it is < grade 2/6

CARDIOLOGY

CONGENITAL HEART DISEASE (CHD)

The most common symptom of **acyanotic defects** is **congestive heart failure.** The most common acyanotic lesions are these:

- **Ventricular septal defect**
- **Atrial septal defect**
- **Atrioventricular canal**

- **Pulmonary stenosis**
- **Patent ductus arteriosus**
- **Aortic stenosis**
- **Coarctation of the aorta**

In infants with **cyanotic defects,** the primary concern is **hypoxia.** The most common defects associated with cyanosis are these:

- **Tetralogy of Fallot**
- **Transposition of the great arteries**

Consider CHD in any child presenting with the following:

- **Shock, tachypnea, cyanosis** (especially if fever is absent): Note that cyanosis and hypoxemia classically do *not* respond to oxygen as is seen in pulmonary conditions.
- Infants: **Feeding difficulty, sweating while feeding, rapid respirations, easy fatigue**
- Older children: **Dyspnea on exertion, shortness of breath, failure to thrive**
- Abnormalities on exam:
  - **Upper extremity hypertension** or **decreased lower extremity blood pressures**
  - **Decreased femoral pulses** (obstructive lesions of the left side of the heart)
  - **Facial edema, hepatomegaly**
  - **Heart sounds:** Pansystolic murmur, grade 3/6 murmurs, PMI at upper left sternal border, harsh murmur, early midsystolic click, abnormal S2

The presence or absence of a heart murmur is *not* used to suggest CHD.

Do *not* be reassured by normal antenatal ultrasounds; the majority of CHD cases are diagnosed after delivery.

Functional closure of the ductus arteriosis may be delayed in CHD. Because of this,

- CHDs that rely on the ductus will present within 1 month;
- infants with left-to-right shunting lesions will present between 2–6 months of age.

Because sepsis and CHD present very similarly, begin antibiotic therapy at the same time as workup for CHD.

Diagnostic Testing

- Best initial tests: **Chest X-ray and ECG.** Increased pulmonary vascular markings are the following:
  - Transposition of the great arteries (TGA)
  - Hypoplastic left heart syndrome
  - Truncus arteriosis
- Most specific test: **Echocardiography**

High-Yield Congenital Heart Defects

Acyanotic lesions	
Heart Defect	**Comments**
Ventricular septal defect	Harsh holosystolic murmur over lower left sternal border ± thrill; loud pulmonic S2
	Almost half of cases have spontaneous closure within the first 6 months.
	Surgical repair if failure to thrive, pulmonary hypertension, or right-to-left shunt > 2:1
Atrial septal defect	Loud S1, wide fixed splitting of S2, systolic ejection murmur along left upper sternal border. Majority are asymptomatic, are of secundum types, and close by age 4.
	Primary and sinus types require surgery.
	Late complications: Mitral valve prolapse, dysrhythmias, and pulmonary hypertension
Atrioventricular canal	Combination of the primum type of atrial septal defect, ventricular septal defect, and common atrioventricular valve
	Presentation similar to ventricular septal defect
	Perform surgery in infancy *before* pulmonary hypertension develops.
Pulmonary stenosis	May be asymptomatic or may result in severe congestive heart failure.
	Give prostaglandin E1 infusion at birth.
	Attempt balloon valvuloplasty.
Patent ductus arteriosus	More common in girls (2:1), babies where maternal rubella infection was present, and premature infants
	Wide pulse pressure, bounding arterial pulses, and characteristic sound of "machinery" (to-and-fro murmur)
	Indomethacin-induced closure helpful in premature infants.
	Term infants often require surgical closure.
Aortic stenosis	Early systolic ejection click at apex of left sternal border
	Valve replacement and anticoagulation may be required.
Coarctation of the aorta	Of all cases, 98 percent occur at origin of left subclavian artery.
	Blood pressure higher in arms than legs, bounding pulses in arms and decreased pulses in legs
	Ductus dependant: Give PGE1 infusion to maintain ductus patent (ensures lower extremity blood flow)
	Surgery repair after stabilization

Cyanotic lesions	
Heart Defect	**Comments**
Tetralogy of Fallot	Most common CHD beyond infancy
	Defects include ventricular septal defect, right ventricular hypertrophy, right outflow obstruction, and overiding aorta
	Substernal right ventricular impulse, systolic thrill along the left sternal border
	Intermittent episodes of hyperpnea, irritability, cyanosis with decreased intensity of murmur
	Treatment: Give oxygen, beta blocker, PGE1 infusion for cyanosis present at birth
	Surgical repair at 4–12 months
Transposition of the great arteries	Most common cyanotic lesion presenting in the immediate newborn period. More common in infant of diabetic mother.
	S2 usually single and loud, murmurs usually absent
	Ductus-dependent: Give PGE1 to keep ductus open.
	Definitive surgical switch of aorta and pulmonary artery needed as soon as possible.

ANTIOBIOTIC PROPHYLAXIS AND PREVENTION OF ENDOCARDITIS

Giving antibiotics prior to dental procedures is no longer recommended *except* with the following:

- Prosthetic valves
- Previous endocarditis
- Congenital heart disease (unrepeaired or repaired with persistent defect)
- Cardiac transplantation patients with cardiac valve abnormalities

Antibiotics prior to genitourinary or gastrointestinal procedures are no longer recommended, *even* in high-risk patients.

HYPERTENSION

Hypertension is defined as **blood pressure > 95 percentile based on normo grams.** Routine blood pressure checks beginning at age 3 are recommended. On exam, be sure to check all 4 extremities (coarctation).

Always work up for secondary hypertension in infants and younger children under the following circumstances:

- **Newborns:** Umbilical artery catheters → renal artery/vein thrombosis.
- **Early childhood:** Renal parenchymal disease, coarctation, endocrine, medications
- **Adolescents:** Essential hypertension is associated with obesity.
  - Evaluate for renal and renovascular hypertension.

- Majority of causes may be due to urinary tract infection (secondary to an obstructive lesion), acute glomerulonephritis, Henoch-Schönlein purpura with nephritis, hemolytic uremic syndrome, acute tubular necrosis, renal trauma, leukemic infiltrates, mass lesions, and renal artery stenosis.

Consider renal causes of hypertension in EVERY pediatric patient presenting with hypertension.

Diagnostic Testing
- Screening tests:
  - **CBC**
  - **Urinalysis**
  - **Urine culture**
  - **Electrolytes**
  - **Glucose**
  - **BUN**
  - **Creatinine**
  - **Calcium**
  - **Uric acid**
  - **Lipid panel** with essential hypertension and positive family history
- **Echocardiogram** for chronicity (left ventricular hypertrophy)
- Evaluating the kidneys:
  - **Renal ultrasound**
  - **Voiding cystourethrogram,** if there is a history of repeated UTIs (especially < 5 years)
  - **24-hour urine collection** for protein excretion and creatinine clearance
  - **Angiography** for plasma renin activity in renal veins and inferior vena cava (IVC)
  - **Plasma renin activity (PRA):** Best screen for renovascular and renal disorders
- Endocrine causes:
  - **Urine and serum catecholamines,** if pheochromocytoma is suspected
  - **Thyroid and adrenal hormone levels**
- **Drug screening** (in adolescents), if drug abuse is suspected

Treatment
- If the patient is obese, order **lifestyle changes:**
  - **Weight control**
  - **Aerobic exercise**
  - **No-added-salt diet**
  - **Monitoring of blood pressure**

- If there is no response to lifestyle changes, give **antihypertensives:**
  - The best initial antihypertensive is a **diuretic** or **beta blocker.**
  - Then add **calcium channel blocker and ACE inhibitor** (good in high-renin hypertension secondary to renovascular or renal disease or high-renin essential hypertension)
  - In the case of an **adolescent with severe hypertension,** *start* with ACE inhibitor and calcium channel blocker.

GASTROINTESTINAL DISEASE

DIARRHEA

Acute Diarrhea

The most common cause of acute diarrhea in infancy is a **rotavirus.** The most common causes of bloody diarrhea are *Campylobacter,* **amoeba** *(E. histolytica), Shigella, E. Coli,* and *Salmonella.*

The best initial test is a stool examination for the following:

- **Stool cultures** with blood, leukocytes, suspected hemolytic uremic syndrome
- *Clostridium difficile* **toxin** if a recent history of antibiotics
- **Ovum and parasites**
- **Enzyme immunoassays for viruses**

The best initial therapy is **hydration and fluid and electrolyte replacement.** Do *not* use antidiarrheals in children. Antibiotics are rarely used (even in bacterial diarrhea), except for the following cases:

- *Shigella:* Trimethoprim/sulfamethoxazole
- *Campylobacter:* Self-limiting. Erythromycin speeds recovery and reduces carrier state and is recommended for patients with severe disease or dysentery.
- *Salmonella:* Treatment indicated only for patients < 3 months old, who are toxic, who have disseminated disease, or who have S. typhi.
- *C. difficile:* Metronidazole or vancomycin and discontinuation of other antibiotics
- *E. histolytica* **or** *Giardia:* Metronidazole
- *Cryptosporidium:* Treat underlying HIV infection by raising CD4 counts with therapy.

Hemolytic Uremic Syndrome (HUS)

- HUS is a complication of acute invasive (bloody) diarrhea, most commonly caused by *E. coli* O157:H7 (also *Shigella, Salmonella, Campylobacter*).
- *Never* give antibiotics in suspected cases of *E. coli* O157:H7—there is an increased risk of developing HUS.
- Young children present 5–10 days after infection with pallor (microangiopathic hemolytic anemia), weakness, oliguria, and acute renal insufficiency or acute renal failure (ARF). (HUS is the most common cause of ARF in young children.)
- Look for anemia, helmet cells, burr cells, fragmented cells, elevated WBCs, negative Coombs, low platelets (< 100,000/ mm3), low-grade microscopic hematuria, and proteinuria.
- Treatment: Supportive care, treatment of hypertension, aggressive nutrition, early dialysis
- Prognosis: More than 90 percent of patients survive the acute stage; a small number develop end-stage renal disease (ESRD).

Chronic Diarrhea

Chronic, nonspecific diarrhea presents with **normal weight, height, and nutritional status with no fat in stool.** History usually includes **excessive intake of fruit juice or carbonated fluids** or **low fat intake.** If there is weight loss and stool with high fat, screen for malabsorption syndromes (see below).

MALABSORPTION

Malabsorption may appear from birth or after introduction of new foods.

Diagnostic Testing
- **Fat malabsorption:**
  - Best initial screening test: **Sudan black stain**
  - Best confirmatory test: **72-hour stool for fecal fat** (gold standard for steatorrhea)
  - **Serum trypsinogen screens** for pancreatic function

- Pancreatic insufficiency presents with prominent steatorrhea. Get a sweat chloride test to rule in/ out cystic fibrosis.
- Giardiasis is the only infection that causes chronic malabsorption. If you suspect giardiasis, order a duodenal aspirate/ biopsy or immunoassay.
- Malrotation can present with malabsorption and incomplete bowel obstruction.

- **Carbohydrate malabsorption:**
  - Best initial test: **Clinitest** (measures reducing substances in stool)
  - Most specific test: **Breath hydrogen test**
- **Protein malabsorption:** *Cannot* be evaluated directly.
  - Best initial test: **Spot stool alpha 1-antitrypsin level**
- **Vitamins/minerals:** Measure serum Fe, folate, Ca, Zn, and Mg and vitamins B12, D, and A.

CELIAC DISEASE

Celiac disease presents with the following within the first 2 years:

- Chronic diarrhea
- Failure to thrive
- Growth retardation
- Anorexia

Symptoms occur with exposure to **gluten, rye, wheat, and barley.** Intolerance is life-long.

Diagnostic Testing

- Best initial diagnostic test: **Antiendomysial and antigliadin antibodies**
- Most specific test: **Histology on biopsy**

Treatment

Celiac disease is managed with a **lifelong strictly gluten-free diet.**

GASTROESOPHAGEAL REFLUX DISEASE (GERD)

A 4-month-old female presents with several weeks of chronic wheeze and apneic episodes 20–30 minutes after feeds. She has been spitting up after feeds since birth. The infant has presented to the office on several occasions with the same complaint despite adjustments in feed technique and formula consistency. She is at the 5th percentile for weight. Which of the following is the most appropriate pharmacological intervention?

a. Erythromycin
b. Fundoplication
c. Metoclopramide
d. Omeprazole
e. Ranitidine

Answer: *The answer is* **E.** *GERD results from incompetent esophageal sphincter tone early in life. Symptoms typically resolve by 12–24 months. Diagnosis is* **clinical.** *However, the best initial test is* **esophageal pH monitoring.** **Endoscopy** *is used to evaluate for erosive gastritis or other complications. The best initial management is a* **change in feeding technique and thickened feeds.** *When this fails, the first-line therapy is an* **H2-receptor antagonist** *(ranitidine, cimetidine, famotidine) because of its safety profile.* **Proton pump inhibitors** *(omeprazole, lansoprazole, pantoprazole) and* **surgical funduplication** *are reserved for severe reflux and esophagitis.*

PYLORIC STENOSIS

A 4-week-old boy presents with recurrent vomiting after feeds. Vomitus is nonbilious in nature. Laboratory findings include chloride 88 mEq, potassium 3.1 mEq, sodium 146 mEq, and pH 7.48. What is the best initial test in the workup of this infant?

a. Abdominal X-ray

b. Barium enema

c. CT scan of the abdomen

d. Esophageal pH monitoring

e. Ultrasound

Answer: *The correct answer is* **E.** *The case will describe a first-born European-Caucasian male with nonbilous projectile vomiting typically in first 6 weeks of life. There is hypochloremic and metabolic alkalosis, and a firm, mobile, 1-inch mass is often palpated in the epigastrium. The best initial test is* **ultrasound of the abdomen.** *Treatment is* **pylorectomy.**

MALROTATION AND VOLVULUS

Look for an infant with **bilious emesis** and **recurrent abdominal pain** with **vomiting.** Always suspect volvulus when the patient has an acute small-bowel obstruction without a history of bowel surgery.

Diagnostic Testing

- Best initial test: **Ultrasound** (inversion of superior mesenteric artery and vein and duodenal obstruction) or **barium enema** (cecum is not in the right lower quadrant)
- Abdominal X-ray is *not* helpful (may only show double-bubble).

Treatment

Treatment is with **surgery.**

HEMATOCHEZIA

A 2-year-old boy is brought to the office because his mother has noticed bleeding in his diaper for 1 week. The child has had no complaints. Physical examination is unremarkable. Which of the following is the best initial test?

a. Guiac exam
b. Push enteroscopy
c. Red blood cell tagged scan
d. Tc-99m pertechnetate scan
e. Upper endoscopy

*Answer: The answer is **D**. The Tc-99m pertechnetate scan is also known as the Meckel radionuclide scan, the diagnostic exam for **Meckel's diverticulum**. Intermittent, painless rectal bleeding is the classic presentation due to acid-related bleeding of aberrant mucosa (remnant of embryonic yolk sac). May present with intussusception (remnant may become a lead point) or diverticulitis or look like acute appendicitis.*

A 16-month-old child is seen for cramping and colicky abdominal pain for the past 12 hours. He has a 1-week history of diarrhea but developed episodes of vomiting and passed black-bloody stool today. Physical examination is remarkable for a lethargic child; abdomen is tender to palpation. Temperature is 101.3°F. White blood count is 18,000. Which of the following is the most important next step in management?

a. Antibiotic prophylaxis
b. Bowel resection
c. Electrolyte replacement
d. Embolectomy
e. Reduction of bowel

*Answer: The answer is **E**. Reduction of telescoped bowel is the priority of management in patients presenting **intussusception**.*

INTUSSUSCEPTION

Intussusception is the **telescoping of bowel that classically occurs in children < 2 years**, often following gastrointestinal or upper respiratory infection, or it may occur spontaneously in patients with a "lead point" (Meckel's diverticulum, polyp, neurofirbroma, hemangioma) or with a history of Henoch-Schönlein purpura.

The case will describe **sudden paroxysms of colicky abdominal pain in a lethargic child along with shock and fever.** The classic **"black currant jelly"** stool results from mucosal necrosis due to venous obstruction.

Diagnostic Testing and Treatment

- Best initial test: **Plain film of the abdomen** to rule out obstruction
- Next steps: **Air enema,** which is both diagnostic and curative. **Manual reduction** may be needed if radiographic reduction is not successful.

RENAL AND UROLOGIC DISORDERS

URINARY TRACT INFECTIONS (UTIS) IN PEDIATRICS

UTIs are more common in **males ≤ 1 year,** more common in **girls > 2.** Most girls develop their first UTI by age 5 (peak is during infancy and toilet-training). The most common causative agent is **gram-negative rods.** Diagnosis is the same as with adults.

Treatment

- **Cystitis (dysuria):** Amoxicillin, trimethoprim-sulfamethoxazole
- **Pyelonephritis (fever, flank pain):** IV ceftriaxone or ampicillin plus gentamicin

Do *not* give the following:

- Sulfonamides or nitrofurantoin in infants < 1 month old (Give ceftriaxone.)
- Tetracyclines in children < 7 years
- Quinolones in children < 16 years

Note that children are at greatest risk of **kidney damage,** including kidney scars, poor kidney growth, poor kidney function, and high blood pressure, especially if an underlying urinary tract abnormality exists.

Follow up treatment with these tests:

- **Do urine culture** 1 week after stopping antibiotics to confirm sterility; do periodic reassessment for next 1–2 years.
- **Obtain voiding cystourethrogram (VCUG) and renal ultrasound** in the following patients:
  - All males
  - All females < 5 years or females > 5 years with second UTI
  - Any patient with UTI with fever

VESICOURETERAL REFLUX (VUR)

A 2-year-old girl presents with a urinary tract infection. She has had multiple urinary tract infections since birth but has never had any follow-up studies to evaluate these infections. Physical examination is remarkable for an ill-appearing child who has a temperature of 40°C (104°F) and is vomiting. Voiding cystourethrogram reveals abnormal urinary backflow from the bladder. Which of the following is the most important step to prevent permanent damage?

a. ACE inhibitors
b. Amoxicillin
c. NSAIDs
d. Regular creatinine measurement
e. Surgical reconstruction

*Answer: The correct answer is **B**. Antibiotic prophylaxis (amoxicillin, trimethoprim-sulfamethoxazole, or nitrofurantoin) is used for the 1st year following diagnosis for any grade of VUR, particularly in younger infants, to prevent kidney scarring from recurrent infections.*

*VUR predisposes the child to **pyelonephritis**, which leads to **scarring**, which leads to **reflux nephropathy** (hypertension, proteinuria, renal insufficiency to end-stage renal disease [ESRD], impaired kidney growth).*

Diagnostic Testing

Perform a **Voiding Cystourethrogram (VCUG) and renal scan.** If scarring is present, follow creatinine periodically.

Treatment

- **Antibiotic prophylaxis**
- **Surgery** under the following conditions:
  - Any breakthrough UTI
  - New scars
  - Failure to resolve

OBSTRUCTIVE UROPATHY

The first presentation of obstructive uropathy is often infection or sepsis. The most common causes of obstructive uropathy are the following:

- **Boys: Posterior urethral valves** are the most common cause of bladder obstruction. Look for walnut-shaped mass (bladder) above pubic symphysis and weak urinary stream.
- **Newborns: Hydronephrosis and polycystic kidney disease** are the most common causes of a palpable abdominal mass.

The best initial diagnostic tests are **VCUG and renal ultrasound.**

HEMATURIA

Acute Poststreptococcal Glomerulonephritis (APGN)

A 10-year-old boy presents with lower extremity swelling. He has had a sore throat for 2 weeks and fever. His mother has noticed very dark, brownish-red urine over the past couple of days. He has no known allergies. On physical examination, his blood pressure is 185/100 mm Hg. Which of the following is indicated for management?

a. ACE inhibitors
b. Diuretics
c. Erythromycin
d. Oral prednisone
e. Penicillin

*Answer: The answer is **E**. The most appropriate therapy for **APGN** is antibiotics to eradicate the underlying infection. Penicillin is the drug of choice. Erythromycin is used on patients who are penicillin-allergic.*

APGN presents in **children 5–12 years old, 1–2 weeks after strep pharyngitis or 3–6 weeks after skin infection (impetigo).** The classic triad of symptoms is **edema, hypertension, and hematuria.**

Diagnostic testing is as follows:

- **Urinalysis:** RBCs, RBC casts, protein, polymorphonuclear cells
- **Low C3** (Returns to normal in 6–8 weeks.)
- Need **positive throat culture** or **increasing antibody titer to streptococcal antigens**
- Most specific test: **Anti-DNase antigen**

Treat with the following:

- **Penicillin** (erythromycin if penicillin-allergic)
- **Supportive care:** Sodium restriction, diuresis, fluid and electrolyte management
- Antihypertensives are *not* indicated in acute management.
- Steroids do *not* have a role in management.

There is complete recovery in > 95 percent of patients.

Other Conditions Presenting with Hematuria

- **IgA nephropathy (Berger disease):** This is the most common chronic glomerular disease worldwide. The case will describe a patient in her **20s or 30s** with **gross hematuria after upper respiratory infection or gastrointestinal infection.** There will be **mild proteinuria and hypertension** and a *normal* C3 on lab workup. The most important step in management is **blood pressure control.**

- **Alport syndrome:** This will present in a **young boy** with **hearing difficulties** and **asymptomatic microscopic hematuria and intermittent gross hematuria after upper respiratory infections.** Family history is significant for males with renal problems and sesorineural hearing loss. Look for **ocular abnormalities** in workup.

POLYCYSTIC KIDNEY DISEASE: AUTOSOMAL-RECESSIVE TYPE (INFANTILE)

Polycystic kidney disease is suggested when an infant presents with **bilateral flank masses and hypoplasia.** Look for the following in the case:

- **Hypertension**
- **Oliguria**
- **Acute renal failure**

Diagnostic Testing

Perform an **ultrasound of the kidneys** (cysts through cortex and medulla) and **the liver** (bile duct proliferation and hepatic fibrosis).

Treatment

Treatment is with **dialysis and transplantation.** Of all patients, 80 percent have 10-year survival.

PROTEINURIA

- **Transient:** From **fever, exercise, dehydration, or cold exposure**
- **Orthostatic:** This is the most common form of persistent proteinuria in school-aged children and adolescents. Look for history of **normal proteinuria in supine position but greatly increased proteinuria in upright position.** Rule this out *before* any other evaluation is done.
- **Glomerular or tubular disorders:** Suspect a glomerular disorder with **proteinuria > 1 g/24 hours** or if the case describes **hypertension, hematuria, or renal dysfunction.**

Nephrotic Syndrome: Minimal Change Disease

A 3-year-old child presents to the physician with puffy eyes. The mother reports diarrhea 2 weeks ago. On physical examination, there is no erythema or evidence of trauma, insect bite, cellulitis conjunctival injection, or discharge. Urinalysis reveals 3+ proteinuria. Laboratory profile is significant for albumin 2.1 mg/dL, creatinine is 0.9, and C3 and C4 are normal. Which of the following is the next step in management?

a. Outpatient prednisone
b. Hospitalize and observe
c. Heparin
d. High-dose methylprednisone
e. Intravenous antibiotics

*Answer: The answer is **A**. Outpatient prednisone is the first step in management of patients presenting with **mild cases of minimal change disease**. Prednisone is continued daily for 4–6 weeks, then tapered to alternate days for 2–3 months without initial biopsy.*

Nephrotic syndrome is most common between 2–6 years, often arising after minor infections. It presents with the following:

- **Proteinuria** (> 40 mg/m2/hour) (Creatinine is usually normal.)
- **Hypoalbuminemia** (< 2.5 g/dL)
- **Edema** (initially around eyes and lower extremities)
- **Hyperlipidemia**
- C3 and C4 are normal.

Treat this condition as follows:

- **Supportive care:** Sodium restriction, fluid restriction
- **Oral prednisone**
- Relapses on steroids may indicate that patient is steroid dependent or resistant). The patient should receive **cyclophosphamide, cyclosporine, high-dose pulsed methylprednisolone.**

Following are possible complications of nephrotic syndrome:

- **Infection:** Most frequent is spontaneous bacterial peritonitis. You *must* immunize against *Pneumococcus* and *Varicella*.
- Increased risk of **thromboembolism** due to increased prothrombotic factors and decreased fibrinolytic factors

ENDOCRINE DISORDERS

CONGENITAL ADRENAL HYPERPLASIA (CAH)

CAH refers to a group of autosomal recessive disorders that result in inadequate cortisol and/or aldosterone synthesis. The most common is **21-Hydroxylase deficiency** in which

- decreased production of cortisol →
- increased ACTH →
- adrenal hyperplasia →
- shunting to androgen synthesis →
- masculinization of external genitalia in females.

CAH presents in an infant with the following signs:

- **Vomiting**
- **Dehydration**
- **Hyponatremia** (salt losing)
- **Hypoglycemia**
- **Hyperkalemia**
- Females have **ambigious genitalia** at birth.

Diagnostic Testing

- Best initial test: **Increased 17-OH progesterone** (Also find low cortisol levels, increased renin, and decreased aldosterone.)
- Definitive diagnostic test: 17-**OH progesterone before and after an intravenous bolus of ACTH.**

Treatment

- **Hydrocortisone**
- **Fludrocortisone** if salt losing
- Increased doses of both hydrocortisone and fludrocortisone in times of stress
- **Corrective surgery for females**

RHEUMATIC AND VASCULITIC DISORDERS

KAWASAKI DISEASE

An 18-month-old presents with a fever for 1 week and a rash on his hands with desquamation that developed today. On examination, he is noted to have conjunctival injection, erythematous tongue, cracked lips, and edema of the hands. He has palpable and painful lymph nodes in the neck. What is the next step in management?

a. Anticoagulation
b. Echocardiogram
c. IVIg
d. Methylprednisolone
e. Prednisone

*Answer: The answer is **C**. **Kawasaki disease** is an acute vasculitis of medium-sized arteries and the leading cause of acquired heart disease in the United States and Japan. IVIG and high-dose aspirin should be started immediately to prevent coronary artery involvement (reduces risk from 25 percent to < 5 percent). Echocardiogram should be performed at diagnosis for baseline measurement; however, coronary artery abnormalities occur in 2nd to 3rd week.*

Of patients with Kawasaki disease, 80 percent are < 5 years. The condition presents with **fever for ≥ 5 days, plus 4 of the following 5 criteria:**

- **Bilateral bulbar conjunctivitis without exudate**
- **Intraoral erythema, strawberry tongue, dry and cracked lips**
- **Erythema and swelling of hands and feet; desquamation of fingertips 1–3 weeks after onset**
- **Nonvesicular rash**
- **Nonsuppurative cervical lymphadenitis**

Diagnostic Testing

- Increased ESR, C–reactive protein (CRP) at 4–8 weeks
- Platelets increase in weeks 2–3 (often > 1 million)
- Cardiac findings:
  - Early myocarditis, pericarditis
  - Coronary artery aneurysms in the 2nd to 3rd week

Treatment

- **Best initial step:** Intravenous immunoglobulin (IVIg) and high-dose aspirin as soon as possible, based on clinical diagnosis
- **2D echocardiogram and ECG:** Get baseline at diagnosis; repeat at 2–3 weeks and at 6–8 weeks
- Steroids have *not* shown benefit
- Add **anticoagulant (warfarin)** for high-risk thrombosis (e.g., when platelet count is very high)

The prognosis is as follows:

- Only IVIg has been shown to reduce incidence of cardiovascular complications.
- There is a 1–2 percent mortality due to coronary artery thrombosis secondary to coronary artery aneurysms.

HENOCH-SCHÖNLEIN PURPURA (HSP)

HSP is the diagnosis when the case describes a young child (2–8 years) with the following:

- **Maculopapular lesions** (purpura) on the legs and buttocks
- **Fever**
- **Abdominal pain**
- A recent history of **upper respiratory viral illness**

There is IgA-mediated vasculitis of small vessels (IgA and C3 deposit in skin, kidneys, and gastrointestinal tract).

HSP is associated with the following conditions:

- **Intussusception**
- **Arthritis**
- One-fourth of patients develop **glomerulonephritis/nephrosis.**

Diagnostic Testing

Diagnosis is from the clinical presentation. Tests show the following:

- **Increased platelets, WBCs, ESR, anemia**
- **Increased IgA, IgM**
- **Anticardiolipin** or **antiphospholipid antibodies**
- Urine: **RBCs, WBCs, casts, albumin**
- Definitive diagnosis: **Skin biopsy** (rarely done)

Treatment

Treatment is **supportive:**

- Intestinal or renal complications are treated with **corticosteroids,** which help prevent renal insufficiency and bowel perforation.
- Give **aspirin** (acetylsalicylic acid, ASA) if anticardiolipin or antiphospholipid antibodies are positive and/or thrombotic events occur.

HEMATOLOGY

ANEMIA

When Is Anemia Considered Physiological?

- In **term infants,** normal hemoglobin nadir occurs at **12 weeks at 9–11 mg/dL.** The anemia results from a progressive drop in RBC production (due to erythropoietin suppression at birth) until tissue oxygen needs are greater than at delivery. *No* treatment is needed.
- Response is exaggerated and earlier in **preterm infants.** In preterms, hemoglobin nadir occurs at **3–6 weeks** at **7–9 mg/dL.** Some patients may require transfusions.

Iron-Deficiency Anemia

A normal newborn has sufficient stores of iron to meet requirements for 4–6 months, but iron stores and absorption are variable.

Breast milk has less iron than most formulas but has higher bioavailability. Iron in breast milk is more readily absorbed in the proximal intestine.

- Placenta previa occurs when the placenta is implanted in the **lower uterine segment.** As the lower uterine stretches, placental villi dislodge and painless vaginal bleeding results.
- If placenta previa occurs over a previous uterine scar, the **villi may invade** into the deeper layers of the decidua basalis and myometrium (called placenta accreta, increta, or percreta). In this scenario, intractable bleeding may require a **cesarean hysterectomy.**

The 3 forms of placenta accreta are distinguised by the depth of penetration:

- **Placenta accreta:** does not penetrate the entire thickness of the endometrium
- **Placenta increta:** extends further into the myometrium
- **Placenta percreta:** when the placenta penetrates the entrie myometrium to the uterine serosa

VASA PREVIA

- Vasa previa is **life-threatening for the fetus.** It occurs when vilamentous cord insertion results in umbilical vessels crossing the placental membranes over the cervix. When membranes rupture, the fetal vessels are torn, and blood loss is from the fetal circulation. **Fetal exsanguination** and **death** occur rapidly.
- The classic triad is as follows:

  1) **Rupture of membranes**

  2) **Painless vaginal bleeding**

  3) **Fetal bradycardia**

- **Emergency cesarean section** is *always* the first step in management.

If the question describes an antenatal Doppler sonogram showing a vessel crossing the membranes over the internal cervical os, do *not* perform amniotomy. Amniotomy may rupture the fetal vessels and cause fetal death.

UTERINE RUPTURE

Uterine rupture is the diagnosis when there's a **history of a uterine scar** with sudden-onset **abdominal pain** and **vaginal bleeding** associated with a **loss of electronic fetal heart rate, uterine contractions,** and **recession of the fetal head.**

	Abruptio Placenta	**Placenta Previa**	**Vasa Previa**	**Uterine Rupture**
Pain	Yes	No	No	Yes
Risk factors	Previous abruption Hypertension Trauma Cocaine abuse	Previous previa Multiparity Structural abnormalities (e.g. fibroids) Advanced maternal age	Velamentous insertion of the umbilical cord Accessory lobes Multiple gestation	Previous classic uterine incision Myomectomy (fibroids), Excessive oxytocin Grand multiparity
Diagnosis: Sonogram	Placenta in normal position +/- retroplacental hematoma	Placenta implanted over the lower uterine segment	Vessel crossing the membranes over the internal cervical os	N/A
Management	1. Emergent C-section: Best choice for placenta previa or if patient/fetus is deteriorating. 2. Vaginal delivery if ≥ 36 weeks or continued bleeding. May be attempted in placenta previa if placenta is > 2 cm from internal os. 3. Admit and observe if bleeding has stopped, vitals and Fetal Heart Rate (FHR) stable, or < 34 weeks.		Immediate C-section	Immediate surgery and delivery
Complication	Disseminated Intravascular coagulation	Placenta accreta/increta/percreta → hysterectomy	Fetal exsanguination	Hysterectomy for uncontrolled bleeding

PERINATAL INFECTIONS

Group B β-Hemolytic Streptococci (GBS)

A 28-year-old woman presents at 36 weeks gestation with rupture of membranes. On examination she is found to have 7cm cervical dilatation. She received all of her prenatal care, and her only complication was a course of antibiotics for assymptomatic bacteruria. GBS screening was negative. Her first baby was hospitalized for 10 days after delivery for GBS pneumonia and sepsis. What is the most appropriate management?

a. Administer intrapartum IV penicillin.

b. Administer intramuscular azithromycin.

c. Rescreen for group B streptococci.

d. Schedule cesarean section.

e. No intervention is needed.

*Answer: The correct answer is **A**. Intrapartum IV penicillin is indicated because the patient's previous birth was complicated with neonatal GBS sepsis.*

- Thirty percent of women have **asymptomatic vaginal colonization** with GBS.
- Vertical transmission results in **pneumonia** and **sepsis in the neonate** within hours to days of birth.
- There is a **50 percent mortality rate** with neonatal infection.

GBS-related meningitis occurs after the first week and is a hospital-acquired infection that is unrelated to vertical transmission.

Treatment is as follows:

- Intrapartum IV penicillin G
- Penicillin allergy: IV cefazolin, clindamycin, or erythromycin

---

When are antibiotics the answer?

- GBS (+) urine, cervical, or vaginal culture at any time during pregnancy
- Presence of high-risk factors:
  - Preterm delivery
  - Membrane rupture > 18 hours
  - Maternal fever
  - Previous baby with GBS sepsis

When are antibiotics NOT the answer?

- **Planned C-section without rupture** of membranes (even if culture is [+])
- Culture (+) on a previous pregnancy, but **culture (–) in the current pregnancy**

Toxoplasmosis

- Infection with *Toxoplasma gondii* parasite is the most common diagnosis when the case describes a patient handling **cat feces or litter boxes,** drinking **raw goat milk,** or eating **raw meat.**
- Vertical transmission only occurs with **primary infection of the mother.** Most serious infections occur during the first trimester.

The CMU except intracranial calcifications not the CMV Periventricular not the CMV

- Suspect primary infection of toxoplasmosis when the question gives a history of a **mild mononucleosis-like syndrome** and **presence of a cat** in the household. Intrauterine growth retardation may be seen on ultrasound.

Prevention is as follows:

- The most important preventitive measure is to advise pregnant women to avoid handling cat feces, raw goat milk, and undercooked meat.
- **Spiramycin** is given to the mother to prevent vertical transmission.

Treatment is as follows:

- Give **pyrimethamine** and **sulfadiazine** for the treatment of serologically confirmed fetal/neonatal infection.

> Classic triad of congenital toxoplasmosis:
> 1. Chorioretinitis
> 2. Intracranial calcifications
> 3. Hydrocephalus

Varicella

A 29-year-old woman (G2 P1) is at 34 weeks gestation. She complains of uterine contractions every 5 minutes. Her previous records are not available. During the last few days, she has developed diffuse pruritic vesicles on her neck, which appear to be also developing on her chest and breasts. She has a fever and complains of malaise. Which of the following is the next step in management?

a. Oral acyclovir
b. RhoGAM
c. Varicella zoster antibody assay
d. Varicella vaccine
e. Varicella zoster immunoglobulin

Answer: The correct answer is C. Varicella antibodies is seen in 90 percent of pregnant women due to prior infection. Varicella antibodies are protective, and no therapy is necessary.

- Transplacental infection results from **primary *varicella* infection** in the mother (25–40 percent infection rate).
- The greatest risk to the fetus is if a **rash** appears in the mother **between 5 days antepartum and 2 days postpartum.**
- Neonatal infection presents with "zigzag" skin lesions, limb hypoplasia, microcephaly, microphthalmia, chorioretinitis, and cataracts.

Prevention is as follows:

- **Vaccination:** Live-attenuated varicella virus (Varivax III) to **nonpregnant** women.
- **Postexposure prophylaxis: VariZIG** (antivaricella antibodies) or **Varicella Zoster immunoglobulin** within 96 hours of exposure. VariZIG/VZIG does not prevent infection but only attenuates the clinical effects of the virus.

Treatment is as follows:

- **Maternal *varicella*: VariZIG** to mother *and* neonate
- **Congenital *varicella*: VariZIG *and* IV acyclovir** to the neonate

Rubella

- Vertical transmission of rubella virus (causative virus of German measles) occurs with primary infection during pregnancy (70–90 percent).
- Neonates with congenital rubella present with **congenital deafness** (most common sequelae), congenital heart disease (e.g., patent ductus arteriosus, or PDA), **cataracts, mental retardation, hepatosplenomegaly, thrombocytopenia,** and **"blueberry muffin" rash.** Adverse effects occur with primary infection in the first 10 weeks

Prevention is as follows:

- Perform **first-trimester screening** and have mother **avoid infected individuals.**
- Immunize seronegative women *after* delivery.
- No postexposure prophylaxis is available.

A 24-year-old child-care worker is 29 weeks pregnant and is currently working. One of the children was diagnosed with rubella last week. Rubella antigen testing is performed and her IgG titer is negative. What is the risk of neonatal transmission in this patient? What is the next step in management?

a. Give anti-rubella antibodies
b. Give betamethasone
c. Give rubella vaccine now
d. Give rubella vaccine after delivery
e. Ultrasound of the fetus

*Answer: The correct answer is **D.** There is no postexposure prophylaxis available, and immunization during pregnancy is contraindicated (live vaccine). The only correct management is to await normal delivery and give vaccination to the mother after delivery.*

Cytomegalovirus (CMV)

- Congenital CMV syndrome is the *most* common congenital viral syndrome in the United States. CMV is the *most* common cause of sensorineural deafness in children. CMV is spread by **infected body fluid secretions.**
- The greatest risk for vertical transmission occurs with **primary infection** (infection rate is 50 percent).
- Most mothers develop **asymptomatic infections** or describe **mild, mononucleosis-like symptoms.** About 10 percent of infants with congenital CMV infection are symptomatic at birth.

- Manifestations include **intrauterine growth restriction, prematurity, microcephaly, jaundice, petechiae, hepatosplenomegaly, periventricular calcifications, chorioretinitis,** and **pneumonitis.**

Diagnosis is as follows:

- Perform a viral culture from urine or other body fluids in first 2 weeks of life.
- May consider PCR.

Prevention is as follows:

- Follow universal precautions with all body fluids. Avoid transfusion with CMV-positive blood.

Treatment is as follows:

- Antiviral therapy with **ganciclovir** prevents viral shedding and prevents hearing loss but does not cure the infection.

Herpes Simplex Virus (HSV)

A 21-year-old multipara is admitted to the birthing unit at 39 weeks gestation in active labor at 6 cm dilation. Membranes are intact. She has a history of genital herpes preceding the pregnancy. Her last outbreak was 8 weeks ago. She now complains of pain and pruritis. On examination, she had localized, painful, ulcerative lesions on her right vaginal wall. Which of the following is the next step in management?

a. Administer IV acyclovir
b. Administer terbutaline
c. Obtain culture of ulcer
d. Proceed with vaginal delivery
e. Schedule cesarean section

*Answer: The correct answer is **E**. Active genital herpes is an indication for cesarean section. The only other infection-related indication for cesarean section is HIV sero-positive status of the mother.*

- The *most* common cause of transmission is **contact with maternal genital lesions** during an active HSV episode.
- Transplacental infection can also occur with **primary infections** during pregnancy (50 percent risk). *Greatest risk* is primary infection in the third trimester.
- Suspect primary HSV infection if the case describes **fever, malaise,** and **diffuse genital lesions** during pregnancy.
- Neonatal infection acquired during delivery has **50 percent mortality rate.**
- Surviving infants develop meningoencephalitis, mental retardation, pneumonia, hepatosplenomegaly, jaundice, and petechiae.

Diagnosis is as follows:

- (+) HSV culture from vesicle fluid or ulcer or HSV PCR of maternal blood (not screened routinely)

Prevention is as follows:

- Perform C-section in women with **active genital HSV lesions** at the time of labor.
- Do *not* use fetal scalp electrodes for monitoring (increased risk of HSV transmission).
- Manage expectantly for premature rupture of membranes (PROM) or prolonged rupture of membranes (ROM) (i.e., > 8–12 hours).
- Advise standard precautions (avoid intercourse if partner has active lesions, avoid oral sex in presence of oral lesions, avoid kissing neonate in presence of oral lesions).

Treatment is as follows:

- **Acyclovir** to patient for primary infection during pregnancy

Human Immunodeficiency Virus (HIV)

A 24-year-old HIV positive female (G2 P1) presents in her 16th week of pregnancy. Her previous child was diagnosed HIV positive after vaginal delivery. What is the most effective method of decreasing the risk of vertical transmission?

a. Avoidance of artificial rupture of membranes
b. Avoidance of breastfeeding
c. Antiretroviral triple therapy
d. Cesarean section
e. Zidovudine monotherapy

*Answer: The correct answer is **E**. All of the strategies are recommended, however. Zidovudine (ZDV) monotherapy is the **most effective** in decreasing the risk of HIV transmission to the fetus (25% to 8%). Triple antiretroviral therapy is indicated for more effective management of HIV in the mother when viral load is >1,000; or women with load <1,000 may take ZDV monotherapy alone. Cesarean section (**before rupture of membranes**), avoidance of breastfeeding or intrapartum invasive procedures (articficial ROM, fetal scalp electrodes) also decreases transmission rate. Combination of all of the above strategies listed above reduces the transmission rate to 1%.*

> Continue antiretrovirals in pregnancy for HIV (+) patients with low CD4 counts and/or high viral load.

- Major route of vertical transmission is contact with infected genital secretions at the time of vaginal delivery. Without treatment, the vertical transmission rate is 25–30 percent.
- Elective cesarean is of most benefit in women with low CD4 counts and high RNA viral loads (> 1,000). All neonates of HIV-positive women will have positive HIV tests from transplacental passive IgG passage.

Prevention and treatment are as follows:

- **Triple-drug therapy** (which *must* include ZDV):
  - Starting at 14 weeks and continuing throughout pregnancy
  - Intravenous intrapartum ZDV
  - PO ZDV for the infant for 6 weeks after delivery
- Give the infant prophylaxis against **pneumocystis pneumonia** (trimethoprim-sulfamethoxazole) after 6 weeks of AZT therapy.
- Schedule C-section at 38 weeks *unless* < 1,000 viral copies/mL.
- Advise the mother **not to breastfeed** (breast milk transmits the virus).
- **Avoid invasive procedures** (e.g., artificial rupture of membranes, fetal scalp electrodes).

Syphilis

- If the case describes a previously treated syphilis infection, *never* assume immunity. There is **no immunity** from prior infection with syphilis, and reinfection can occur over and over again.
- Transplacental infection results from primary and secondary infection (60 percent risk of transmission). The lowest risk of transmission is with latent or tertiary infection.
- **Early acquired (first trimester) congenital syphilis** includes the following symptoms/outcomes:
  - Nonimmune hydrops fetalis
  - Maculopapular or vesicular peripheral rash
  - Anemia, thrombocytopenia, and hepatosplenomegaly
  - Large and edematous placenta
  - Perinatal mortality rates ~ 50 percent
- **Late-acquired congenital syphilis** is diagnosed after 2 years of age and includes the following symptoms:
  - Hutchinson teeth
  - "Mulberry" molars
  - "Saber" shins
  - "Saddle" nose
  - Deafness (cranial nerve 8 palsy)

Diagnosis is as follows:

- VDRL or RPR screening in first trimester. Confirm (+) screen with FTA-ABS or MHA-TP.
- Screening test will be falsely negative in primary syphilis.
  - When the case describes a woman with a painless genital ulcer, order **darkfield microscopy** for diagnosis of primary syphilis.

[handwritten margin note: False (+) VDRL or RPR: Varicella, measles, lymphoma, TB, malaria, connective tissue disease + pregnancy :)]

> Always order an HIV test in any pregnant patient who has tested positive for an STD.

> C-section will not prevent vertical transmission of syphilis, because it happens through the placenta before birth.

- With sustained hypertension, the fetus may be **growth restricted** and **hypoxic** and is at risk for **abruptio placentae.**

Diagnosis is as follows:

- **Chronic hypertension** is the diagnosis when there is a **history of elevated blood pressure before pregnancy** or **before 20 weeks gestation.**
- **Gestational hypertension** is the diagnosis when blood pressure develops after **20 weeks gestation** and **returns to normal baseline by 6 weeks** postpartum. It occurs more commonly in multifetal pregnancy.
- **Preeclampsia** is the diagnosis when there is **proteinuria** and/or **presence of "warning signs."**

Mild preeclampsia is indicated with the following:

- Sustained BP elevation > **140/90 mm Hg**
- Proteinuria of **1–2+** (on dipstick) or > **300 mg** (on a 24h urine)

Severe preeclampsia is indicated by mild preeclampsia plus one of the following:

- Sustained BP elevation >**160/110 mm Hg**
- Proteinuria of **3–4+** (on dipstick) or > **5 g** (on 24h urine)
- Presence of **"warning signs"**

Risk factors are as follows:

- **Primiparas** are *most* at risk. Other risk factors are multiple gestation, hyatidiform mole, diabetes mellitus, age extremes, chronic hypertension, and chronic renal disease.

A 19-year-old primigravida presents at 32 weeks gestation for routine follow-up. She denies headache, epigastric pain, or visual disturbances. She has gained 2 pounds since her last visit 2 weeks ago. On examination, her blood pressure is 155/95, which is persistent on repeat BP check 10 minutes later. She has only trace pedal edema. Which of the following is the next step in management?

a. Begin methyldopa.
b. Begin labetalol.
c. Perform an electrocardiogram.
d. Perform a fetal ultrasound.
e. Perform urinalysis.

Answer: The correct answer is E. Always rule out preeclampsia in a hypertensive pregnant patient. Even if she is asymptomatic, proteinuria indicates preeclampsia and a worse prognosis.

- **Chronic hypertension with superimposed preeclampsia** is the diagnosis when there is chronic hypertension with **increasingly severe hypertension, proteinuria,** and/or **"warning signs."**
- **Eclampsia** is the diagnosis when the case describes **unexplained grand mal seizures** in a **hypertensive** and/or **proteinuric** pregnant woman in the last

---

Warning signs of maternal jeopardy:
- Hallmark symptoms:
  - Headache
  - Epigastric pain
  - Changes in vision
- Signs: Pulmonary edema, oliguria (Peripheral edema is *not* a warning sign.)
- Labs: Thrombocytopenia, elevated liver enzymes

half of pregnancy. Patients present with same signs and symptoms as in pre-eclampsia with the addition of unexplained tonic-clonic seizures. Seizures from **severe diffuse cerebral vasospasm** cause cerebral perfusion deficits and edema.

- **HELLP syndrome** is the diagnosis when there is hemolysis (H), elevated liver (EL) enzymes, and low platelets (LP)

Laboratory:

- Order **CBC, chem-12 panel, coagulation panel,** and **urinalysis with urinary protein**
- Labs will show the following:
  - **Hemoconcentration:** ↑hemoglobin, ↑hematocrit, ↑blood urea nitrogen (BUN), ↑serum creatinine, and ↑serum uric acid
  - **Proteinuria**
  - In severe preeclampsia, **disseminated intravascular coagulation** and **liver enzyme elevation**

Treatment is as follows:

- **Blood pressure control:**
  - Don't treat *unless* BP > 160/100 mm Hg (antihypertensives decrease utero-placental blood flow)
  - Goal SBP is 140–150 mm Hg and DBP is 90-100 mm Hg
  - **Maintenance therapy:**
    - ∘ First line therapy is methyldopa.
    - ∘ Second line therapy is β-blockers (labetolol, atenolol). Watch out for Intrauterine Growth Retardation (IUGR), which is associated with β-blocker use in pregnancy.
  - **Acutely elevated BP**/treatment of severe preclampsia or eclampsia:
    - ∘ Intravenous hydralazine or labetolol
  - *Never* give ACE inhibitors or start thiazide diuretics during pregnancy.
- **Seizure management and prophylaxis:**
  - Protect the patient's airway and tongue
  - **Give IV MgSO4 (magnesium sulfate)** bolus for seizure and infusion for continued prophylaxis
- **Monitoring:**
  - Serial sonograms (evaluate for Intrauterine Growth Retardation (IUGR)
  - Serial BP monitoring and urine protein
- **Labor:**
  - Induce labor if ≥ 36 weeks with mild preeclampsia: attempt vaginal delivery with IV oxytocin if mother and fetus are stable.

Seizure disorder is *not* a risk factor for eclampsia.

The *only* definitive cure is delivery and removal of all fetal-placental tissue.

- Aggressive, prompt delivery is the best step for severe/superimposed pre-eclampsia or eclampsia at *any* gestational age.
- Give intrapartum IV MgSO4 and hydralazine and/or labetalol to manage BP.

A 32-year-old multigravida at 36 weeks gestation was found to have BP 160/105 on routine prenatal visit. Previous BP readings were normal. She complained of some right-upper-quadrant abdominal pain. Urinalysis showed 3+ proteinuria. She is emergently induced for labor and delivers an 8 lb. 3 oz. boy. Two days after delivery, routine labs reveal elevated total bilirubin, lactate dehydrogenase, alanine aminotransferase (AST), and aspartate aminotransferase (ALT). Platelet count is 85,000. Postpartum evaluation reveals that she has no complaints of headache or visual changes. Which of the following is the most likely diagnosis?

a. Cholecystitis
b. HELLP syndrome
c. Hepatitis
d. Idiopathic thrombocytopenia
e. Preeclampsia

*Answer: The correct answer is **B**. Patient has evidence of hemolysis (elevated LDH), elevated liver enzymes, and thrombocytopenia.*

HELLP SYNDROME

HELLP syndrome occurs in 5–10 percent of preeclamptic patients. It typically presents in the **third trimester** but may occur in the postpartum period, commonly presenting **2 days after delivery.** Risk factors differ from preeclampsia, since HELLP syndrome is more common in whites, multigravids, and women of older maternal age.

Management is as follows:

- Schedule **immediate delivery** at any gestational age.
- Give **IV corticosteroids** (dexamethasone) when platelets < 100,000/mm^3 *both* antepartum and postpartum; continue until platelet count is > 100,000/mm^3 and liver function normalizes.
- Give **platelet transfusion** if platelet count < 20,000/mm^3 *or* platelet count < 50,000/mm^3 if cesarean section will be performed.
- **IV MgS04** for seizure prophylaxis, even if BP is normal.
- Steroids may also need to be considered for assistance with fetal lung maturation if prior to 36 weeks.

Complications are as follows:

- DIC
- Abruptio placenta
- Fetal demise
- Ascites
- Hepatic rupture

MEDICAL COMPLICATIONS IN PREGNANCY

CARDIAC ABNORMALITIES

- Heart disorders account for about **10 percent of maternal obstetric deaths.**
- Women with high-risk disorders (e.g., pulmonary hypertension, Eisenmenger syndrome, severe valvular disorders, prior postpartum cardiomyopathy) should be advised *not* to become pregnant due to risk of sudden death.
- Cardiovascular changes in pregnancy (30–50 percent ↑ Cardiac Output (CO) may unmask or worsen underlying cardiac conditions. These changes are maximal at **28 and 34 weeks gestation.**

PERIPARTUM CARDIOMYOPATHY

- Heart failure with no identifiable cause can develop between the last month of pregnancy to 5 months postpartum.
- Risk factors include multiparity, age ≥ 30, multiple gestations (i.e., twins or triplets, etc.), and preeclampsia.
- The 5-year mortality rate is 50 percent.

MANAGEMENT OF SPECIFIC CARDIAC CONDITIONS

Heart Failure

- Risk of maternal or fetal death is associated with class III or IV heart failure.
- *Never* use an ACE inhibitor or aldosterone antagonist in pregnancy.
- Loop diuretics, nitrates, and β-blockers may be continued.
- Digoxin may be used in pregnancy to improve symptoms, but it does not improve outcome.

Arrhythmias

- Continue rate control as with nonpregnant patients.
- Do *not* give amiodarone or warfarin.

Endocarditis Prophylaxis

- Indications are the same as for nonpregnant patients (see "Endocarditis" in Infectious Disease).
- Give daily prophylaxis in patients with rheumatic heart disease.
- Do *not* give prophylactic antibiotics during uncomplicated vaginal/cesarean delivery in patients with valvular disease or prosthetic valves.

Valvular Disease

- Regurgitant lesions are well tolerated and do *not* require therapy.
- Stenotic lesions have an increased risk of maternal/fetal morbidity and mortality.
- Mitral stenosis has an increased risk of pulmonary edema and atrial fibrillation.

Hypercoagulable States

- **Pulmonary embolus** is the leading cause of maternal death in the United States. Fifty percent of pregnant women who develop thromboemboli have an underlying thrombophilic disorder.
- When is anticoagulation the answer on the test?
  - **DVT** or **PE** in pregnancy
  - Atrial fibrillation (AF) **with underlying heart disease,** but not atrial fibrillation alone
  - **Antiphospholipid syndrome**
  - **Severe heart failure** (Ejection Fraction (EF) < 30 percent)
  - **Eisenmenger syndrome**
- The anticoagulant of choice is **LMWH,** which does not cross the placenta (warfarin does cross the placenta and is contraindicated in pregnancy) and isn't associated with osteopenia (unfractionated heparin causes osteopenia).
  - Warfarin is contraindicated, as it causes fetal abnormalities and even death.
- Patients with a history of **DVT** or **PE** in a previous pregnancy or a history of **underlying thrombophilic condition** should receive **prophylactic LMWH** throughout pregnancy, **unfractionated heparin** during labor and delivery, and warfarin for 6 weeks postpartum.
- **Thrombolytics** are used in pulmonary embolism with the same indications as in the nonpregnant patient.

THYROID DISORDERS

- Hyperthyroidism in pregnancy causes **fetal growth restriction** and **stillbirth.**
- Hypothyroidism in pregnancy causes **intellectual deficits** in offspring and **miscarriage.**
- Pregnancy does *not* change the symptoms of hypothyroidism or hyperthyroidism or the normal values and ranges of free serum thyroxine (T4) and thyroid-stimulating hormone (TSH).
- Continue hormone replacement in patients with hypothyroidism during pregnancy.
- **Beta blockers** are the drug of choice for symptomatic hyperthyroidism. Radioactive iodine is never given in pregnancy

Graves' Disease

- **Propylthiouracil (PTU)** is the drug of choice (methimazole is the second line therapy). PTU crosses the placenta and may cause goiter and hypothyroidism in the fetus. Congenital Graves' disease in the fetus may be **masked until 7 to 10 days after birth,** when the drug's effect subsides.

- Maternal thyroid-stimulating immunoglobulins (Igs) and thyroid-blocking Igs can cross the placenta and cause **fetal tachycardia, growth restriction,** and **goiter.**

DIABETES IN PREGNANCY

- Target values of **FBS < 90 mg/dL** and **< 120 mg/dL** 1 hour after a meal.

- **Gestational diabetes (GDM)** is managed with **diet alone.** Glyburide, though controversial, has been used by some in pregnancy.

- **Diabetes mellitus** is managed with **insulin.** Insulin requirements increase throughout the course of the pregnancy but decrease as soon as the placenta is delivered.

- Avoid oral hypoglycemics while breastfeeding, as they can cause hypoglycemia in neonates.

Routine Monitoring in Diabetic Patients

- **HbA1c in each trimester.** If HbA1c elevated in first trimester,
  - obtain fetal echocardiogram at 22–24 weeks to assess for congenital heart disease; and
  - obtain targeted ultrasound at 18–20 weeks to look for structural anomalies.

- **Triple-marker screen at 16–18 weeks** to assess for Neural Tube Defects (NTD)

- **Monthly sonograms** to assess fetal macrosomia or IUGR

- **Monthly biophysical profiles**

- **Start weekly Nonstress Test (NST) and Amniotic Fluid Index (AFI) at 32 weeks** if taking insulin, macrosomia, previous stillbirth, or hypertension.

- **Start NSTs and AFIs at 26 weeks** if small vessel disease is present or there is poor glycemic control.

- For Gestional Diabetes Mellitus (GDM) patients, order a **2-hour 75g OGTT** 6–12 weeks postpartum to determine if diabetes has resolved.
  - Thirty-five percent of women with GDM will develop overt diabetes within 5 to 10 years after delivery.

- **Caudal regression syndrome** is an uncommon congenital abnormality associated with overt DM.

Congenital malformations (especially NTDs) are strongly associated with HbA1c > 8.5 in the first trimester.

GDM is *not* associated with congenital anomalies, since hyperglycemia is not present in the first half of pregnancy.

Labor in Diabetic Patients

- Target delivery gestational age is **40 weeks** because of delayed fetal maturity.
- Induce labor at **39–40 weeks if < 4,500 g** or earlier if there is poor glycemic control. A lecithin/sphingomyelin (L/S) ratio of 2.5 and presence of phosphatidyl glycerol ensures fetal lung maturity.
- Schedule cesarean section if **> 4,500 g** because of the risk of **shoulder dystocia.**
- Maintain maternal blood glucose levels between **80 and 100 mg/dL** using 5 percent dextrose in water and an insulin drip.
- Turn off any insulin infusion after delivery, because insulin resistance decreases with rapidly falling levels of hPL after delivery of the placenta. Maintain blood glucose levels with a sliding scale.

Neonatal Problems

- **Hypoglycemia** (maternal hyperinsulinemia) and **hypocalcemia** (PTH synthesis failure)
- **Polycythemia** (hypoxia) and **hyperbilirubinemia** (excessive neonatal RBCs breakdown)
- **Respiratory distress syndrome** (delayed surfactant production)

LIVER DISEASES

A 31-year-old primigravida woman presents at 20 weeks' gestation with dizygotic twins of different genders. She is of Swedish descent and complains of intense skin itching. Her sister experienced similar complaints when she was pregnant and delivered her baby prematurely. No identifiable rash is noted on physical examination. She states that her urine appears dark colored.

Answer: The diagnosis is **intrahepatic cholestasis of pregnancy.** *It occurs in genetically susceptible women (of European heritage) and is associated with multiple pregnancies.*

- *Symptoms: Classic symptoms include* **intractable nocturnal pruritus** *on the palms and soles of the feet without skin findings.*
- *Diagnosis: 10- to 100-fold increase in serum* **bile acids**
- *Treatment:* **Ursodeoxycholic acid** *is the treatment of choice. Symptoms may be relieved by antihistamines and cholestyramine.*

A 29-year-old primagravida is at 33 weeks gestation. She is brought to the maternity unit by her husband, who states she is becoming confused. She developed nausea, vomiting, and anorexia three days ago associated with a lack of appetite. Fundal height is 30 cm. Fetal heart rate is 145/min with nonreactive nonstress test. Mother's BP is 150/95 mm Hg. Random blood glucose is 52 mg/dL. Platelet count is 75,000. PTT is prolonged at 64.7 seconds. Creatinine is 2.1 mg/dL. Uric acid is 11.9 mg/dL, LDH is 1063 U/l, ALT is 220 U/l, AST is 350 U/l, total bilirubin is 8.4 mg/dL. Serum ammonia is elevated. Urine protein dipstick is 3+.

*Answer: The diagnosis is **acute fatty liver**. This rare condition is related to disordered metabolism of fatty acids by mitochondria in the fetus. Hypertension, proteinuria, and edema can mimic preeclampsia.*

- *Diagnosis: **Elevated liver enzymes** (e.g., ALT, AST, GGT), **hyperbilirubinemia, DIC.** Hypoglycemia and increased serum ammonia are unique laboratory abnormalities.*

- *Treatment: Admit to the ICU for **aggressive IV fluid treatment** and **prompt delivery.***

URINARY TRACT INFECTIONS, PYELONEPHRITIS, AND BACTERIURIA

Assymptomatic Bacteriuria	Acute Cystitis	Pyelonephritis
1. Urine culture (+) 2. No urgency, frequency, or burning 3. No fever	1. Urine culture (+) 2. Urgency, frequency, or burning 3. No fever	1. Urine culture (+) 2. Urgency, frequency, or burning 3. Fever and CVA tenderness
Tx: *Outpatient* PO antibiotics (Nitrofurantoin is drug of choice; Alt: Cephalexin or amoxicillin)		**Tx:** Admit to hospital; IV hydration, IV cephalosporins or gentamicin, and tocolysis
Cx: 30% of cases develop acute pyelonephritis when untreated		**Cx:** Preterm labor and delivery; Severe cases → sepsis, anemia, and pulmonary dysfunction

ECTOPIC/TUBAL PREGNANCY, CERVICAL INCOMPETENCE

INDUCED ABORTION

The more advanced the gestation, the higher the rate of complications.

First-Trimester Methods

- **Dilation and curettage (D&C)** is the *most* common first trimester abortion procedure and is performed **before 13 weeks gestation.** Give prophylactic antibiotics, conscious sedation, and paravertebral block local anesthetic. Rarely complicated by endometritis (outpatient antibiotic) and/or retained products of conception (repeat curettage).

- **Medical abortion** through the use of **oral mifepristone** (Mifeprex, a progesterone antagonist) and **oral misoprostol** (Cytotec, prostaglandin E1) is an alternative to surgical abortion. It may only be used in the **first 63 days of amenorrhea.** Approximately 2 percent abort incompletely and require D&C. *Clostridium sordellii* sepsis can occur in rare cases.

Second-Trimester Methods

- **Dilation and evacuation (D&E)** is the most common second-trimester abortion method.
- **An intact dilation and evacuation (D&E) ("partial birth")** is used for more advanced pregnancies. Wide cervical dilation is induced, followed by assisted breech delivery of the fetus under ultrasound guidance.

Complications

- The most common immediate complication is **retained placenta.** Other complications include uterine perforation, retained tissue, hemorrhage, infection, and, rarely, disseminated intravascular coagulation.
- The most common delayed complication is **cervical trauma** and **cervical insufficiency.**

SPONTANEOUS ABORTION/FETAL DEMISE/ECTOPIC PREGNANCY

Death of an embryo or fetus has various different terms based on the gestational age or weight at the time of in utero death.

- **Spontaneous abortion** is the expulsion of an embryo/fetus **< 500 g** or **< 20 weeks** gestation. It most commonly initially presents with uterine pain and vaginal bleeding.
- **Fetal demise** is the in utero death of a fetus **after 20 weeks** gestation. The most common symptom is a **loss of fetal movements.**

A 27-year-old pregnant female at 7 weeks gestation presents with vaginal bleeding and pelvic pain.

a. What is the diagnosis?

*Answer: A woman with amenorrhea, vaginal bleeding, and pelvic pain is diagnosed with **threatened abortion.***

b. What is the first step in management?

Answer: The first step in management in any patient presenting with early pregnancy vaginal bleeding is a speculum exam. If the pregnancy is advanced far enough, ultrasound or Doppler should be done to evaluate fetal cardiac activity.

c. The mother is concerned about her baby and asks you: What is the risk to my baby?

Answer: Half of pregnancies complicated by threatened abortion continue to term.

- When the case describes painful cramps, continued bleeding, and a dilated cervix on exam, the abortion is **inevitable.**
  - **Treatment: Emergency suction D&C** should be performed to prevent further blood loss and anemia.
- When the case describes loss of early pregnancy symptoms (eg, nausea, breast tenderness) and loss of fetal cardiac activity, the diagnosis is **missed abortion.**
  - **Diagnosis:** Nonviable fetus seen on ultrasound with retention of the pregnancy. The cervix is usually closed on physical examination.
- When the case describes bleeding, uterine cramping, and cervical dilation with expulsion of the products of conception (POC), the next step in management is a **sonogram** to look for **retained products of conception.**
  - If the sonogram shows intrauterine debris, the abortion is **incomplete,** and **emergency suction D&C** needs to be done.
  - If the sonogram does not show intrauterine debris (i.e., **complete abortion**), **serial β-hCG titers** need to be taken weekly until negative to make sure an ectopic pregnancy has not been missed.

Etiology

- **Chromosomal abnormalities of the embryo or fetus** are the most common cause of spontaneous abortion. Risk factors are strongly related to advanced maternal age, previous spontaneous abortion, and maternal smoking.
- **Fetal demise is most commonly idiopathic.** Risk factors include antiphospholipid syndrome, overt maternal diabetes, maternal trauma, severe maternal isoimmunization, and fetal infection.

Diagnosis

1. **Speculum exam** to evaluate for cervical/vaginal sources of bleeding and presence of vaginal dilation Speculum exam is never the first step in management of late trimester bleeding because of the risk of bleeding in a low implanted placenta; and the
2. **ultrasound** to evaluate fetal cardiac activity and +/- of products of conception

Complications

- When the case describes prolonged fetal demise (> 2 weeks), the most serious complication to look out for is **disseminated intravascular coagulation (DIC),** resulting from release of **tissue thromboplastin** from deteriorating fetal organs.

Always rule out coagulopathy by ordering platelet count, D-dimer, fibrinogen, PT, and PTT in patients presenting with fetal demise. If DIC is identified, immediate delivery is needed.

A 24-year-old woman visits the clinic with left-sided abdominal and flank pain and vaginal spotting. Her last menstrual period was 7 weeks ago. She denies fevers, nausea or vomiting. She has one prior pregnancy with spontaneous vaginal delivery. She has used OCPs in the past but currently uses and intrauterine device for contraception. Pelvic examination, reveals a slightly enlarged uterus, closed cervix. No palpable adnexal mass is identified however there is tenderness on bimanual exam. A quantitative serum ß-hCG value is 2,650 mIU. What is the diagnosis?

a. Ectopic pregnancy
b. Hydatidiform mole
c. Incomplete abortion
d. Missed abortion
e. Threatened abortion

*Answer: The correct answer is **A**. The classic presentation of ectopic pregnancy is 1) amenorrhea, 2) vaginal bleeding and 3) unilateral pelvic-abdominal pain. When the case also describes, abdominal guarding or rigidity, hypotension and tachycardia, **ruptured eptopic pregnancy** is the diagnosis.*

Risk Factors

- The *most* common risk factor is **pelvic inflammatory disease** (PID).
- Any cause of tubal scarring or adhesions: infectious (PID, IUD), history of surgery (tubal ligation, tubal surgery), or congenital risks (diethylstilbestrol [DES] exposure)
- One percent of pregnancies are ectopic pregnancies. Incidence increases to 15 percent if the patient has had a previous ectopic pregnancy.

Diagnosis

- Diagnosis is presumed when
  - β-hCG > 1,500 mIU; and
  - no intrauterine pregnancy is seen on vaginal sonogram.
- Note: The absence of an adnexal mass does *not* rule out ectopic pregnancy.
- Presume ectopic pregnancy has **ruptured** when the patient is unstable (hypotension, tachycardia) and there are symptoms of peritoneal irritation (abdominal guarding or rigidity).

You cannot rule out a normal intrauterine pregnancy when ß-hCG is < 1,500 mIU. The next step is to repeat ß-hCG and repeat the sonogram when ß-hCG is > 1,500 mIU.

Management

- Ruptured ectopic (look for an unstable patient): Immediate **laparotomy/salpingectomy**
- Unruptured ectopic: **Methotrexate** or **laparoscopy** (salpingostomy)
- Give **RhoGAM** to Rh negative women

> Intrauterine pregnancy is normally seen on the following:
> - **Vaginal sonogram** at 5 weeks gestation when serum ß–hCG > 1,500 mIU
> - **Abdominal sonogram** at 6 weeks gestation when ß–hCG > 6,500 mIU

> Indications for methotrexate are as follows:
> - Pregnancy mass < 3.5 cm diameter
> - Absence of fetal heart motion
> - ß-hCG level < 6,000 mIU
> - No history of folic supplementation

Follow-Up

- Follow β-hCG to ensure there has been complete destruction of the ectopic trophoblastic villi.

CERVICAL INSUFFICIENCY

A 29-year-old primigravida presents to the emergency department at 19 weeks' gestation with lower pelvic pressure without contractions. She reports increased clear vaginal mucus discharge. Fetal membranes are found to be bulging into the vagina, and the cervix cannot be palpated. Fetal feet can be felt through the membranes. What is the next step in management?

a. Abdominal cerclage
b. Prophylactic antibiotics
c. Tocolysis
d. Vaginal cerclage
e. Rule out chorioamnionitis

*Answer: The answer is E. Although emergency cerclage (vaginal or abdominal) is indicated in women who present with cervical dilation in the absence of labor or abruption, **it can only be performed when choramionitis is first ruled out**. Tocolysis is not appropriate in management of cervical insufficiency. Prophylactic antibiotics and tocolytics are not recommended.*

Risk Factors

Risk factors are a history of any of the following:

- Second-trimester abortion
- Cervical laceration during delivery
- Deep cervical conization
- Diethylstilbestrol (DES) exposure

Management

- Perform **elective cerclage placement** at 13–16 weeks gestation for patients with ≥ 3 unexplained midtrimester pregnancy losses.
- Only perform **urgent cerclage** after first ruling out labor and chorioamnionitis.
- Perform **cerclage removal** at 36–37 weeks after fetal lung maturity.

What is the next step in management of an assymptomatic woman with no prior history of preterm labor, found to have short cervix on routine transvaginal ultrasound before 16–20 weeks?

Answer: Transvaginal ultrasound surveillance to evaluate for persistent cervical shortening, and to evaluate for changes in cervical dilation, however cerclage is not indicated unless dilation is present and chorioamnionitis or signs of labor are not present. Repeat the exam after 20 weeks if short cervix is still present.

DISPROPORTIONATE FETAL GROWTH

Intrauterine Growth Restriction (IUGR)

- **IUGR** is the diagnosis when the estimated fetal weight (EFW) is < **5–10 percentile** for gestational age or < **2,500 grams** (5 lb, 8 oz). Accurate, early pregnancy dating is essential for making the diagnosis.

- An **early sonogram** (< 20 weeks) is the next step in management if accurate dates are not known.

- *Never* change the gestational age based on a late sonogram.

	Symmetric IUGR	Asymmetric IUGR	
	Fetal Causes	**Maternal Causes**	**Placental Causes**
	↓ *growth potential*	↓ *placental perfusion*	
Etiology	– Aneupleidy – Infection (e.g. TORCH) – Structural anomalies (e.g., congenital heart disease, NTD, ventral wall defects)	– Hypertension – Small vessel disease (e.g. SLE) – Malnutrition – Tobacco, alcohol, street drugs	– Infarction – Abruption – Twin-twin transfusion – Velamentous cord insertion
Ultrasound	↓ *in all measurements*	↓ *abdomen measurements; normal head measurements*	
Workup	– Detailed sonogram – Karyotype – Screen for fetal infections	– Monitor with serial sonograms, nonstress test, AFI, biophysical profile, and umbilical artery dopplers – AFI is often decreased, especially with severe uteroplacental insufficiency	

MACROSOMIA

Macrosomia is indicated by a fetus with estimated fetal weight (EFW) > 90–95 percentile for gestational age or birth weight of 4,000–4,500 grams.

Risk factors include the GDM, overt diabetes, prolonged gestation, obesity, ↑ ↑ in pregnancy weight gain, multiparity, and male fetus.

Complications include the following:

- **Maternal:** Injury during birth, postpartum hemorrhage, and emergency cesarean section
- **Fetus:** Shoulder dystocia, birth injury, asphyxia
- **Neonate:** Hypoglycemia, Erb palsy

Management: Elective cesarean (if EFW > 4,500 g in diabetic mother or > 5,000 g in nondiabetic mother)

LABOR, DELIVERY, AND THE POSTPARTUM PERIOD

Intrapartum fetal testing:

- **Obstetric ultrasound**
  - Crown rump length determines gestational age at 10–13 weeks.
  - High-resolution ultrasonography is indicated when maternal serum markers are abnormal or there is a family history of congenital malformations.
- **Chorionic villous sampling (CVS)**
  - Performed at 12–14 weeks.
  - Chorionic villi is sampled for karyotyping.
  - Pregnancy loss rate is 0.7 percent.
- **Amniocentesis**
  - Performed after 15 weeks with ultrasound guidance.
  - Amniocytes are used for karyotyping.
  - AF-AFP and acetylcholinesterase from amniotic fluid screens for neural tube defects.
  - Pregnancy loss rate is 0.5 percent.
- **Percutaneous umbilical blood sample**
  - Involves ultrasound guided aspiration of fetal blood from the umbilical vein after 20 weeks gestation.
  - Is both diagnostic (e.g., blood gases, karyotype, IgG and IgM antibodies) and therapeutic (e.g., intrauterine transfusion with fetal anemia).
  - Pregnancy loss rate is 1–2 percent.
- **Fetoscopy**
  - Transabdominal fiberoptic scope performed after 20 weeks under regional or general anesthesia.
  - Indications include intrauterine surgery or fetal skin biopsy (icyhthosis).
  - Pregnancy loss rate is 2–5 percent.
- **Cervical cerclage**
  - Performed between 14 and 24 weeks.
  - Suture encircles the cervix to prevent the cervical canal from dilating.
  - Indicated electively or emergently in cervical insufficiency.

> ## Stepwise approach to nonreassuring fetal tracings:
>
> 1. Examine the Electronic Fetal Monitoring (EFM) strip: Look for nonreassuring patterns.
> 2. Identify nonhypoxic causes that can explain the abnormal findings. (Most common are medications, particularly β-agonists or β-blockers.)
> 3. Begin intrauterine resuscitation as follows:
>   a. Discontinue medications (e.g., oxytocin)
>   b. Give IV normal saline bolus
>   c. Provide high-flow oxygen
>   d. Change patient's position (left lateral)
>   e. Vaginal exam to rule out prolapsed cord
>   f. Perform scalp stimulation to observe for accelerations (reassuring)
> 4. Prepare for delivery if the EFM tracing does not normalize.

OPERATIVE OBSTETRICS

Forceps- or Vacuum-Assisted Delivery

When is it the answer?

- Prolonged second stage (most common indication)
- Nonreassuring EFM strip in absence of contraindications
- To avoid maternal pushing when mother has cardiac and/or pulmonary conditions that would increase her risk.

When is it not the answer?

- Mother has small pelvis
- Cervix is not fully dilated
- Membranes have not ruptured
- Fetal head is not engaged
- Orientation of the head is not certain

Cesarean Delivery

- The cesarean section rate is approximately **29 percent** in the United States (including both primary and repeat procedures).
- **Risks** include the following: Increased risk of hemorrhage, infection, visceral injury (bladder, bowel, ureters), and DVTs.

- **Low segment transverse incision:** This is the most common procedure. It can only be performed with longitudinal lie of the fetus.
- **Classic vertical incision:** Can be performed with any fetal lie. Because of the increased risk of uterine rupture in subsequent pregnancies, cesarean must be initiated before labor begins.

When is it the answer?

- **Cephalopelvic disproportion (CPD):** With failure of progression or arrest in labor
- **Fetal malpresentation:** Most commonly preterm breech and nonfrank breech
- **Nonreassuring EFM strip**
- **Placenta previa** (unless placental edge > 2 cm from internal os)
- **Infection:** Mother who is HIV-positive or has active vaginal herpes
- **Uterine scar:** Prior myomectomy (fibroid) or prior classic incision C-section

Trial of vaginal birth after cesarean (VBAC) should be attempted in patients in the absence of C-section indications when the previous cesarean was a low segment uterine incision. The success rate is 80 percent.

External cephalic version

When is it the answer?

- Is first attempted in patients with transverse lie or breech presentation.
- The optimum time for external version is 37 weeks gestation, and success rates are 60–70 percent.

> External cephalic version (ECV) is done to change a baby from breech or other non-cephalic presentation cephalic. The physician pushes on the baby through the mother's abdomen, to attempt to roll the baby into position.

POSTPARTUM HEMORRHAGE

- **Utrine atony:** Is the *most* common cause of excessive postpartum bleeding. Consider in rapid or protracted labor, chorioamnionitis, medications (MgSO4, halothane), and overdistended uterus. Management is as follows: **Uterine massage** and **uterotonic agents** (e.g., oxytocin, methylergonovine, or carboprost).
- **Lacerations:** Management involves **surgical repair.**
- **Retained placenta:** Associated with accessory placental lobe or abnormal uterine invasion. Suspect with any missing placental cotyledons. Management is as follows: **Manual removal** or **uterine curettage** under ultrasound guidance. **Placenta accrete/increta/percreta** is the diagnosis when the examination shows placental villi infiltration. Placental villi may be infiltrated to the deeper layers of the endometrium (accrete), myometrium (increta), or serosa (percreta). **Hysterectomy** may be needed to control the bleeding.
- **DIC:** Most commonly related to abruption placenta. Also associated with severe preeclampsia, amniotic fluid embolism, or prolonged retention of

dead fetus. Suspect when there is generalized oozing or bleeding from IV or laceration sites in the presence of a contracted uterus.

- **Uterine inversion:** Suspected when there is a beefy-appearing bleeding mass in the vagina and failure to palpate the uterus. Management is as follows: **Uterine replacement,** followed by **IV oxytocin.**

- **Urinary retention** may occur with a hypotonic bladder: If residual volume is > 250 mL, give bethanechol (Urecholine). If this fails, urinary catheterize for no more than 2–3 days.

POSTPARTUM CONTRACEPTION

- **Breastfeeding:** Contraceptive use may be deferred for 3 months in women who are breastfeeding because of temporary anovulation.

- **Diaphragm and IUD placement:** Fitting and placement is deferred until the 6-week postpartum visit.

- **Combined estrogen-progestin formulations** (e.g., pills, patch, vaginal ring): These are not started until 3 weeks postpartum to prevent hypercoagulable state and risk of DVT. They are not used in breastfeeding women because of diminished lactation.

- **Progestin contraception** (e.g., mini-pill, Depo-Provera, Implanon) can safely be used during breastfeeding. They can be begun immediately after delivery.

POSTPARTUM FEVER

PP Day	Diagnosis	Risk Factors	Clinical Findings	Management
0	Atelectasis	General anesthesia with incisional pain Cigarette smoking	Mild fever with mild rales Patient is unable to take deep breaths	Incentive spirometry and ambulation Chest X-rays are unnecessary
1	UTI	Multiple catheterizations and vaginal exams	High fever, CVA tenderness, (+) urinalysis, (+) urine culture	Single-agent intravenous antibiotics
2–3	Endometritis		Moderate-to-high fever, uterine tenderness, (-) peritoneal signs	Multiple-agent IV antibiotics (e.g., gentamycin and clindamycin)
4–5	Wound infection	Emergency C-section after PROM	Persistent spiking fever despite antibiotics Wound erythema, fluctuance, or drainage	IV antibiotics Wet-to-dry wound packing Closure by secondary intention

PP Day	Diagnosis	Risk Factors	Clinical Findings	Management
5–6	Septic thrombophlebitis	Prolonged labor	Persistent wide fever swings despite broad-spectrum antibiotics	IV heparin for 7–10 days
7–21	Infectious mastitis	Nipple trauma and cracking	Unilateral breast tenderness, erythema, and edema	PO cloxacillin Breast feeding can be continued

SECTION 7
GYNECOLOGY

THE BREAST

Benign Breast Disease	Malignant Breast Disease (i.e., Breast Cancer)
1. Fibroadenoma	1. Ductal carcinoma in situ (DCIS)
2. Fibrocystic disease	2. Lobular carcinoma in situ (LCIS)
3. Intraductal papilloma	3. Ductal carcinoma
4. Fat necrosis (think of this with trauma to the breast)	4. Lobular carcinoma
	5. Inflammatory breast cancer
5. Mastitis (inflamed, painful breast in women who are breastfeeding)	6. Paget's disease of the breast/nipple

NIPPLE DISCHARGE

History will describe bilateral discharge with compression, but keep prolactinoma in the back of your mind.

Most Common Cause

The most common cause is **intraductal papilloma.** If a palpable mass is also present, the likelihood of cancer is greater. Further workup is needed when discharge is **unilateral, spontaneous, bloody,** or **associated with a mass.**

- Bloody discharge = Likely intraductal papilloma

Next Steps

- **Mammogram:** Look for underlying masses or calcifications.
- **Surgical duct excision:** Perform this for definitive diagnosis.
- Cytology is *not* helpful in the diagnosis and is never the answer for nipple discharge.

Surgical duct excision is *never* the answer for bilateral, milky nipple discharge. These patients should undergo workup for **prolactinoma**.

BREAST MASS

Fibrocystic Disease

This classically presents with **bilateral painful breast lump(s).** A clue to the diagnosis is that the **pain will vary with the menstrual cycle.** A simple cyst will have sharp margins and posterior acoustic enhancement on ultrasound. It will collapse on fine-needle aspiration FNA.

Treatment is **oral contraceptive pills/medications (OCP).**

Fibroadenoma

This classically presents as a **discrete, firm, nontender, and highly mobile breast nodule.** A clue to the diagnosis is a **mass that's highly mobile** on clinical exam. FNA will show epithelial and stromal elements.

Diagnostic testing: The steps in diagnosis of any patient (including pregnant women) with a breast mass are as follows:

1. Clinical **breast examination** (CBE)
2. Imaging: **Ultrasound or diagnostic mammography** (if patient > 40)
3. Fine-needle aspiration (FNA) **biopsy**

Treatment is **surgery,** which can be diagnostic and curative, but it is not necessary.

> *Never* diagnose a simple cyst on clinical exam alone. You must confirm the diagnosis with either ultrasound or FNA.

A 30-year-old woman complains of bilateral breast enlargement and tenderness, which fluctuates with her menstrual cycle. On physical examination, the breast feels lumpy, and there is a painful, discrete 1.5 cm nodule. A fine-needle aspiration is performed, and clear liquid is withdrawn. The cyst collapses with aspiration. Which of the following is the next step in management?

a. Clinical breast exam in 6 weeks
b. Core needle biopsy
c. Mammography
d. Repeat FNA in 6 weeks
e. Ultrasound in 6 weeks

*Answer: The correct answer is **A**. Clinical breast exam in 6 weeks is appropriate follow-up for a cystic mass that disappears after FNA. If the mass recurs on the 6-week follow-up, FNA may be repeated, and a core biopsy can be performed.*

When do you answer the following?

- **Ultrasound:**
  - First step in workup of **a palpable mass that feels cystic** on exam.

- **Fine-needle aspiration:**
  - First step in workup of a **palpable mass.** May be done **after ultrasound or instead of ultrasound.**
- **Mammography (> 40 years old) and biopsy (or biopsy alone if < 40 years old):**
  - Cyst recurs > twice within four to six weeks.
  - There is bloody fluid on aspiration.
  - Mass does not disappear completely upon FNA.
  - There is bloody nipple discharge (excisional biopsy).
  - There are skin edema and erythema suggestive of inflammatory breast carcinoma (excisional biopsy).
- **Cytology:**
  - Any aspirate that is grossly bloody must be sent for cytology.

- **Observation with repeat exam in 6–8 weeks:**
  - Cyst disappears on aspiration, and the fluid is clear.
  - Needle biopsy and imaging studies are negative.

A 47-year-old woman completes her yearly mammogram and is told to return for evaluation. The mammogram reveals a "cluster" of microcalcifications in the left breast. What is the most appropriate next step in management?

a. Excision biopsy
b. Needle biopsy
c. Repeat screening mammogram in 6 months
d. Repeat screening mammorgram in 12 months
e. Ultrasound

*Answer: The correct answer is **B**. Needle biopsy. A cluster of microcalcifications are mostly benign, however approximately 15–20% represent early cancer. The next step in workup is needle biopsy under mammographic guidance.*

BREAST CANCER

Preinvasive Diseases

Both **ductal carcinoma in situ (DCIS)** and **lobular carcinoma in situ (LCIS)** increase the risk of invasive disease. If biopsy reveals

- **DCIS,** then schedule **surgical resection with clear margins** (lumpectomy; i.e., breast conserving surgical resection) and **give RT and/or tamoxifen** to prevent invasive disease.
- **LCIS,** then **tamoxifen alone** can be administered. It is *not* necessary to perform surgery.

Note that LCIS is classically seen in premenopausal women.

Invasive Breast Diseases

Ductal carcinoma is the most common form of breast cancer (85 percent of all cases).

- It is **unilateral.**
- It metastasizes to **bone, liver, and brain.**

Lobular carcinoma accounts for 10 percent of breast carcinomas.

- It tends to be **multifocal** (within the same breast) and is bilateral in 20 percent of cases.

Inflammatory breast cancer is uncommon, grows rapidly, and metastasizes early.

- Look for a **red, swollen, and warm breast and pitted, edematous skin** (classic *peau d'orange* appearance).

Paget's disease of the breast/nipple presents with a pruritic, erythematous, scaly nipple lesion. It's often confused with dermatosis like eczema or psoriasis.

- Look for an **inverted nipple** or **discharge.**

Breast cancer screening guidelines per the U.S. Preventive Services Task Force (USPTF):

- Women ≥ 40 years old: Screening mammography every 1–2 years, with or without clinical breast examination (CBE)
- Mammography has the greatest benefit for women ≥ 50 years and women with family history of premenopausal breast cance.r
- BRCA genetic testing is *not* used for screening.

> ## Established risk factors for breast cancer:
>
> - Age ≥ 50 years old
> - Benign breast disease, especially cystic disease, proliferative types of hyperplasia, and atypical hyperplasia
> - Exposure to ionizing radiation
> - First childbirth after age 30 or nulliparity
> - Higher socioeconomic status
> - History of breast cancer
> - History of breast cancer in a first-degree relative
> - Hormone therapy
> - Obesity (BMI ≥ 30 kg per m^2)

Treatment of **invasive carcinoma:**

- Primary treatment when tumor size < 5 cm is **lumpectomy + radiotherapy +/– adjuvant therapy +/– chemotherapy.**
- **Sentinal node biopsy** is preferred over axillary node dissection.
- *Always* test for the following:
  - Estrogen and progesterone receptors
  - HER2 protein
- Primary treatment of inflammatory, tumor size > 5cm, and metastatic disease is systemic therapy.

A 68-year-old woman visits her primary care physician with a solid peanut-shaped hard mass in the upper outer quadrant of the left breast. A biopsy of the lesion is done, revealing "infiltrating ductal breast cancer." What is the next step in management?

a. Lumpectomy plus radiotherapy

b. Modified radical mastectomy

c. Modified radical mastectomy plus radiotherapy

d. Neoadjuvant chemotherapy plus lumpectomy plus radiotherapy

e. Tamoxifen and radiotherapy

*Answer: The correct answer is **A**. Breast conserving surgical therapy(lumpectomy) plus radiotherapy is the standard of care for invasive disease. There is no survival benefit with modified radical mastectomy.*

When are **BRCA 1 and BRCA 2 gene testing** indicated?

- Family history of early-onset breast cancer or ovarian cancer
- Breast and/or ovarian cancer in the same patient
- Family history of male breast cancer
- Ashkenazi Jewish heritage

When is **breast-conserving therapy** *not* the answer?

- Pregnancy
- Prior irradiation to the breast
- Diffuse malignancy or $\geq$ 2 sites in separate quadrants
- Positive tumor margins
- Tumor > 5 cm

When is adjuvant hormonal therapy included in management?

- In *any* hormone receptor-positive tumors, *regardless* of age and regardless of menopausal status, stage, or type of tumor

There is the **greatest benefit** when both ER+ and PR+ receptors are present. Therapy is **nearly as good** when there are only ER+ estrogen receptors. Therapy has the **least benefit** when only PR+ receptors are present.

- **Tamoxifen** competitively binds estrogen receptors.
  - 5-year treatment → 50 percent decrease in the recurrence, 25 percent decrease in mortality.
  - May be used in pre- or postmenopausal patients.

- **Aromatase inhibitors** (anastrozole, exemestane, letrozole) block peripheral production of estrogen.
  - This is the standard of care in HR+ postmenopausal women (more effective than tamoxifen).
  - Does *not* cause menopausal symptoms but *does* increase the risk of osteoporosis.

- **LHRH analogues** (e.g., goserelin) or **ovarian ablation** (surgical oophorectomy or external beam RT) is an alternative or an addition to tamoxifen in premenopausal women.

Benefits of Tamoxifen	Adverse Effects of Tamoxifen
• ↓ incidence of contralateral breast cancer • ↑ bone density in postmenopausal women • ↓ fractures • ↓ serum cholesterol • ↓ cardiovascular mortality risk	• Exacerbates menopausal symptoms • ↑↑ risk of endometrial cancer (1% in postmenopausal women after 5 yrs therapy)
	TIP: All women with a history of tamoxifen use and vaginal bleeding need evaluation & endometrial biopsy.

When is **chemotherapy** included in management?

- Tumor size > 1 cm
- Node-positive disease

When is **trastuzumab** included in management?

- It is indicated for metastatic breast cancer overexpressing HER2/neu.
- Trastuzumab is a monoclonal antibody directed against the extracellular domain of the HER2/neu receptor and is used to treat and control visceral metastatic sites.

If the case describes invasive breast cancer in an

- **HR-negative, pre- or postmenopausal woman** → Give chemotherapy alone.
- **HR-positive, premenopausal woman** → Give chemotherapy + tamoxifen.
- **HR-positive, postmenopausal woman** → Give chemotherapy + aromatase inhibitor.

UTERUS

ENLARGED UTERUS

An enlarged uterus may be caused by the following:

1. **Pregnancy** (discussed in Section 6: Obstetrics)
2. **Leiomyoma**
3. **Adenomyosis**

> Always make sure that the pregnancy (beta-HCG/urine pregnancy test) is *negative* before considering leiomyoma or adenomyosis.

Leiomyoma

Leiomyoma of the uterus is a **smooth muscle growth of the myometrium** and is the most common benign uterine tumor. The case will describe an **African-American woman** (the disease is 5 times more common in African Americans) of childbearing age with an **enlarged, firm, asymmetric, nontender** uterus. **Beta-hCG is negative.** Look for increased tumor growth and symptoms during pregnancy (growth corresponds to estrogen stimulation) and tumor shrinkage in menopause. It is most commonly asymptomatic (intramural location), but when symptomatic, it presents as one of the following:

- **Intermenstrual bleeding and menorrhagia** (submucosal location) with distortion of the uterine cavity seen on saline ultrasound (see image).

- **Bladder, rectum or ureter compression symptoms** (subserosal location). This type may become "parasitic" (i.e., break away from the uterus and obtain its blood supply from momentum, intestinal mesentery).

- **Acute-onset pain in a pregnant woman** as tumor outgrows blood supply and degenerates.

Intracavitary Leiomyoma

> - Asymmetric and nontender uterus = Leiomyoma

Adenomyosis

Adenomyosis is the **abnormal location of endometrial glands and stroma within the myometrium of the uterine wall.** When symptomatic, it causes **dysmenorrhea** and **menorrhagia**. The uterus feels **soft, globular, symmetrical, and tender.** Unlike leiomyoma, there is no change with high or low estrogen states.

The first test to order in a patient with an enlarged uterus is ß-hCG.

Diagnosis	Leiomyoma	Adenomyosis
Symptoms	Secondary dysmenorrhea and menorrhagia +/- symptoms of bladder, ureter, or rectal compression	Secondary dysmenorrhea and menorrhagia
1. Pelvic Exam	**Asymmetrically enlarged, firm, NONtender** uterus	**Symmetrically enlarged, soft, TENDER** uterus May be tender immediately before and during menses
2. Sonogram	Large intramural or subserosal myomas; saline infusion can show submucosal myomas	Diffusely enlarged uterus **with cystic areas** within the myometrial wall
3. Hysteroscopy	Direct visualize tumors	N/A
4. Histology	Definitive diagnosis	

Management	Leiomyoma	Adenomyosis
Observation/ Medical	Serial pelvic exams & observation for most	Levonorgestrel intrauterine system (IUS), may decrease heavy menstrual bleeding
Presurgical shrinkage	Tx: GnRH analog 3–6 months → ↓ size by 70% → regrowth after stopping GnRH cannot be used indefinitely	N/A
Myomectomy	Preserves fertility Laparotomy, laparoscopy **Must deliver next pregnancies by cesarean section because of increased risk of scar rupture in labor**	N/A
Embolization of vessels	Preserves uterus Invasive radiology	N/A
Hysterectomy	Best choice when fertility is completed Definitive therapy: Trans abdominal or transvaginal hyesterectomy	

- Symmetric and tender uterus = Adenomyosis

POSTMENOPAUSAL BLEEDING

A 65-year-old obese patient complains of vaginal bleeding for 3 months. Her last menstrual period was at age 52. She has no children. She has type 2 diabetes and chronic hypertension. Physical examination is normal with a normal-sized uterus and with no vulvar, vaginal, or cervical lesions. What is the next step in management?

a. Begin progestin therapy.
b. Begin estrogen and progestin therapy.
c. Perform an endometrial biopsy.
d. Perform a PAP smear and endocervical sampling.
e. Prescribe topical estrogen cream.

*Answer: The correct answer is **C**. The most common cause of postmenopausal bleeding is vaginal or endometrial atrophy, but the most important diagnosis to rule out is endometrial carcinoma (the most common gynecologic malignancy). Endometrial biopsy is the first step in management of any patient with postmenopausal bleeding.*

> *Never* give estrogen alone to a woman with a uterus. Always combine with progestins to prevent unopposed endometrial stimulation.

The most important risk factors for **endometrial carcinoma** are **unopposed estrogen states** (obesity, nulliparity, late menopause/early menarche, chronic anovulation).

All postmenopausal bleeding is suspected endometrial carcinoma until proven otherwise.

> All reproductive age women with chronic anovulation (e.g., PCOS) are at high risk of endometrial carcinoma. Give **progestins** to prevent endometrial hyperplasia and cancer.

Diagnosis	Management
1. Pelvic Exam	If the endometrial biopsy reveals **atrophy and no cancer,** no further workup is needed Give HRT (estrogen **PLUS** progesterone)
	If the endometrial biopsy reveals **adenocarcinoma → perform surgery staging:** (TAH and BSO, pelvic and para-aortic lymphadenectomy, and peritoneal washings) + *Radiation therapy if:* lymph node metastasis, >50% myometrial invasion, positive surgical margins, or poorly differentiated + *Chemotherapy if:* metastasis
2. Hysteroscopy	Identifies endometrial or cervical polyps as source of bleeding
3. Ultrasonography	Measures thickness of endometrial lining In postmenopausal patients the endometrial lining stripe should < 5 mm thick

TAH: Total abdominal hysterectomy; BSO: bilateral salpingo-oophorectomy; HRT: hormone replacement therapy

OVARIES: OVARIAN ENLARGEMENT

Ovarian enlargement may be found incidentally on physical exam or may present with symptoms. The following conditions should be considered.

SIMPLE CYST: PHYSIOLOGIC CYSTS (LUTEAL OR FOLLICULAR CYSTS)

This is the most common cyst that occurs during the reproductive years. It is **asymptomatic,** unless torsion has occurred (occurs with large cysts). The **β-hCG is negative;** ultrasound shows **fluid-filled simple cystic mass.**

Management is as follows:

- **Follow-up exam in 6–8 weeks** (resolves spontaneously). Steroid contraception prevents new cysts.
- **Laparoscopic removal** if
  - cyst is > **7 cm diameter;** or
  - there has been **previous steroid contraception without resolution** of the cyst.

COMPLEX CYST: BENIGN CYSTIC TERATOMA (DERMOID CYSTS)

These are benign tumors. They can contain cellular tissue from all 3 germ layers. Rarely, squamous cell carcinoma can develop. The **β-hCG is negative;** ultrasound shows a complex mass.

Management is as follows:

- **Laparoscopic/laparotomy removal,** either
  - **cystectomy** (to retain ovarian function); or
  - **oophorectomy** (if fertility is no longer desired).

BILATERAL OVARIAN ENLARGEMENT: POLYCYSTIC OVARIAN SYNDROME (PCOS)

See PCOS later in this section. PCOS is associated with **valproic acid.**

OVARIAN HYPERTHECOSIS

This refers to **nests of luteinized theca cells** in the ovarian stroma that produce **high levels of androgens.** The case will usually describe a postmenopausal woman (she may also be premenopausal) with **severe hirsutism** and **virilization.**

Management is as follows:

- **OCPs (both estrogen and progestin)** to suppress androgen production (by reducing LH stimulation of the theca cells) and to decrease free androgens (by stimulating sex hormone binding globulin).

DURING PREGNANCY

Luteoma of Pregnancy

This is a rare, nonneoplastic, tumorlike mass of the ovary that **emerges during pregnancy** and **regresses spontaneously** after delivery. It is found incidentally during a cesarean section or postpartum tubal ligation. It can be hormonally active and produce androgens, resulting in **maternal and fetal hirsutism and virilization.** No treatment is needed.

Theca Lutein Cysts

These benign neoplasms are caused by **high levels of FSH and β-hCG.** They are associated with **twins** and **molar** pregnancies. They **spontaneously regress** after pregnancy.

> The initial workup of an ovarian mass involves the following:
> - ß–hCG
> - Ultrasound
> - Laparoscopy/laparotomy if complex or > 7 cm

A 31-year-old woman is taken to the emergency department complaining of severe, sudden lower abdominal pain that started 3 hours ago. On examination, the abdomen is tender, no rebound tenderness is present, and there is an adnexal mass in the cul-de-sac area. An ultrasound evaluation shows an 8 cm left adnexal mass. Beta-hCG is negative. What is the next step in management?

a. Appendectomy
b. Give high-dose estrogen and progestin
c. Laparoscopic evaluation of ovaries
d. Observation
e. Perform oophorectomy

*Answer: The correct answer is **C**. Sudden onset of severe lower abdominal pain in the presence of an adnexal mass is presumed to be **ovarian torsion**. Laparoscopy and **detorsioning** of the ovaries is needed. If blood supply Is not affected, **cystectomy** can be done. If there is necrosis, **oophorectomy** is needed. She should then receive a 4-week follow-up and yearly evaluation to ensure there is complete resolution.*

PREPUBERTAL OR POSTMENOPAUSAL OVARIAN MASS

Any ovarian enlargement in prepubertal or postmenopausal women is always suspicious for an **ovarian neoplasm.**

Risk Factors	Protective Factors

• *BRCA1 gene*
• Positive family history
• High # of lifetime ovulations
• Infertility
• Use of perineal talc powder
	• Conditions that decrease # of ovulations
	  - oral contraceptive pills (OCPs)
	  - chronic anovulation
	  - breast-feeding
	  - short reproductive life

A 68-year-old woman presents with weakness and bloated feeling in her abdomen. She is found to have abdominal distention shifting dullness and a large right adnexal mass. Pelvic ultrasound reveals a 7-cm irregular and solid mass in the right ovary. Which of the following is the next step in the management?

a. Abdominal paracentesis

b. CT of the abdomen

c. Endometrial biopsy

d. Laparoscopy

e. Laparotomy

*Answer: The correct answer is **B**. In a postmenopausal woman with abdominal distension, an ovarian mass, the first step is CT of the abdomen to evaluate the mass and confirm the presence of ascities (indicating peritoneal seeding). If ascites is present, the next step is **laparotomy, oophorectomy and surgical staging**. Oophorectomy may be done by laparoscopy if no ascites is present.*

Diagnosis

Which cancer should you suspect in the following cases? What tumor markers will you order?

A 9-year-old girl presents with right adnexal pain and complex cystic mass on ultrasound

*Answer: **Germ cell tumor**: These are most common in **young women** and present in early-stage disease. The most common malignant epithelial cell type is **dysgerminoma**.*

Tumor markers: *LDH, ß-hCG, a-FP*

A 67-year-old woman presents with progressive weight loss, distended abdomen, and left adnexal mass.

*Answer: **Epithelial tumor**: This is the most common ovarian cancer in postmenopausal women. The most common malignant subtype is serous.*

Tumor markers: *CA-125, CEA*

A 58-year-old woman presents with postmenopausal bleeding. Endometrial biopsy shows endometrial hyperplasia. Pelvic ultrasound reveals a right ovarian mass.

*Answer: **Granulosa-theca** (stromal tumor): This ovarian tumor **secretes estrogen** and can cause **endometrial hyperplasia**.*

Tumor markers: *Estrogen*

A 48-year-old woman complains of increased facial hair and deepening of her voice. An adnexal mass is found on examination.

*Answer: **Sertoli-Leydig cell** (stromal tumor): This ovarian tumor secretes **testosterone**. Patients present with **masculinization syndromes**.*

Tumor markers: *Testosterone*

A 84-year-old woman presents with history of gastric ulcer and recent worsening dyspepsia presents with weight loss and abdominal pain. An adnexal mass is found.

Answer: **Metastatic gastric cancer** *to the ovary* **(Krukenberg tumor)**

Tumor markers: *Mucin-producing tumor from the stomach*

Management

- **Sonogram** (and CT scan for postmenopausal women)
- **Biopsy** via laparoscopy for simple cysts (no septations or solid components) or postmenopausal without ascites
- **Tumor markers**
- **Cystectomy** for benign tissue
- Premenstrual women: **Salpingoophorectomy**
- Postmenopausal women: **Total abdominal hysterectomy** (TAH); bilateral salpingoopherectomy (BSO) and postoperative chemotherapy for malignant tissue

CERVIX: CERVICAL NEOPLASIA

ETIOLOGY

- HPV 16, 18, 31, 33, and 35 are the most common HPV types associated with **cervical cancer.**
- HPV 6 and 11 are **benign condyloma acuminata.**

PAP smear classifications are as follows:

- Indeterminate smears:
  - **Atypical squamous cells of undetermined significance (ASCUS)**
- Abnormal smears:
  - **Low-grade squamous intraepithelial lesion (LSIL):** HPV, mild dysplasia, or CIN 1
  - **High-grade squamous intraepithelial lesion (HSIL):** Moderate dysplasia, severe dysplasia, CIS, CIN 2 or 3
  - **Cancer:** Invasive cancer

RISK FACTORS AND SCREENING

- Early age of intercourse
- Multiple sexual partners

- Cigarette smoking
- Immunosuppression

When is screening started?
- **Three years after onset of sexual activity or age 21,** whichever occurs first

What screening is used?
- **Conventional method:** 50 percent sensitivity
- **Liquid-based prep:** Sensitivity is increased to 75–80 percent
- **HPV DNA testing:** Useful in management of ASCUS

Frequency of screening?
- If < 30 years old, annually for conventional Pap or every 2 years for liquid-based.
- If > 30 years old, screen every 2 to 3 years if > 3 consecutive negative Pap smears.

A 35-year-old woman is referred because of a Pap smear reading of ASCUS. The patient states that her last Pap smear, done approximately 1 year ago, was negative. She has been sexually active, using combination oral contraception pills for the last 4 years. A repeat Pap smear after 3 months again reveals ASCUS. Which of the following is the next step in evaluation?

a. Endocervical curettage
b. Colposcopy and biopsy
c. HPV DNA typing
d. Repeat Pap smear in 6 months
e. Repeat Pap smear in 12 months

*Answer: The correct answer is **B.** ASCUS is most commonly inflammation due to **early HPV infection.** Approx 10–15 percent of patients with ASCUS have premalignant or malignant disease. Two Pap smears revealing ASCUS must be followed up with colposcopy and biopsy.*

Management of abnormal Pap smears is a commonly tested exam topic.

MANAGEMENT OF ATYPICAL SQUAMOUS CELLS OF UNDETERMINED SIGNIFICANCE (ASCUS)
- If the case describes a patient with ASCUS on Pap smear and follow-up is *certain*, **repeat the Pap smear in 3–6 months** or **order HPV DNA typing.** If the result is negative, follow-up is routine. If the repeat Pap smear is again ASCUS, or HPV 16 and 18 are found, then order **colposcopy and biopsies.**
- If the case describes a patient with ASCUS on Pap smear and follow-up is *uncertain*, order **colposcopy and biopsies.**

WORKUP OF AN ABNORMAL PAP

Step in Workup	When is this step the answer?	Next Step
Repeat Pap	– First ASCUS Pap	Repeat Pap at 4- to 6-month intervals until there are 2 consecutive, negative Paps If a repeat Pap is again ASCUS or worse, refer for colposcopy
HPV DNA testing	– First ASCUS Pap	If liquid-based cytology was used on the initial Pap, use specimen for DNA testing If conventional methods were used, a second Pap needs to be performed Colposcopy is then performed only if HPV 16 and 18 identified
Colposcopy and ectocervical biopsy	– An abnormal Pap smear – Two ASCUS Pap smears	Colposcopy is a magnification of the cervix (10–12 times) Abnormal lesions (e.g., mosaicism, punctation, white lesions, abnormal vessels) are biopsied and sent for histology
Endocervical curettage (ECC)	– All NONpregnant patients with an abnormal Pap smear	All nonpregnant patients undergoing colposcopy for an abnormal Pap smear must undergo an ECC to rule out endocervical lesions
Cone biopsy	– Pap smear worse than histology (suggests abnormal cells were not biopsied) – Abnormal ECC histology – An endocervical lesion – A biopsy showing microinvasive carcinoma of the cervix	NOTE: Deep cone biopsies can result in an *incompetent cervix* or *cervical stenosis*.

MANAGEMENT OF ABNORMAL HISTOLOGY

Step in Management	When is this step the answer?	Details
Observation and follow-up	– CIN 1 – CIN 2 or 3 after ablation or excision	– *Follow-up repeat Pap smears, colposcopy + Pap smear, or HPV DNA testing every 4 to 6 months for 2 years*
Ablative modalities	– CIN 2 or 3	– Cryotherapy – Laser vaporization – Electrofulguration
Excisional procedures	– CIN 2 or 3	– LEEP (loop electrosurgical excision procedure) – Cold-knife conization
Hysterectomy	– **Biopsy-confirmed** – **recurrent CIN 2 or 3**	

INVASIVE CERVICAL CANCER

The average age of diagnosis is 45 years.

Diagnosis

- **Cervical biopsy:** The most common diagnosis is squamous cell carcinoma.
- **Metastatic workup** is the next step in evaluation: Includes pelvic exam, chest X-ray, IV pyelogram, cystoscopy, and sigmoidoscopy.
- Imaging studies are *not* indicated. Invasive cervical cancer is the *only* gynecologic cancer that is not staged clinically. Do *not* order an abdominal/pelvic CT/MRI for clinical staging.

Management

- Management is simple hysterectomy or modified radical hysterectomy.
- Adjuvant therapy (radiation therapy and chemotherapy) is given when any of the following conditions is present:
    - Metastasis to lymph nodes
    - Tumor size > 4 cm
    - Poorly differentiated lesions
    - Positive margins
    - Local recurrence

CERVICAL NEOPLASIA IN PREGNANCY

A 25-year-old woman with a 15 week pregnancy by dates is found to have HGSIL (high-grade squamous intraepithelial lesion) on a recent pap smear. On pelvic examination there is a gravid uterus consistent with 15 weeks size, and the cervix is grossly normal to visual inspection. What is the next step in management?

a. Colposcopy and biopsy
b. Cone biopsy
c. Endocervical curettage
d. Hysterectomy
e. Repeat Pap after pregnancy

*Answer: The correct answer is **A**. A woman with abnormal pap smear is managed in the same way as a non-pregnant woman with the exception of endocervical curettage which is not performed because of increased cervical vascularity. An abnormal Pap smear is evaluated with colposcopy and biopsy. Pregnancy does not predispose to abnormal cytology and does not accelerate precancerous lesion progression into invasive carcinoma.*

MANAGEMENT OF ABNORMAL HISTOLOGY DURING PREGNANCY	
Stage	**Management**
CIN/dysplasia	– *Pap smear and colposcopy every 3 months during pregnancy* – *Repeat Pap and colposcopy 6–8 weeks postpartum. Any persistent lesions are then definitively treated postpartum*
Microinvasive cervical cancer	– *Cone biopsy to ensure no frank invasion* – *Deliver vaginally, reevaluate and treat 2 months postpartum*
Invasive cancer	*Diagnosed before 24 weeks:* – Definitive treatment (radical hysterectomy or radiation therapy) *Diagnosed after 24 weeks:* – Conservative management up to 32–33 weeks – Cesarean delivery and begin definite treatment

PREVENTION OF CERVICAL DYSPLASIA BY VACCINATION

- Give **quadrivalent HPV recombinant vaccine (Gardasil®)** to all females 8–26 years of age.
- Protects against the **4 HPV types (6, 11, 16, 18)** that cause 70 percent of cervical cancer and 90 percent of genital warts.
- Testing for HPV before vaccination is *not* needed.
- Sexually active women can receive the vaccine.
- Women with previous abnormal cervical cytology or genital warts can receive the vaccine, but it may be less effective.
- It can be given to patients with previous CIN, but benefits are limited.
- The vaccine is *not recommended* for pregnant, lactating, or immunosuppressed women.
- Females who have been vaccinated for HPV must still follow Pap smear recommendations.

PELVIC PAIN

The main differentials for a woman with pelvic pain are cervicitis, acute salpingoophoritis, chronic PID, and tuboovarian abscess.

> ## The initial workup for pelvic pain involves the following steps:
>
> 1. Pelvic exam
> 2. Cervical culture
> 3. Laboratory: ESR (sedimentation rate), WBC (include blood culture if fever is present)
> 4. Sonogram

CERVICITIS

This is the diagnosis when cervical discharge is found on routine exam, usually without other symptoms. Get cervical cultures (for chlamydia and gonorrhea). Manage by giving a single dose of **oral cefixime** *and* **azithromycin.**

ACUTE SALPINGOOPHORITIS

This is suspected when there is **cervical motion tenderness** on exam and the patient complains of **lower pelvic pain after menstruation.**

- Cervical cultures will be positive.
- WBC and ESR are elevated.
- Rule out pelvic abscess with sonogram.

Management is as follows:

- Outpatient: **Two oral antibiotics** (ofloxacin *and* metronidazole)
- Inpatient: **Three intravenous antibiotics** (IV cefoxitin or cefotetan *and* IV doxycycline or clindamycin *and* gentamicin)

CHRONIC PELVIC INFLAMMATORY DISEASE

This classically presents with **infertility** or **dyspareunia.** May also have a history of ectopic pregnancy or abnormal vaginal bleeding. Cervical cultures and laboratory tests will be **negative.** Sonogram will show **bilateral cystic pelvic masses** (hydrosalpinges).

Management involves the following:

- Lysis of tubal adhesions, which may be helpful for infertility
- Severe, unremitting pelvic pain may require a pelvic clean-out (TAH, BSO)

TUBOOVARIAN ABSCESS

This advanced form of pelvic inflammatory disease is diagnosed when the case describes an **ill-appearing woman** with **severe, lower abdominal/pelvic pain, back pain, and rectal pain,** with **systemic signs** and symptoms (nausea, vomiting, fever, tachycardia). **WBC and ESR are markedly elevated,** there is **pus on culdocentesis,** and sonogram shows a **unilateral pelvic mass** that appears as a multilocular, cystic, complex adnexal mass. Blood cultures will grow **anaerobic organisms.**

Management is as follows:

1. Admit to the hospital and give **IV clindamycin *and* IV gentamicin.**
2. If no response within 72 hours or if there is abscess rupture, perform an **exploratory laparotomy** +/– TAH and BSO or percutaneous drainage.

When are outpatient antibiotics the answer?

- All cases of **cervicitis**
- **Acute salpingoophoritis** when there is no systemic infection or pelvic abscess

When are inpatient antibiotics the answer?

- **Acute salpingoophoritis in a nulligravida or adolescent patient, previous outpatient treatment failure, intrauterine device (IUD) in place, presence of fever, or pelvic abscess**
- All cases of **tuboovarian abscess**

A 21-year-old female presents to the emergency department with lower abdominal pelvic pain starting 1 day ago. Symptoms began after her menstrual period completed. She is sexually active but using no contraception. Speculum examination reveals mucopurulent cervical discharge. Bimanual pelvic examination shows bilateral adnexal tenderness and cervical motion tenderness. She is afebrile. Her qualitative urinary β-hCG test is negative. Complete blood cell count (CBC) shows a WBC of 14,000. ESR is elevated. What is the most appropriate management?

a. Outpatient PO cefixime and azithromycin

b. Inpatient IV cefotetan, clindamycin, and gentamicin

c. Inpatient IV clindamycin and gentamicin

d. Exploratory laparotomy

e. Percutaneous drainage

*Answer: The correct answer is **B**. This patient has acute salpingo-oophoritis. Her nulligravid status is an indication for inpatient IV antibiotic triple-therapy.*

DYSMENORRHEA

PRIMARY DYSMENORRHEA

- Primary dysmenorrhea is the diagnosis when the case describes **recurrent, crampy lower abdominal pain** along with **nausea, vomiting, and diarrhea during menstruation.** Symptoms begin **2–5 years after onset of menstruation** (ovulatory cycles). There is no pelvic abnormality.
- Symptoms are related to **excessive endometrial prostaglandin F2,** which causes uterine contractions and acts on gastrointestinal smooth muscle.

Management is as follows:

- **NSAIDs** are the first line of therapy.
- **Combination oral contraceptives** are the second line.

SECONDARY DYSMENORRHEA

Secondary dysmenorrhea presents similar symptoms as primary dysmenorrheal but is due to another disorder. Most commonly, secondary dysmenorrhea occurs due to endometriosis. However, other pathology such as **adenomyosis, leiomyomas,** etc., can also be the underlying pathology.

Endometriosis

This involves endometrial glands outside the uterus. It classically presents in women over 30 with **dysmenorrhea, dyspareunia, dyschezia** (painful bowel movements), and **infertility.**

- The most common site is **the ovary,** causing adnexal enlargements (endometriomas), also known as a **chocolate cyst.**
- The second most common site is the **cul-de-sac**, causing **uterosacral ligament nodularity** and **tenderness on rectovaginal examination.** This location is associated with bowel adhesions and a fixed, retroverted uterus.
- Investigations: CA-125 may be elevated. Sonogram may show endometriomas. Definitive diagnosis is made with **laparoscopic visualization.**

Management is as follows:

- First-line therapy: **Continuous oral progesterone** or oral contraceptive pill (OCP)
- Second-line therapy: **Testosterone derivatives** (Danocrine or danazol) or **GnRH analogs** (Lupron or leuprolide)
- Laparoscopic lysis adhesions, laser vaporization of lesions can improve fertility.
- TAH and BSO can be done for severe symptoms when fertility is not desired.

VAGINAL BLEEDING AND ITS ABSENCE

PREMENARCHAL VAGINAL BLEEDING

This is bleeding that occurs before menarche. The average age at menarche is 12. Causes are as follows:

- The most common cause is the **presence of a foreign body.**

- You must *rule out* **sarcoma botryoides** (cancer of vagina or cervix suggested by a grapelike mass arising from the vaginal lining or cervix), **tumor** of the pituitary adrenal gland or ovary, and sexual abuse.

Diagnosis

- Perform **pelvic exam under sedation.**

- Order **CT or MRI of pituitary, abdomen, and pelvis** to look for estrogen-producing tumor.

- If workup is *negative*, the diagnosis is **idiopathic precocious puberty.**

Abnormal Vaginal Bleeding

A 31-year-old woman complains of 6 months of metromenorrhagia. The patient states that she started menstruating at age 13 and that she has had regular menses until the past 6 months. The pelvic examination, including a Pap smear, is normal. She has no other significant personal or family history. What is the next step in management?

a. Obtain ß-hCG
b. Obtain LH, FSH levels
c. Perform a pelvic ultrasound
d. Recommend oral contraceptive pill
e. Recommend progestin-only pill

*Answer: The correct answer is **A**. Irregular bleeding in reproductive age should always be evaluated first for pregnancy. If pregnancy is ruled out, workup for anatomical causes of bleeding or anovulation can be started.*

PRIMARY AMENORRHEA

Primary amenorrhea is diagnosed with **absence of menses at age 14 *without* secondary sexual development or at age 16 *with* secondary sexual development.**

Workup

- Physical exam and ultrasound:

  - Are **breasts** present or absent? Breasts indicate adequate estrogen production.

  - Is a **uterus** present or absent on ultrasound?

- Karyotype, testosterone, FSH

	Uterus Present	Uterus Absent

Breasts Present	**Workup as secondary amenorrhea**
	• Imperforate hymen
	• Vaginal septum
	• Anorexia nervosa
	• Excessive exercise
	• Pregnancy before the first menses
		Order testosterone levels and karyotype
		• Müllerian agenesis
		  – *XX karyotype, normal testosterone for female*
		• Complete androgen insensitivity (testicular feminization)
		  – *XY karyotype, normal testosterone for male*

Breasts Absent	**Order FSH level and karyotype**
	• Gonadal dysgenesis (Turner syndrome)
	  – *X0 karyotype, FSH elevated*
	• Hypothalamic–pituitary failure
	  – *XX karyotype, FSH low*
		RARE
		• Not clinically relevant

A 17-year-old girl is brought to the clinic by her mother concerned because her daughter has never had a menstrual period. She reports that her daughter has good grades, studies hard but seems stressed out most of the time which is why she believed her period was delayed. On examination she seems to be well-nourished, with adult breast development and pubic hair present. Pelvic examination reveals a foreshortened vagina. No uterus is seen on ultrasound. What is the most appropriate advice?

a. CT scan of the brain is indicated to evaluate a pituitary tumor.

b. Estrogen and progesterone supplementation is indicated.

c. Invitro fertilization is an option for future fertility.

d. Surgical removal of intrabdominal testes is recommended.

e. Vaginal reconstruction may be performed.

*Answer: The correct answer is E. This patient has **Müllerian agenesis** resulting in an absence of uterus, cervix, upper vagina. Ovaries are intact and normal levels of estrogen are present. Vaginal reconstruction may be performed to elongate the vagina for satisfactory sexual intercourse.*

Müllerian Agenesis

This is the diagnosis when karyotype reveals **normal female secondary sexual characteristics** and **normal estrogen and testosterone levels** (ovaries are intact). The only abnormality is **absence of all Müllerian duct derivatives** (fallopian tubes, uterus, cervix, and upper vagina).

Management involves the **surgical elongation of the vagina** for satisfactory sexual intercourse.

Androgen Insensitivity

This is the diagnosis when there is **no pubic or axillary hair,** a karyotype reveals **male genotype,** and ultrasound reveals **testes.** The testes produce *both* normal levels of estrogen for a female and normal levels of testosterone for a male.

Management involves the **removal testes before age 20** because of increased risk of testicular cancer. Estrogen replacement will then be needed.

Gonadal Dysgenesis (Turner Syndrome, XO)

This is the diagnosis when karyotyping reveals **absence of one X chromosome (45, X), absence of secondary sexual characteristics,** and **elevated FSH.** Because the second X chromosome is essential to the development of normal ovarian follicles, streak gonads develop.

Management involves **estrogen and progesterone replacement** for development of secondary sexual characteristics.

Hypothalamic-Pituitary Failure

This is the diagnosis when there are **no sexual characteristics** but the **uterus is normal on ultrasound** and **FSH levels are low.** It may be due to stress, excessive exercise, or anorexia nervosa. **Kallman syndrome** is the likely diagnosis when the case also describes **anosmia** (hypothalamus doesn't produce GnRH). CNS imaging (CT head) will rule out a brain tumor.

Management involves **estrogen and progesterone replacement** for development of secondary sexual characteristics.

SECONDARY AMENORRHEA

Secondary amenorrhea is diagnosed when one of the following conditions presents:

- Regular menses are replaced by an **absence of menses for 3 months.**
- Irregular menses are replaced by an **absence of menses for 6 months.**

STEPS IN THE WORKUP OF SECONDARY AMENORRHEA	
Steps in the Workup	**Next Step in Management**
1. Pregnancy Test (ß-hCG)	
2. Thyrotropin (TSH) (rule out hypothyroidism)	An elevated TRH in primary hypothyroidism → ↑ prolactin. Treat hypothyroidism with thyroid replacement for rapid restoration of menstruation

3. Prolactin (rule out elevation)	*If elevated:*
	
	1) *Review medications:* Antipsychotics have antidepressants have anti-dopamine side effect → ↑ prolactin
	
	2) *CT or MRI of head to rule out pituitary tumor*
	  – Tumor <1 cm: give bromocriptine (dopamine agonist)
	  – Tumor >1 cm: treat surgically
	
	3) If the cause of elevated prolactin is idiopathic, treat with bromocriptine.

4. Progesterone Challenge Test (PCT)	• *Positive PCT:* Any withdrawal bleeding is *diagnostic of* **anovulation.** – *Treatment:* Cyclic progesterone to prevent endometrial hyperplasia. Clomiphene ovulation induction is done if pregnancy is desired. • *Negative PCT:* inadequate estrogen or outflow tract obstruction

5. Estrogen–Progesterone Challenge Test (EPCT)	• 3 weeks of oral estrogen followed by 1 week of progesterone
	• *Positive EPCT:* Any withdrawal bleeding is *diagnostic of* **inadequate estrogen.** **Next step is to get an FSH level.**
	  – ↑ *FSH is ovarian failure.* Y chromosome mosaicism may be the cause if patient is < 25 years. Order a **karyotype** for confirmation.
	  – ↓ *FSH is hypothalamic–pituitary insufficiency.* Order a **brain CT/MRI** to rule out a tumor. Give estrogen-replacement therapy to prevent osteoporosis and cyclic progestins to prevent endometrial hyperplasia.
	• *Negative EPCT:* Diagnostic of an outflow tract obstruction or endometrial scarring (e.g., *Asherman syndrome*). Order a **hysterosalpingogram** to identify the lesion. Management: Adhesion lysis followed by estrogen stimulation of the endometrium. An inflatable stent prevents re-adhesion of the uterine walls.

PREMENSTRUAL SYNDROME

Premenstrual Tension

This is defined as distressing physical, psychological, and behavioral symptoms recurring at the same phase of the menstrual cycle and disappearing during the remainder of the cycle.

Premenstrual Dysphoric Disorder (PMDD)

This is more severe, involving major disruptions to daily functioning and relationships.

Management

- **SSRI**s are the treatment of choice.
- Low doses of **vitamin B6 (pyridoxine)** may improve symptoms.
- Diuretics have shown mixed results in the management of premenstrual fluid retention.

ENDOCRINE DISORDERS

- **Hirsutism:** Excessive male-pattern hair growth in a woman.
- **Virilization:** Excessive male-pattern hair growth in a woman *plus* other masculinizing signs, such as clitoromegaly, baldness, lowering of voice, increasing muscle mass, and loss of female body contours.

Almost all cases of hirsutism are either **PCOS** or **idiopathic.** More serious causes of hirsutism (androgen-secreting tumors) need to be *excluded* in the workup.

Initial steps in workup involve the following lab work:

- Testosterone
- DHEAS
- LH/FSH
- 17-hydroxyprogesterone

POLYCYSTIC OVARIAN SYNDROME (PCOS)

This is the diagnosis when there is **gradual onset hirsutism, obesity, acne, irregular bleeding,** and **infertility.** There are chronic anovulatory cycles and **infertility.** Diagnosis is mostly clinical. However, an **elevated LH/FSH ratio** is used for confirmation. **Bilaterally enlarged ovaries** will be found on exam and ultrasound.

- **Anovulation** → no corpus luteum production of progesterone → unopposed estrogen → hyperplastic endometrium and irregular bleeding → **predisposition to endometrial cancer.**
- **Increased testosterone:** ↑LH levels → ↑theca cell production of androgens → hepatic production of SHBG is suppressed → ↑**total testosterone and** ↑**free testosterone.**
- **Ovarian enlargement:** Ultrasound shows a necklacelike pattern of multiple peripheral cysts (20–100 cystic follicles in each ovary). ↑androgens → multiple follicles in various stages of development, stromal hyperplasia, and a thickened ovarian capsule → **bilaterally enlarged ovaries.**

> **Anovulation** classically presents with a **history of amenorrhea** followed by **unpredictable bleeding** (prolonged unopposed estrogen stimulates the endometrium). Consider the following diagnoses:
> - Polycystic ovary syndrome (PCOS)
> - Hypothyroidism
> - Pituitary adenoma
> - Elevated prolactin
> - Medications (e.g., antipsychotics, antidepressants)

Diagnosis

- LH:FSH ratio = **3:1** (normal is 1.5:1).
- Testosterone level is **mildly elevated.**
- Pelvic ultrasound shows **bilaterally enlarged ovaries with multiple subcapsular small follicles and increased stromal echogenicity.**

Management

- **Oral contraceptive pill** treats irregular bleeding and hirsutism. The progestin component prevents endometrial hyperplasia.
- **Spironolactone** may also be used to suppress hair follicles.
- **Clomiphene citrate** or **human menopausal gonadotropin** (HMG) is the treatment of choice for infertility.
- **Metformin** enhances ovulation and manages insulin resistance.

ADRENAL OR OVARIAN TUMOR

This is the diagnosis when the question describes **rapid onset hirsutism** and **virilization** *without* a family history. **DHEAS is markedly elevated** in an adrenal tumor; **testosterone is markedly elevated** in an ovarian tumor. The next step is to order an **ultrasound** (adnexal mass) or CT (adrenal mass).

Management involves **surgical removal** of the tumor.

CONGENITAL ADRENAL HYPERPLASIA (21-HYDROXYOLASE DEFICIENCY)

This is the diagnosis when the question describes **gradual-onset hirsutism** *without* virilization in the **second or third decade** that is associated with **menstrual irregularities** and **anovulation. Serum 17-hydroxyprogesterone** level is markedly elevated. Precocious puberty with short stature is common. Family history may be positive.

Management involves **corticosteroid replacement,** which will arrest the signs of androgenicity and restore ovulatory cycles.

IDIOPATHIC HIRSUTISM

This is the diagnosis when there is **no virilization** and **all laboratory tests are normal.** It is the most common cause of hirsutism.

Management is as follows:

- **Spironolactone** is the treatment of choice.
- **Eflornithine (Vaniqa)** is the first-line topical drug for the treatment of unwanted facial and chin hair.

Diagnosis	Testosterone	DHEAS	LH/FSH	17-OHP	Next Step in Management
	Produced by ovary & adrenal gland	Produced by adrenal glands		Precursor in cortisol synthesis & converted peripherally to androgens	
Polycystic ovary syndrome	↑	NL /↑	↑LH ↓FSH	NL	**Ultrasound** to rule out other disorders/ tumors Screen lipids and fasting blood glucose
Congenital adrenal hyperplasia	NL/↑	NL /↑	NL/NL	↑↑	**ACTH stimulation** confirms the diagnosis
Ovarian tumor	↑↑	NL	NL/NL	NL	**Ultrasound/CT** to image tumor
Adrenal tumor	↑	↑↑	NL/NL	NL	**Ultrasound/CT** to image tumor

MENOPAUSE DISORDERS

- *Menopause* is defined as **3 months of amenorrhea** with **elevation of FSH and LH.** The mean age is 51 years. Smokers experience menopause up to 2 years earlier.
- Diagnose with **serial levels of elevated gondaotropins.**
- If menopause occurs between ages 30 and 40, it is **premature menopause.** It is most often idiopathic but can also occur after radiation therapy or surgical oophorectomy.
- If menopause occurs before age 30, it is **premature ovarian failure** and may be associated with autoimmune disease or Y chromosome mosaicism.

The following menopausal symptoms are related to a **lack of estrogen:**

- **Amenorrhea:** Menses become anovulatory and decrease in the 3- to 5-year period known as perimenopause.
- **Hot flashes:** This is unpredictable, profuse sweating and heat that occurs in 75 percent of women. Obese women are less likely to undergo hot flashes (due to peripheral conversion of androgens to estrone).
- **Reproductive tract:** Decreased vaginal lubrication, increased vaginal pH, and increased vaginal infections can occur.
- **Urinary tract:** Increased urgency, frequency, nocturia, and urge incontinence can occur.

- **Psychic:** Depressed mood, emotional lability, and sleep disorders can occur.
- **Cardiovascular disease:** This is the most common cause of mortality (50 percent) in postmenopausal women.
- **Osteoporosis**

OSTEOPOROSIS

- The most common site of symptomatic osteoporosis is in the **vertebral bodies,** leading **to crush fractures, kyphosis,** and **decreased height.** Hip and wrist fractures are the next most frequent sites.
- The most common risk factor is **positive family history in a thin, white female.** Other risk factors are **steroid use, low calcium intake, sedentary lifestyle, smoking,** and **alcohol.**
- Prevent with calcium and vitamin D, weight-bearing exercise, and elimination of cigarettes and alcohol.

Diagnosis

- **Bone density** is assessed with a **DEXA scan** (dual-energy X-ray absorptiometry). The results are reported as a T-score: a T-score ≥ -2.5 indicates the presence of osteoporosis.
- **Calcium loss** is assessed with a **24-hour urine hydroxyproline** or **NTX** (N-telopeptide, a bone breakdown product).

Management

- First-line therapy is **bisphosphonates** and **SERMs.**
  - Bisphosphates (e.g., alendronate, risedronate) **inhibit osteoclastic activity.**
  - Selective estrogen receptor modulators (SERMs) **increase bone density.**
    - **SERMs** are protective against the heart and bones but are *not* effective for vasomotor symptoms of menopause.
    - **Tamoxifen (Nolvadex)** has endometrial and bone agonist effects but breast antagonist effects.
    - **Raloxifene (Evista)** has bone agonist effects but endometrial antagonist effects.
- **Calcitonin** and **fluoride** are second-line therapy.
- Estrogen is *never* the primary treatment of osteoporosis because of associated risks.

HORMONE REPLACEMENT THERAPY (HRT)

When is HRT the answer?	When is HRT NOT the answer?
Treatment of:	*Treatment of:*
• Menopausal vasomotor symptoms (hot flashes)	• Osteoporosis
• Genitourinary atrophy	*When the case describes a history of:*
• Dyspareunia	• Estrogen-sensitive cancer (breast or endometrial)
	• Liver disease
	• Active thrombosis
	• Unexplained vaginal bleeding

- Women *without* a uterus can be given **continuous estrogen.**
- All women *with* a uterus must also receive progestin therapy to prevent endometrial hyperplasia.

Benefits of HRT	Risks of HRT
↓ Rate of osteoporotic fractures	↑ Risk of DVT
↓ Rate of colorectal cancer	↑ Risk of heart attacks and breast cancer in combination therapy
	Risk of breast cancer is only associated with therapy > 4 yrs

GUIDELINES FOR HORMONE REPLACEMENT THERAPY

- *Only* start HRT for vasomotor symptoms.
- *Never* give HRT for the prevention of cardiovascular disease.
- Use the *lowest dose* of HRT to treat symptoms.
- Use the *shortest duration* of HRT to treat symptoms; reevaluate annually.
- Do not exceed 4 years of therapy (increased risk of breast cancer after 4 years of therapy).

CONTRACEPTION

Low-dose contraceptive pills do *not* increase the risk of cancer, heart disease, or thromboembolic events in women with no associated risk factors (hypertension, diabetes, or smoking).

	Examples	Absolute Contraindication	Relative Contraindication	Benefits
Barrier Methods	Condoms Vaginal diaphragm +/- spermicides	N/A	N/A	– Protective against STDs
Steroid Contraception	Combination (estrogen + progesterone) Progestin only (OCP called "mini-pill", injectable, implant, morning after pill)	– Pregnancy – Acute liver disease – Vascular disease (e.g., thrombo-embolism, DVT, CVA, SLE) – Hormone dependent cancer (e.g., breast CA) – Smoker >35 – Uncontrolled hypertension – Migraines with aura – DM with vascular disease – Thrombophilia	– Migraines – Depression – DM – Chronic HTN – Hyperlipidemia	– ↓ovarian and endometrial CA – ↓dysmenorrhea – ↓dysfunctional uterine bleeding – ↓ectopic pregnancy
Intrauterine Devise	– Levonorgestrel-impregnated – Copper-banded	– Pregnancy – Pelvic malignancy – Salpingitis	– Abnormal uterine size or shape – Immune suppression (including steroid therapy) – Nulligravidity – Abnormal Pap smears – History of ectopic pregnancy	

INFERTILITY

A 35-year-old woman comes to the gynecologist's office complaining of infertility for 1 year. She and her husband have been trying to achieve pregnancy for > 1 year and have been unsuccessful. There is no previous history of pelvic inflammatory disease, and she had used oral contraception medication for 6 years. The pelvic examination is normal. Semen analysis is low volume and shows decreased sperm density and low motility. What is the next step in management?

a. *Administer testosterone*

b. *Measure serum testosterone*

c. *Measure thyroid hormone*

d. *Repeat semen analysis*

e. *Refer for intrauterine insemination*

*Answer: The correct answer is **D**. Because semen samples are variable, an abnormal semen analysis is repeated in 4–6 weeks to confirm findings.*

Infertility is defined as inability to achieve pregnancy after 12 months of unprotected and frequent intercourse.

The steps in workup are as follows:

1. The first step is **semen analysis**.
2. If semen analysis is normal, work up for **anovulation**.
3. If semen analysis is normal and ovulation is confirmed, work up for **fallopian tube abnormalities.**

Step	Diagnosis	Management
1. Semen Analysis	Normal values: • Volume > 2 ml; pH 7.2–7.8; sperm density > 20 million/ml; sperm motility > 50%; and sperm morphology > 50% normal.	• If values are abnormal, repeat the semen analysis in 4–6 weeks. • *Abnormal semen analysis:* Intrauterine insemination, intracytoplasmic sperm injection (ICSI) and invitro fertilization (IVF) are fertility options. • *No viable sperm:* Artificial insemination by donor may be used.
2. Anovulation	• Basal body temperature (BBT) chart: NO midcycle temperature elevation • Progesterone: Low • Endometrial biopsy: Proliferative histology	• Hypothyroidism or hyperprolactinemia are causes of anovulation that can be treated. • *Ovulation induction:* – *Clomiphene citrate* is the agent of choice. – Human menopausal gonadotrophin (hMG) is used if clomiphene fails – *Most common side effect* = ovarian hyperstimulation. Ovarian size must be monitored during induction.
3. Tube Abnormalities: Hysterosalpinogram and Laparoscopy	• *Chlamydia Antibody:* A negative IgG antibody test for chlamydia rules out infection-induced tubal adhesions.	• *Hysterosalpingogram* (HSG): No further testing is performed if the HSG shows normal anatomy. • Laparoscopy: Performed with an abnormal HSG to visualize the oviducts and attempt reconstruction (tuboplasty). If tubal damage is severe, IVF should be planned.

UNEXPLAINED INFERTILITY

The **semen analysis** is normal, **ovulation** is confirmed, and **patent oviducts** are noted. **No treatment** is indicated, and approximately 60 percent of patients with unexplained infertility will achieve a spontaneous pregnancy within the next 3 years.

IN VITRO FERTILIZATION

1. Eggs are aspirated from the ovarian follicles using an ultrasound-guided transvaginal approach.
2. They are fertilized with sperm in the laboratory, resulting in the formation of embryos.
3. Multiple embryos are transferred into the uterine cavity with a cumulative pregnancy rate of 55 percent after 4 IVF cycles.

GESTATIONAL TROPHOBLASTIC DISEASE (GTN)

This is an **abnormal proliferation of placental tissue** involving both the cyto-trophoblast and/or syncytiotrophoblast. It can be either benign or malignant.

- GTN is most common in **Taiwan** and the **Philippines.** Other risk factors are **maternal age extremes** (< 20 years old, > 35 years old) and **folate deficiency.**
- The most common symptom is **bleeding < 16 weeks gestation** and **passage of vesicles from the vagina.** Other symptoms of a molar pregnancy include hypertension, hyperthyroidism, and hyperemesis gravidarum and no fetal heart tones appreciated.
- The most common signs are **fundus larger than dates, absence of fetal heart tones, bilateral cystic enlargements of the ovary** (theca-lutein cysts).
- The most common site of distant metastasis is the **lungs.**

Benign: H. Mole		Malignant		
Complete	Incomplete	Nonmetastatic	Metastatic: Good prognosis	Metastatic: Poor prognosis
Empty egg	Normal egg	Uterus only	Pelvis or lung	Brain or liver
46,XX (dizygotic ploidy)	69,XXY (*triploidy*)	100% cure	> 95% cure	65% cure
Fetus absent	Fetus nonviable	Single-agent chemotherapy until after ß-hCG (–) for 3 weeks		Multiple agent chemotherapy until after ß-hCG (–) for 3 weeks
20% → malignancy	10% → malignancy	f/up for 1 year on OCP		f/up for 5 years on OCP
No chemotherapy; serial ß-hCG titers until (-); f/up for 1 year on OCP				

A 32-year-old Filipino woman is 15 weeks pregnant by dates. She presents with painless vaginal bleeding associated with severe nausea and vomiting. Her uterus extends to her umbilicus but no fetal heart tones can be heard. Her blood pressure is 162/98 mm Hg. A dipstick urine shows 2+ proteinuria. Which of the following is the most likely diagnosis?

a. Chronic hypertension

b. Chronic hypertension with superimposed preeclampsia

c. Eclampsia

d. Molar pregnancy

e. Preeclampsia

*Answer: The correct answer is **D**. This patients presentation is typical for a molar pregnancy. Absence of fetal heart tones eliminates the other options.*

Diagnosis

Sonogram reveals **homogenous intrauterine echoes without a gestational sac or fetal parts** ("snowstorm" ultrasound).

Management

- **Baseline quantitative β-hCG titer**
- **Chest X-ray** (rule out lung metastasis)
- **Suction dilation and currettage (D&C)** (to evacuate the uterine contents)
- Place the patient on **effective contraception** (oral contraceptive pills) to ensure no confusion between rising β-hCG titers from recurrent disease and normal pregnancy

SECTION 8
RADIOLOGY

CHOOSING AN IMAGING STUDY

WHEN IS CT THE BEST ANSWER ON THE TEST?

- **Noncontrast head CT:** This is the best initial test to **rule out hemorrhage** when the case describes trauma or acute neurological change.
- **Contrast head CT:** This is appropriate when you want to evaluate for **AV malformations** or **primary or metastatic tumors.**
- This is the best test to evaluate **retroperitoneal structures:** pancreatitis or pancreatic masses or nodal metastasis from colon, prostate, testicular, or renal malignancies.
- **High-resolution CT scan of chest:** This is the test of choice to evaluate **parenchymal lung disease** (interstitial fibrosis). It is also the best test to evaluate **bony structures.**

WHEN IS MRI THE BEST ANSWER ON THE TEST?

- MRI is the test of choice for evaluating **demyelinating diseases** (e.g., multiple sclerosis and some dementias).
- It is the best test to evaluate the **posterior fossa, base of the skull, and the orbit.**
- It is the best test to evaluate **acoustic neuromas, pituitary tumors, and small intraparenchymal brain tumors.**
- It is the test of choice for **bone tumors, bone and soft tissue infections** (e.g., osteomyelitis), **joint spaces, and aseptic necrosis of femoral head.**
- It is the test of choice for evaluating **disease of the spinal cord and spinal column** (e.g., herniated discs, degenerative disc disease, and spinal tumors).

> Keep the following in mind regarding CT scans:
> - Do *not* order CT with contrast in patients with renal disease (creatinine $\geq$ 1.5).
> - *Always* discontinue metformin before doing a CT scan with IV contrast and only resume metformin 48 hours after the scan, when renal failure has been ruled out.
> - Do *not* order MRI with contrast in patients with renal disease (creatinine $\geq$ 1.5) due to the risk of nephrogenic systemic fibrosis.

WHEN ARE NUCLEAR SCANS THE ANSWER ON STEP 3?

- **HIDA (hepatobiliary) scan:** This is used for **evaluating biliary obstruction versus acute cholecystitis** and the **evaluation of biliary leaks postoperatively.** It is also the test of choice to evaluate **congenital abnormalities of the biliary tract,** including biliary atresia. It is *not* the test of choice for evaluating gallbladder stones.

- **Bone scan:** This is used for evaluating **metastatic bone lesions** (prostate, breast, kidney, thyroid, lung), **evaluating delayed fractures,** and **evaluating osteomyelitis and avascular necrosis of the femoral head.**

- **Adrenal scan:** This is the test of choice to **localize pheochromocytoma** when a MRI/CT scan is nondiagnostic.

- **V/Q scan:** This is the initial test of choice to evaluate for **pulmonary embolism** (PE). (A normal study rules out PE. An indeterminate scan requires further workup with CT angiogram. A perfusion defect with normal ventilation quite probably indicates PE.) Do *not* order a V/Q scan in a patient with COPD or extensive lung disease.

- **Gallium scan:** This is the test of choice for **localizing abscesses, staging lymphomas, and melanomas.**

WHEN IS ULTRASOUND THE ANSWER ON THE TEST?

- It is the best initial test to **evaluate the gallbladder for stones** when a patient presents with right upper-quadrant pain.

- It is the best initial test for **assessing the uterus, adnexa, and ovaries** (with the *exception* of cervical carcinoma).

- It is the best initial test to **evaluate the prostate;** it also aids in **obtaining biopsy.**

- It is the best test to **evaluate for deep venous thrombosis (DVT).**

IMAGES YOU MUST BE ABLE TO RECOGNIZE ON THE EXAM

Pneumothorax

Pneumomediastinum

Pneumoperitoneum

COPD

Pleural Effusions

Bilateral Pleural Effusions

Pulmonary Embolism

Lobar Pneumonia

Aortic Dissection

Aortic Aneurysm

Small Bowel Obstruction

Cecal Volvulus

Toxic Megacolon

Carcinoma of the Colon

Epidural Hemorrhage

Subdural Hemorrhage

Thalamic Hemorrhage

Cholecystitis

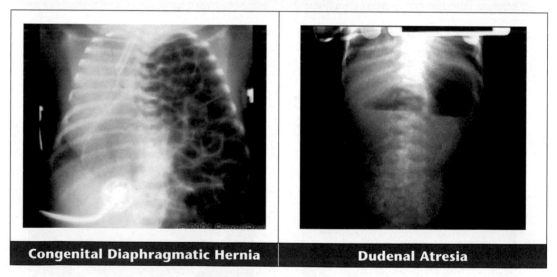

Congenital Diaphragmatic Hernia

Dudenal Atresia

Foreign Body

Child Abuse: gastric perforation and intraperitoneal air and bilateral healing rib fractures (diagnostic of abuse)

OTHER RADIOLOGY KNOWLEDGE FOR THE EXAM

When you see...	Think of...
Bones	
Lytic bone lesions on X-ray films	Multiple myeloma Primary bone tumor Metastasis (most common: lung, renal or thyroid, breast)
Blastic bone lesions on X-ray films	Metastasis (most common: breast, prostate, lymphoma) Paget's disease Medulloblastoma in pediatrics
Chest	
Large mediastinum	Aortic aneurysm Lymphadenopathy
Lung infiltrated with an effusion	Staphylococcus pneumonia Streptococcus pneumonia Lung infarct Tuberculosis

Abdomen/Pelvis	
Small bowel obstruction	Adhesions Hernia Intussusception (pediatrics) Gallstone ileus Carcinoma
Large bowel obstruction	Carcinoma Hernia Diverticulitis Intussusceptions (pediatrics)
Gas in biliary system	Gallstone ileus Gas forming infection Instrumentation
Small kidney(s)	Renal artery disease Chronic hydronephrosis Chronic glomerulonephritis Chronic pyelonephritis
Large kidney(s)	Acute pyelonephritis Acute glomerulonephritis Renal vein thrombosis Carcinoma (unilateral) Wilms' tumor (pediatrics)
Brain/Neurology	
Ring-enhancing lesion in brain	Immunocompetent patients: • Metastatic tumors • Demyelinating disease • Pyogenic abscess Immunocompromised patients: • Toxoplasma encephalitis *(T. gondii)* • Primary CNS lymphoma (Epstein-Barr virus) • Tuberculosis (in endemic areas)
Hemorrhage into basal ganglia, cerebellum, or pons	Hypertensive brain hemorrhage
Hemorrhage into the cerebral hemispheres	Arteriovenous malformation Aneurysm Trauma Metastatic lesions Other causes: vasculitis, cocaine, coagulation abnormalities

Section 9
Psychiatry

Psychotic Disorders

Psychotic disorders present with a combination of positive and/or negative symptoms. The key differentiating feature is the **duration** of symptoms.

SYMPTOMS OF PSYCHOSIS

Positive Symptoms	Negative Symptoms
Associated with dopamine receptors	Associated with muscarinic receptors
• Delusions (mostly bizarre) • Disorganized speech/behavior • Hallucinations • Agitation	• Flattened affect • Social withdrawal • Anhedonia • Apathy • Poverty of thought
	Tip: Atypical antipsychotics are the most effective treatment for negative symptoms.

- **Schizophrenia** is the diagnosis when there are positive psychosis symptoms that affect social and occupational function for **longer than 6 months.** Schizophrenia presents at a younger age in males than in females (15–24 years versus 25–34 years).
- When symptoms are present for < **6 months but** > **1 month**, the diagnosis is **schizophreniform disorder.**
- When symptoms are present for < **1 month** and the question states that there is a return to baseline, the diagnosis is **brief psychotic disorder** (look for a stressful life event that precipitates it).

- When there is a history of symptoms for many years with **no impairment of baseline functioning,** think of
    - delusional disorder (key is that **delusions are nonbizarre);** and
    - **personality disorders** (especially **schizotypal personality disorder,** which presents with peculiar thinking and social isolation but does *not* involve psychosis).

These patients do *not* respond to antipsychotics. **Psychotherapy** is the preferred therapy.

Rule out other forms of psychosis that aren't schizophrenia:

- Get a drug screen to rule out substance abuse.
- Look for signs or symptoms of seizure. Temporal lobe epilepsy can present with hallucinations (auditory and olfactory distortions), feeling of *déjà vu,* or dissociation from surroundings.

Watch out for **suicidal ideation** in schizophrenia patients and schizophreniform patients. Fifty percent of schizophrenia patients attempt suicide in their lifetimes, and 10 percent of these attempts are successful. Schizophreniform patients are at greater risk of depression and suicide *after* the episode of psychosis resolves. The first step in management is *always* to hospitalize if there is any risk of suicide.

> The first step in management of any acute psychiatric condition is to determine if the patient needs hospitalization. Hospitalize if the patient is at risk of harm to self or to others. You may hospitalize against the patient's will if the patient has suicidal or homicidal ideation.

What is the greatest risk factor for progression to schizophrenia?

- **Schizophreniform disorder.** Two thirds eventually progress to schizophrenia.

Prognosis

- In general, **females** have a better prognosis and respond better to treatment than males.
- Patients with **paranoid schizophrenia** are more responsive to treatment than those with other kinds.

> When the case describes any of the following features, the prognosis is poor:
>
> - Early age of onset
> - Negative symptoms
> - Poor premorbid functioning
> - Family history of schizophrenia
> - Disorganized or deficit subtype

MANAGEMENT

The initial steps in the management of acute psychotic disorders are as follows:

1. If the case describes bizarre or paranoid symptoms, **hospitalize the patient.**
2. Give **benzodiazepines** for agitation and start **antipsychotics.**
    - Antipsychotic medications are given for 6 months and are the *most effective* therapy to prevent further episodes.
    - Long-term antipsychotics are *only* given when there is a history of repeat episodes.

3. Initiate **long-term psychotherapy.**

Antipsychotics

Antipsychotics have an immediate **quieting effect** in acute psychotic attacks of any cause (e.g., schizophrenia, depression with psychotic features, mania in bipolar disorder). They also delay relapses.

There are two other indications for antipsychotics:

1. For **sedation** when benzodiazepines are contraindicated or as an adjunct during anesthesia
2. For **movement disorders: Huntington's disease** and **Tourette disorder** (to suppress tics and vocalization)

Antipsychotics are chosen based on side effect profile, *not* efficacy.

	Conventional Antipsychotics		Atypical Antipsychotics
	High Potency	Low Potency	
Examples	Fluphenazine, haloperidol	Thioridazine, chlorpromazine	Risperidone, olanzapine, quetiapine, clozapine
Advantages	Less sedating Fewer anticholinergic effects Less hypotension Useful as depot injections (e.g., haloperidol decanoate) for noncompliant patients Give IM route for acute psychosis when patient is unable or unwilling to take PO.	Less likely to cause EPS	Drug of choice for initial therapy Greater effect on negative symptoms Little or no risk of EPS
Disadvantages	Greatest association with extrapyramidal systems (EPS)	Greater anticholinergic effects More sedation More postural hypotension	Clozapine is reserved for treatment-resistant patients because of risk of agranulocytosis.

- **Low-potency antipsychotics** have the highest risk of causing **orthostatic hypotension** (alpha blockade), **acute urinary retention, dry mouth, blurry vision, and delirium** (anticholinergic effect). Change to an atypical antipsychotic if these symptoms are present.

> Clozapine is associated with **agranulocytosis.** *Always* check CBC when starting clozapine.

- **Thioridazine** is associated with **prolonged QT and arrhythmias.** *Always* get an EKG if the case describes **chest pain, shortness of breath,** or **palpitations** in a patient taking thioridazine. Thioridazine is also associated with **abnormal retinal pigmentation** after many years of use. Routine eye exam is needed for chronic therapy.
- **Impotence** and **inhibition of ejaculation** (α-blocker effect) are common reasons for noncompliance in males.
- **Weight gain** (due to hyperprolactinemia) is a common reason for noncompliance in females. Also ask about galactorrhea and amenorrhea.

a. A newly diagnosed schizophrenic patient complains of insomnia. What is the most appropriate antipsychotic to initiate therapy?

b. A schizophrenic patient has been maintained on olanzapine for the past 6 months. He complains of daytime sedation, and he has lost 2 jobs in the past month because of impaired performance. What is the next step in management?

Answers:

a. Olanzapine, quetiapine, ziprasidone, aripiprazole are first-choice medications when insomnia is a problem.

b. Drescribe risperidone, a first-choice medication for the treatment of schizophrenia when sedation is a problem.

MOVEMENT DISORDERS

Extrapyramidal symptoms (EPS) are the most common reason for failure to comply with therapy. Be able to identify a patient with a medication-related movement disorder and know how to minimize the symptoms.

Acute Dystonia	Bradykinesia (Parkinsonism)	Akathisia	Tardive Dyskinesia	Neuroleptic Malignant Syndrome
Occurs in the first week	Within weeks	Weeks to chronic use	Months to years	Anytime
Muscle spasms (eg. torticollis), difficulty swallowing *TIP: Young men are at higher risk*	Bradykinesia, tremors, rigidity and other signs of parkinsonism. *TIP: Elderly are at higher risk*	Motor restlessness. Do not mistake for anxiety for agitation. *TIP: Always review medication list*	Choreoathetosis and other involuntary movements after chronic use. Often irreversible	Muscle rigidity, hyperthermia, volatile vital signs, altered LOC, ↑ WBC & CK
-Reduce the dose -Rx: Anticholinergics • benztropine • diphenhydramine • trihexyphenidyl	-Reduce the dose -Rx: Anticholinergics • benztropine • diphenhydramine • trihexyphenidyl	-Reduce the dose -Add benzodiazepines or beta-blockers Switch to newer antipsychotics	-Stop older antipsychotics -Switch to newer antipsychotics (e.g. clozapine), *TIP: Symptoms commonly worsen after medication discontinuation.*	-Stop antipsychotic *TIP: Transfer to ICU for monitoring, mortality rate is 20%*

A 35-year-old male presents with poor adherence to chlorpromazine and haloperidol. He complains of tics and other uncontrolled movements. His wife reports that even when he takes his medications, they don't appear to help his paranoia. What is the next step in management?

a. Add risperidone

b. Add diphenhydramine

c. Change to clozapine

d. Increase the dose of chlorpromazine

e. Increase the dose of haloperidol

Answer: The correct answer is C. The case describes two main problems in management, poor response to therapy prescribed and movement disorder as a side effect from the regimen. Clozapine is the most effective antipsychotic for schizophrenia and also has no incidence of movement disorders. It is a second-line therapy because of the risk of seizures and agranulocytosis. Remember to monitor CBC to watch for bone marrow suppression.

A 78-year-old male with a slow-growing stomach tumor in palliative care is brought in by the family, who has noticed increased sedation and difficulty eating. They are concerned because he continues to lose more weight. On examination, he has repetitive movements of his lips and tongue. He has limited facial expression. His medications include morphine, metoclopramide, and hydrochlorothiazide. Which of the following is the most appropriate management?

a. Decrease morphine
b. Discontinue metoclopramide
c. Start omeprazole
d. Start prochlorperazine
e. Place NG tube for supplemental feedings

*Answer: The correct answer is **B**. Chronic use of dopamine antagonists, including antimetics (metoclopramide, prochlorperazine), can result in **tardive diskinesia**. Management includes discontinuing the offending drug and, if indicated, begin a newer antipsychotic.*

ANXIETY DISORDERS

Anxiety disorders are characterized by anxiety that interferes with daytime functioning and is not be due to any other identifiable causes of symptoms. Other conditions that may present as an anxiety disorder include the following:

- **Medical causes:** Hyperthyroidism, pheochromocytoma, excess cortisol, heart failure, arrhythmias, asthma, and COPD
- **Drugs:** Corticosteroids, cocaine, amphetamines, and caffeine, as well as withdrawal from alcohol and sedatives

ADJUSTMENT DISORDER

This is a normal psychological reaction (anxiety, depression, irritability) that occurs soon after profound changes in a person's life, such as divorce, migration, or birth of a handicapped child. Symptoms are not severe enough to be classified in another category. Adjustment disorder is *not* a true anxiety disorder.

Treatment

Do *not* treat these patients with medications; instead provide **counseling** to help with the patient adjust to the life stressor.

PANIC DISORDER

Panic disorder is the diagnosis when the case describes **brief attacks of intense anxiety with autonomic symptoms (e.g., tachycardia, hyperventilation, dizziness, and sweating).** Episodes occur **regularly,** without an obvious precipitant and in the absence of other psychiatric illness.

Treatment

Treatment is **cognitive-behavioral therapy** and/or **relaxation training and desensitization.** Relaxation and desensitization may be more useful when agoraphobic symptoms are present. Medications include SSRIs (e.g., fluoxetine), benzodiazepines (e.g., alprazolam, clonazepam), imipramine, and MAOIs (e.g., phenelzine).

PHOBIC DISORDERS

Phobic disorder is the diagnosis when the case describes a **persistent, unreasonable, intense fear of situations, circumstances, or objects.** It is differentiated from post traumatic stress disorder (PTSD) and acute stress disorder (ASD), which has a **history of a traumatic event** (threat to life or limb). There are no known eliciting events in phobic disorders associated with the onset of symptoms.

Agoraphobia

Fear or avoidance of places due to anxiety about not being able to escape (public places, being outside alone, public transportation, or crowds). Agoraphobia is more common in women.

Social Phobia

Fear of humiliation or embarrassment in either general or specific social situations (e.g., public speaking, "stage fright," urinating in public restrooms). In social phobia, the patient knows that the response is excessive and unreasonable.

- Differentiate from **avoidant personality disorder,** where the person does not believe the avoidance is excessive or unreasonable.

Specific Phobias

Most common phobia: Fear or avoidance of **objects or situations** other than those involved in agoraphobia or social phobia. Commonly involves animals (e.g., carnivores, spiders), natural environments (e.g., storms), injury (e.g., injections, blood), and situations (e.g., heights, darkness).

- Treatment: **Exposure therapy** (involves increasing exposure to stimulus in order to induce habituation and decreased anxiety). **Benzodiazepines** and **beta-blockers** are helpful when given prior to exposure.

A 19-year-old ballet dancer presents because of extreme anxiety on stage. She reports that she fell 3 months ago at a national ballet competition and since then suffers extreme anxiety, trembling, diaphoresis and breathlessness when she has to go on stage. She denies any problems with ballet practice and has no other medical problems. Which of the following is the most likely diagnosis?

a. Acute stress disorder
b. Adjustment disorder with anxious mood
c. Panic disorder
d. Social phobia

*Answer: The correct answer is **C**. Panic disorder presents with a clear precipitating event which subsequently results in anxiety in similar circiumstances. Panic disorder is differentiated from social phobia which has no clear precipitating cause..*

OBSESSIVE-COMPULSIVE DISORDER (OCD)

OCD is the diagnosis when the case describes **recurrent obsessions or compulsions.** The case must also describe that the **individual recognizes that the behavior is unreasonable and excessive** (i.e., there is insight). **Obsessions** are anxiety provoking; thoughts are intrusive and are commonly related to contamination, doubt, guilt, aggression, and sex. **Compulsions** are peculiar behaviors that reduce the anxiety and are most commonly habitual hand washing, organizing, checking, counting, and praying. Patients with Tourette syndrome often also have OCD. **Depression** and **substance abuse** are common in OCD.

Treatment

Behavioral psychotherapy and pharmacotherapy (**SSRIs** and **clomipramine**).

Obsessive symptoms in psychotic disorders may be misdiagnosed as OCD. You can differentiate psychosis from OCD by looking for a lack insight and loss of contact with reality.

ACUTE STRESS DISORDER (ASD) AND POSTTRAUMATIC STRESS DISORDER (PTSD)

These disorders involve severe anxiety symptoms that follow a life-threatening event. ASD is diagnosed when symptoms **last less than 1 month and occur within 1 month of stressor.** PTSD is diagnosed when symptoms **last longer than 1 month.**

Following are three key symptom groups:

1. **Re-experiencing of the traumatic event:** Dreams, flashbacks, or intrusive recollections
2. **Avoidance of stimuli** associated with the trauma or **numbing** of general responsiveness
3. **Increased arousal:** Anxiety, sleep disturbances, hypervigilance, emotional lability, or impulsiveness

Treatment

Give benzodiazepines acutely for anxiety symptoms. SSRIs and other antidepressants can be helpful for long-term therapy.

A school bus is involved in a major collision. Two children are killed, and seven others are injured. What is the most important therapy to prevent PTSD?

a. Diazepam
b. Fluoxetine
c. Group counseling
d. Haloperidol
e. Individual psychotherapy

Answer: The correct answer is **C.** Group counseling is the most effective therapy to prevent PTSD following a traumatic event.

GENERALIZED ANXIETY DISORDER (GAD)

Excessive, poorly controlled **anxiety that occurs daily for more than 6 months. No single event or focus** is related to the anxiety. It often coexists with major depression, specific phobia, social phobia, and panic disorder.

Treatment

Treatment consists of **supportive psychotherapy,** including relaxation training and biofeedback. Medications include **SSRIs, venlafaxine, buspirone, and benzodiazepines.**

Distinguish GAD from panic attack or social phobia by what is causing the anxiety. If the question describes persistent worry of a panic attack or social encounter, then GAD is not the answer. In GAD, multiple life circumstances, not just one, are causing the anxiety.

ANXIOLYTIC MEDICATIONS

Anxiolytics prescribed for anxiety disorders are as follows:

- **Adjustment disorder with anxious mood:** Benzodiazepines with brief psychotherapy
- **Panic disorder:** SSRIs, alprazolam, and clonazepam. These decrease the frequency and intensity of panic attacks.
- **Generalized anxiety disorder:** Venlafaxine, other SSRIs, and buspirone (These decrease overall anxiety.)
- **OCD:** SSRIs and clomipramine (These decrease obsessional thinking.)
- **Social phobia:** SSRIs and buspirone (These decrease fear associated with social situations.)

Benzodiazepines

- Do *not* change dosages abruptly.
- Use the lowest dose in the elderly.
- Advise against using machinery or driving.
- In order from shortest to longest half-life: Alprazolam (Xanax®) < lorazepam (Ativan®) < diazepam (Valium®)

Buspirone

- Therapeutic effect can take up to 1 week
- Can be used safely with other sedative-hypnotics (no additive effect)
- Best option for people with occupations where driving or machinery is involved, as there is no sedation or cognitive impairment
- No withdrawal syndrome

MOOD DISORDERS

MAJOR DEPRESSIVE DISORDER

This disorder is characterized by **depressed mood** or **anhedonia** and depressive symptoms lasting **at least 2 weeks.**

Look for other causes of depression where the first step in management is different, such as the following:

- **Hypothyroidism:**
  - Check TSH
  - First step in management is thyroxine
- **Parkinson's disease:**
  - Treat with anti-Parkinson medications
- **Medications:**
  - Corticosteroids, β-blockers, antipsychotics (especially in the elderly), and reserpine
  - Treat by discontinuing medication and switching to an alternative
- **Substance disorders:**
  - Alcohol (ask CAGE questionnaire), amphetamines
  - Treat with detoxification and antidepressants

Treatment

- **Admit the patient** if there is suicidal/homicidal ideation or paranoia.
- Begin **antidepressant medications** (SSRI is first drug of choice).
- Give **benzodiazepines** if agitated.
- **Electroconvulsive therapy (ECT)** is the best choice if the patient is acutely suicidal (works quicker than antidepressants) or for patients worried about side effects from medications.

SIGECAPS: Major depressive disorder = depressed mood +

S: changes in *sleep*
I: loss of *interests*/pleasure
G: thoughts of worthlessness or *guilt*
E: loss of *energy*
C: trouble *concentrating*
A: changes in *appetite* or weight
P: changes in *psychomotor activity*
S: thoughts about death or *suicide*

DYSTHYMIC DISORDER

Dysthymic disorder is characterized by **low-level depression symptoms** that are **present on most days for at least 2 years.** However the question may describe superimposed acute major depression, which is common in these patients. Do *not* hospitalize these patients unless there's suicidal ideation.

Treatment

Long-term individual, insight-oriented psychotherapy is the best treatment. If this fails, a trial of SSRIs is the next step in management.

Seasonal Affective Disorder

The diagnosis is seasonal affective disorder when the case describes **depressive symptoms in the winter months** (shorter daylight hours) and absence of depressive symptoms during summer months (longer daylight hours). Treatment is **phototherapy** or **sleep deprivation.**

BIPOLAR DISORDER

Bipolar disorder is the diagnosis when the case describes episodes of **depression, mania, or mixed symptoms for at least 1 week** that cause distress or impaired functioning.

Bipolar disorder is the *most commonly missed* diagnosis in the USMLE, because it can easily be mistaken for depression or mania alone. The questions will describe a history of both manic symptoms and depressive symptoms, as well as periods of normal mood. **Rapid cycling bipolar** is indicated by > 4 episodes of mania per year.

Symptoms:

- **Mania symptoms:** Include grandiosity, less need for sleep, excessive talking or pressured speech, racing thoughts or flight of ideas, distractibility, goal-focused activity at home or at work, or sexual promiscuity.
- **Major depressive symptoms:** Include depressed mood or loss of pleasure or interest.

If the history suggests drug use, first get a drug screen to rule out **amphetamine use** as a cause of mania. If the history gives elevated blood pressure or low TSH, consider medical conditions, such as **pheochromocytoma** and **hyperthyroidism.**

Steps in Management of Acute Mania

1) **Hospitalize**

2) **Mood stabilizers** are used to induce remission. Lithium is the drug of choice (takes 1 week for effect).

3) **Antipsychotics** are used until acute mania is controlled. Drug of choice is risperidone.

4) Give **IM depot phenothiazine** in noncompliant, severely manic patients.

5) Give antidepressants *only* when there's a history of recurrent episodes of depression and *only* together with mood stabilizers (to prevent inducing manic episode).

   a. *What is the most common cause of progression to rapid cycling bipolar?*

   b. *How should you manage rapid cycling bipolar?*

   c. *What other medical conditions predispose a patient to rapid cycling bipolar?*

   d. *What drug has been shown to prevent suicidal ideation in bipolar disorder?*

   e. *A 32 year-old known bipolar patient who is undergoing maintenance therapy with lithium presents with a positive pregnancy test. How will you manage this patient's bipolar disorder?*

   Answers:

   a. ***Use of antidepressants:*** *Do not give antidepressants prophylactically unless the question describes previous severe depressive episodes. In that case, antidepressants are only given for a few weeks.*

   b. ***Gradually stop*** *all antidepressants, stimulants, caffeine, benzodiazepines, and alcohol.*

   c. ***Hypothyroidism:*** *Check TSH in any patient with rapid cycling bipolar and replace thyroid hormones if needed.*

   d. ***Lithium***

   e. ***Discontinue lithium*** *(to avoid heart abnormalities): Choose **ECT therapy** for first-trimester patients with manic episodes. **Lamotrogine** may be used in 2nd or 3rd trimester.*

CYCLOTHYMIA

When the patient presents with a history of **recurrent episodes of depressed mood and hypomanic mood for at least 2 years,** the diagnosis is cyclothimia. It resembles a milder form of bipolar affective disorder.

Treatment

Psychotherapy is the first step in management. Many people function without medications and learn to manage their hypomanic dispositions (especially artists). Start **divalproex** when functioning is impaired. Divalproex is more effective in cyclothymia than lithium.

GRIEF AND DEPRESSION

Grief	Depression
Sadness, tearfulness, decreased sleep, decreased appetite, decreased interest in the world	
Symptoms wax and wane	Symptoms are pervasive and unremitting
Shame and guilt are less common	Shame and guilt are common
Suicide is threatened less often	Suicide is threatened more often
Symptoms can last up to one year	Symptoms continue for more than one year
Patient usually returns to baseline level of functioning within 2 months	Patient does not return to baseline functioning
Treatment includes **supportive therapy**	Treatment includes antidepressant medications

A 32-year-old woman who recently gave birth 4 months ago is brought in by her husband because of depressed mood. The husband reports that she has been depressed since the birth of her child, refuses to eat, has trouble sleeping and is unable to concentrate. The woman reports that she has lost interest in everything and sometimes can't even get out of bed. She reports that she's recently had visions of seeing her deceased mother talking to her and criticizing her skills as a new mother. She also admits that she hears her voice talk to her constantly too. She denies homicidal or suicidal ideation. Which of the following is the best initial treatment.

a. Psychotherapy
b. Behavioral therapy
c. Sertraline
d. Respiridone
e. Phenelzine

Answer: The correct answer is **D.** Patients with both mood and psychotic symptoms respond to both antidepressants and antipsychotic medication. However, you must **treat the worst symptom first.** In this case, the antipsychotic would be most indicated to reduce her psychotic symptoms.

A 45-year-old woman presents 2-months after the sudden loss of her son in a car accident. She reports "not being able to cope well." She is constantly teary, has lost her appetite and has decreased 2 dress sizes. She finds herself laying out a dinner plate every night for him. Recently, she believes she has heard his voice and every night she has nightmares about the car accident. She denies suicidal ideation. Which of the following is the most appropriate next step in management?

a. Group therapy
b. Amitriptyline
c. Fluoxetine
d. Zolpidem
e. Supportive therapy

Answer: The correct answer is E. This patient is undergoing normal grief reaction. Auditory hallucinations without other psychotic symptoms are normal in grief reaction. Antidepressants are indicated when symptoms last longer than 6 months and the patient's symptoms can be classified as major depression.

POSTPARTUM DEPRESSION

	Postpartum Blues or "Baby Blues"	Postpartum Depression	Postpartum Psychosis
Onset	After any birth	Usually after 2nd birth	Usually after 1st birth
Mother's emotions toward baby	Cares about baby	Many have thoughts about hurting the baby	Many have thoughts about hurting the baby
Symptoms	Mild depressive	Severe depressive	Look for psychotic symptoms along with severe depressive symptoms.
Treatment	Self-limited; no treatment necessary	Antidepressants	Mood stabilizers or antipsychotics and antidepressants *TIP:* Avoid medications if patient is breastfeeding; instead choose Electro-convulsive Therapy (ECT).

SUICIDE AND SUICIDAL IDEATION

Management of the Suicidal Patient	
Ask about risk factors:	**Emergency Assessment**
• **History of suicide threats and attempts is the most important predictor of suicide** • Family history of suicide • Perceived hopelessness (demoralization) • Schizophrenia/borderline or antisocial PD • Drug use, especially alcohol • Males/Age > 65 • Socially isolated/recently divorced or widowed • Chronic physical illness • Low job satisfaction or unemployment	• Take all suicide threats seriously • Detain and hospitalize (usually a couple of weeks) • Never transport patient to emergency department without medically trained personnel accompanying patient • Do not identify with the patient • Do not leave patient unsupervised • Treatment of choice = psychotherapy + antidepressant medications (SSRIs are first choice) • For acute, severe risk of self-harm, treatment of choice is electroconvulsive therapy (ECT)

INDICATIONS FOR ELECTROCONVULSIVE THERAPY (ECT)

- Major depressive episodes that are unresponsive to medications
- High risk for immediate suicide
- Contraindications to using antidepressant medications
- Good response to ECT in the past

Caution: The biggest complication of ECT is **transient memory loss,** which worsens with prolonged therapy and resolves after several weeks. Use of ECT is *cautioned* in patients with space-occupying intracranial lesions (e.g., brain metastasis), as ECT induces transient intracranial pressure.

ANTIDEPRESSANTS AND MOOD STABILIZERS

Guidelines for Use of Antidepressants

- SSRIs are first-line therapy.
- TCAs are avoided because of risk of toxicity (think: **TCA** may be **T**oxic.).
- MAOIs are more helpful in atypical depressive disorders.
- Choose an antidepressant based on side effect profile.
- Switch to another antidepressant if patient does not respond after 8 weeks or if the patient does not tolerate the side effects.
- Treat patients for 6 months and consider long-term therapy for multiple episodes of depression.
- When the question describes a patient concerned about weight gain or sexual side effects, give **bupropion** (causes modest weight loss). Note: Buprioprion is associated with **seizures.**
- When the question describes a patient who has poor appetite, loss of weight, or insomnia, give **mirtazapine.**
- **Amitriptyline** is used to treat chronic pain.
- **Imipramine** is useful in enuresis.
- **Trazodone** is strongly sedating and is often used to treat depressed patients who have severe insomnia.
- SSRIs and TCAs are **safe in pregnancy** *except* for paroxetine (Paxil®).

SSRIs are first-line therapy for many conditions because of their therapeutic effect and low side effect profile. Always think of SSRIs first in patients with the following disorders:

- Major depressive disorder
- Bipolar disorder
- Anxiety disorders: Panic disorder, OCD, social phobia, generalized anxiety disorder
- Bulimia nervosa

A young male recently started on antidepressants develops prolonged erection. What is the antidepressant he was most likely taking?

Answer: **Trazadone**

An elderly patient presents with depression and agitation. What is the most appropriate medication?

Answer: Give an **antidepressant with sedative effects** *(e.g., doxepin, trazadone). Amitriptyline is also sedating but has anticholinergic effects, which may be problematic in elderly.*

A 25-year-old male with history of seizures is diagnosed with depression. Which medications should be avoided?

Answer: Seizures are common with **TCAs and bupropion,** *and these medications should be avoided in patients with seizure disorders. The best first-line therapy in patients with seizures is SSRIs.*

A middle-aged woman is brought into the ER with confusion and disorientation. An overdose of prescription medications is suspected. Blood pressure is 90/53 mm Hg, HR 111/min. Pupils are dilated, mucous membranes are dry, and she has facial flushing.

a. *What is the most likely cause of acute intoxication?*
b. *What is the most important test to determine severity and prognosis in this patient?*
   a. *EKG*
   b. *EEG*
   c. *Serum sodium*
   d. *Serum tricyclic levels*
   e. *Urinalysis*
c. *EKG is performed and shows PR and QRS prolongation and sinus tachycardia. What is the most appropriate next step in management?*
   a. *Calcium carbonate*
   b. *Diazepam*
   c. *Gastric lavage*
   d. *Insulin and glucose*
   e. *Sodium bicarbonate*

Answers:

a. **Tricyclic antidepressants (TCAs):** *TCAs have anticholinergic effects and are an alpha blocker, causing peripheral vasodilatation and hypotension and also affecting sodium channels in cardiac tissue.*
b. *The correct answer is* **A.** *EKG is the single most important test to guide therapy and prognosis. Watch out for prolonged QRS, QT, and PR intervals. Most serious complication is ventricular tachycardia and fibrillation.*
c. *The correct answer is* **E.** *Sodium bicarbonate attenuates TCA cardiotoxicity by alkalinization of blood, which uncouples TCA from myocardial sodium channels and increases extracellular sodium concentration, thereby improving the gradient across the channel.*

A 42-year-old woman with a history of hypertension, diabetes, and depression presents to the clinic with dry eyes and dry mouth. Her medications include hydrochlorothiazide, metformin, and amitriptyline. Which of the following is the next step in management?

a. Discontinue amitriptyline and change to sertraline
b. Order antinuclear antibodies
c. Order SS-Ro and SS-La
d. Prescribe eye drops
e. Refer to ophthalmologist

*Answer: The correct answer is **A**. Discontinue amitriptyline and switch to another antidepressant medication with little/no anticholinergic effects. Anticholinergic effects are most severe with amitriptyline, but there are almost none with most SSRIs.*

LITHIUM

Lithium is the first-line medication for **bipolar and schizoaffective disorders** and treatment and prophylaxis of mood episodes. Side effects are a major reason for noncompliance. These include the following:

- **Acne and weight gain** are the most common problems.
- **Dose-related tremors, GI distress, and headaches** (decrease the dose)
- **Hypothyroidism** (5 percent)
- **Polyuria** secondary to medication-induced diabetes insipidus
- Do *not* use in first trimester of pregnancy. Lithium causes **cardiac defects.**

DIVALPROEX

Divalproex is the first-line choice for **rapid-cycling bipolar disorder** or when lithium is ineffective, impractical, or contraindicated.

CARBAMAZEPINE

Carbamazepine is the **second-line therapy for bipolar disorder** when lithium and divalproex are ineffective or contraindicated. It is not commonly used because of serious **agranulocytosis** and significant **sedation.**

MEDICATION OVERDOSES

LITHIUM TOXICITY

Suspect lithium toxicity when the question describes an **elderly** patient who takes **lithium** with **renal failure** or **hyponatremia** (may be caused by diuretics, vomiting, dehydration). The question will describe nausea, vomiting, acute disorientation, tremors, increased DTRs, and even seizures. The treatment of choice is **dialysis.**

NEUROLEPTIC MALIGNANT SYNDROME

The question will describe a patient who **recently started taking antipsychotics** (particularly haloperidol) or a Parkinson's patient who has **recently stopped levodopa.** Look for **high fever, tachycardia, muscle rigidity, altered consciousness, and autonomic dysfunction.** This syndrome is unrelated to dosage or previous drug exposure. There is a 20 percent mortality rate.

Treatment

- **Transfer to the ICU**
- **Discontinue antipsychotic**
- Give **bromocriptine** to overcome dopamine receptor blockade
- Give muscle relaxants **dantrolene** or **diazepam** to reduce muscle rigidity

SEROTONIN SYNDROME

Serotonin syndrome is the diagnosis when the case describes a **history of SSRI use** and the **use of migraine medication** (triptans) **or an MAOI.** The patient will present with **agitation, hyperreflexia, hyperthermia, and muscle rigidity with volume contraction** secondary to sweating and insensible fluid loss.

Treatment
- IV fluids
- Cyproheptadine to decrease serotonin production
- Benzodiazepine to reduce muscle rigidity

MAOI-INDUCED HYPERTENSIVE CRISIS

Consider this diagnosis if the history describes a patient with **acute hypertension and a history of MAOI use** and either **antihistamines, nasal decongestants, or consumption of tyramine-rich foods** (cheeses, pickled foods). May also be seen in patients who take a MAOI and a TCA concurrently.

What is the first assessment prior to prescribing antidepressants?

a. *Complete blood count*
b. *Family history of depression*
c. *Previous use of antidepressants*
d. *Suicidal ideation*
e. *Thyroid function tests*

*Answer: The correct answer is **D**. Always assess for suicidal ideation prior to starting antidepressants, as there is an increased risk in suicidal ideation in some patients within the first 2 weeks. Know how to manage acute suicidal ideation. If the patient is acutely suicidal, you must hospitalize and consider electroconvulsive therapy, which can help mood in an acute setting.*

SOMATOFORM DISORDERS

A somatoform disorder is the correct diagnosis when the case describes **physical symptoms without medical explanation.** The symptoms are severe enough to **interfere with the patient's ability to function** in social or occupational activities.

SOMATIZATION DISORDER

This involves multiple symptoms affecting multiple organs with **no medical explanation.** There must be **at least 4 pain symptoms, 2 gastrointestinal symptoms, 1 sexual symptom, and 1 pseudoneurologic symptom** to make a diagnosis.

A 47-year-old woman presents to the clinic with shortness of breath, chest pain, abdominal pain, back pain, double vision, and difficulty walking due to weakness in her legs. She remembers being sick all of the time for the past 10 years. According to her husband, she constantly takes medications for all of her ailments. She has visited numerous physicians and none has been able to diagnose her condition correctly. What is the next step in management?

a. *Order ANA*
b. *Order CT of the abdomen*
c. *Order CT of the head*
d. *Hospitalize*
e. *Schedule regular monthly visits*

*Answer: The correct answer is **E**. Scheduling regular monthly visits to establish a single physician as the primary caregiver is the most important first step in management.*

Steps in Management

1. Maintain a **single physician** as the primary caretaker.
2. Schedule **brief monthly visits.**
3. *Avoid* diagnostic testing or therapies.
4. Schedule **individual psychotherapy.**
5. Do *not* hospitalize the patient.

CONVERSION DISORDER

Conversion disorder is the diagnosis when there are **one or more neurologic symptoms** that **cannot be explained by any medical or neurologic disorder.** Most common symptoms are mutism, blindness, paralysis, and anesthesia/ paresthesias. Look for psychologic factors associated with the onset or exacerbation of symptoms. A clue to diagnosis is that patients often **are unconcerned about their impairment** (*la belle indifference*). You must first rule out other medical conditions.

Treatment

- Supportive physician-patient relationship
- Psychotherapy

Somatization disorder and conversion disorder are *never* the correct diagnosis if symptoms are produced intentionally or feigned.

HYPOCHONDRIASIS

Hypochondriasis is the diagnosis when the patient falsely believes that he **has a specific disease, despite repeated negative medical tests and workup.** Symptoms must have been present for **at least 6 months** and **physician's reassurance has failed to relieve concerns.**

Treatment

- Identify one primary caregiver
- Schedule regular routine visits
- Provide psychotherapy

FACTIOUS AND MALINGERING DISORDERS

In both factitious disorder and malingering, the case will suggest that a patient has **intentionally feigned symptoms.**

- The diagnosis is **factitious disorder** when the case describes a patient that has **seen many doctors** and **visited many hospitals,** has **large amount of medical knowledge** (e.g., health care worker), and **demands treatment.** They are typically agitated and threaten litigation if tests return negative.

- The diagnosis is **factitious disorder by proxy** if the signs and symptoms are **faked by another person,** as in a mother making up symptoms in her child. The motivation is to assume the caretaker role.
- **Malingering** is the diagnosis when obvious gain (shelter, medications, disability insurance) results from feigned symptoms. Malingering patients are more **preoccupied with rewards or gain** than with alleviation of presenting symptoms.

A 23-year-old nursing student presents to the emergency department with fever and chills at home. She has had multiple admissions in other hospitals because of pneumonia and chronic pain problems. She was found to be tampering with the blood culture bottles and dipping her temperature thermometer in hot water. Which of the following is the most likely diagnosis?

a. Conversion disorder
b. Factitious disorder
c. Factitious disorder by proxy
d. Malingering
e. Somatization disorder

*Answer: The correct answer is **B**.*

A 46-year-old homeless man presents to the hospital reporting that he had a seizure this morning. He is adamant that he be admitted, however, he refuses all bloodwork and imaging studies. He cannot answer questions about the seizure and cannot describe his symptoms at the time of the seizure. Instead he demands to be admitted and is wondering why you're taking so long. When you ask about his social history, he admits that he is homeless at the moment as he was "kicked out of the shelter" because of drug-taking and alcohol abuse. Which of the following is the most likely diagnosis?

a. Conversion disorder
b. Factitious disorder
c. Factitious disorder by proxy
d. Malingering
e. Somatization disorder

*Answer: The correct answer is **D**.*

Treatment and Precautions

- **Supportive psychotherapy** is the treatment of choice.
- Do *not* confront or accuse the patient (the patient will become angry, more guarded, and suspicious).
- Only **provide the minimum amount of treatment and workup** needed. Aggressive management of the patient's symptoms only further reinforces the behavior.

Eating Disorders and Other Impulse Control Disorders

EATING DISORDERS

Following are the three main eating disorders that you need to distinguish on the exam:

1. **Anorexia nervosa**
2. **Bulemia nervosa**
3. **Body dysmorphic disorder**

Anorexia Nervosa

The diagnosis is anorexia nervosa when the case describes a **young female** who is **underweight** because of **food restriction and excessive exercise** and **has not had a menstrual period for 3 cycles or more.** The question may also include a **history of purging** (50 percent of anorexia nervosa patients also purge), but the diagnosis will still be anorexia nervosa.

Treatment of anorexia nervosa and bulimia nervosa is as follows:

- **Hospitalize for IV hydration** if electrolyte disturbances are present
- **Olanzapine** in anorexia nervosa helps with weight gain
- **SSRI antidepressants** (especially fluoxetine) prevent relapses
- Prescribe **behavioral psychotherapy**

Bulimia Nervosa

The diagnosis is bulimia nervosa when the case describes a **young female** in **normal weight range** with frequent episodes of **binge eating followed by guilt, anxiety, and self-induced vomiting, laxative, diuretics, or enema use.** Food restriction is *not* a feature of bulimia nervosa. Look for painless parotid gland enlargement and dental enamel erosions. Electrolyte disturbances are common (metabolic alkalosis, hypochloremia, and hypokalemia caused by emesis; metabolic acidosis caused by laxative abuse). There is a risk of cardiomyopathy with excessive syrup of ipecac use.

Body Dysmorphic Disorder

The diagnosis is body dysmorphic disorder when the case describes a **young woman** who is preoccupied with an **imagined or slight defect in appearance, causing distress and impaired ability to function in a social or occupational setting.** The distress is most commonly related to facial features, although any body part may be the focus of anxiety. The patients are often isolated and housebound.

Treatment

- High doses of **SSRIs** are first-line therapy.
- If the only concern is body shape and weight, anorexia nervosa is the more accurate diagnosis.
- If the only concern is sex characteristics, gender identity disorder is the more accurate diagnosis.

IMPULSE CONTROL DISORDERS

These occur in people who are unable to resist impulses. The question will describe anxiety prior to the impulse that is relieved after the patient acts on the impulse.

- **Intermittent explosive disorder:** This is the diagnosis when the case describes episodes of **aggression out of proportion to the stressor.** There may be a history of head trauma. If there is a history of drug intake, intermittent explosive disorder is *not* the diagnosis. Treatment of choice is **SSRIs** and **mood stabilizers.**
- **Kleptomania:** This is the diagnosis when the case describes an individual who **repeatedly steals items to relieve anxiety.** The person does *not* steal because she needs the object, and the individual often secretly replaces the object after stealing it.
- **Pyromania:** This is the diagnosis when the case describes an individual who **repeatedly lights fires.** Pyromania is *not* the diagnosis if the motive is personal gain (i.e., insurance money) or to show anger, which differentiates this from conduct disorder.
- **Pathologic gambling:** This is the diagnosis when the case describes **obsession with gambling despite the consequences.** Treatment of choice is group psychotherapy (e.g., gambling anonymous).

Individuals with impulse control disorders do not believe their actions are excessive or out of proportion (i.e., they lack insight), unlike in OCD.

PSYCHOSOCIAL PROBLEMS

TYPES OF ABUSE

Class	Child Abuse	Adult Maltreatment/ Elder Abuse	Spousal Abuse
Definition of abuse	• **Physical is the most common** (look for bruises, burns, lacerations, broken bones, shaken baby syndrome—do eye exam) • Neglect • Sexual exploitation (STDs) • Mental cruelty	• **Neglect is the most common** (50% of all reported cases) • Physical • Psychological • Financial	• **Physical is the most common**—it is the number one cause of injury to American women • Psychological • Financial
Physician's role in care	1. Mandatory reporting up to age 18. You must report *all* suspected cases. 2. Protect the child (separate from parents) and consider admission to hospital.	1. You must report *all* suspected cases. 2. Protect patient from abuser and consider admission to hospital.	1. Reporting is not indicated. 2. Provide information about local shelters and counseling.
Those at risk	• Younger than 1 year • Stepchildren • Premature children • Very active children • "Defective" children	• Caretaker is the most likely source of abuse; spouses are often caretakers	• More frequent in families with drug abuse, especially alcoholism • Victim often grew up in a violent home (about 50%) • Married at a young age • Dependent personalities • Pregnant, last trimester (highest risk)
Exam points	• Be careful not to mistake benign cultural practices, such as "coining" or "moxibustion," for child abuse. • Treat female circumcision as abuse.		

PERSONALITY DISORDERS (PD)

Personality disorders are pervasive, inflexible, and maladaptive thoughts or behaviors. More males have antisocial and narcissistic PDs; more females have borderline and histrionic PDs.

TREATMENT OF CHOICE

- Psychotherapy
- Use of mood stabilizers and antidepressants is sometimes useful for Cluster B PDs.

FEATURES	EXAMPLES
Cluster A: Peculiar thought processes, inappropriate affect	

Paranoid PD:
 • **Distrust and suspiciousness**
   - Individuals are mistrustful and suspicious of the motivations and actions of others and are often secretive and isolated.
   - They are emotionally cold and odd.
   - They often take legal action against other people.
 • **Often confused with paranoid schizophrenia.**
 • **Main defense mechanism is projection.**
	A 62-year-old man lives in an apartment and constantly accuses his neighbours of stealing his mail and prying into his apartment. He believes that all his neighbors are conspiring to have him removed from the building.

Schizoid PD:
 • **Detachment and restricted emotionality**
   - Individuals are emotionally distant and fear intimacy with others.
   - They are absorbed in their own thoughts and feelings and disinterested.
 • **Main defense mechanism is projection**
	A 68-year-old man lives in the country-side man-ing a lighthouse near a remote village. He is seen in town 2-3 times a year to purchase supplies. He has no known friends or family.

Schizotypal PD: • **Discomfort with social relationships, thought distortion, eccentricity** - Like schizoid PD except they also have magical thinking, clairvoyance, ideas of reference, or paranoid ideation. • **Symptoms aren't severe enough for classification of schizophrenia**	A 28-year-old man lives in a small coastal town attempting to start his own internet herbal business. He believes that the herbs have magical powers and he sells their magical properties of healing for a living. He believes that spirits are guiding him to wealth.
Cluster B: Mood lability, dissociative symptoms, preoccupation with rejection	

• **Histrionic PD:**
   - Colorful, exaggerated behavior and excitable, shallow expression of emotions
   - Use of physical appearance to draw attention to self
   - Sexually seductive
   - Discomfort in situations where not the center of attention.
	A 30-year-old woman presents to the doctor's office dressed in a sexually seductive manner and insists that the doctor comment on her appearance. When the doctor refuses to do so, she becomes upset.

FEATURES	EXAMPLES
Borderline PD: • Unstable affect, mood swings, marked impulsivity, unstable relationships, recurrent suicidal behaviors, chronic feelings of emptiness, identity disturbance, and inappropriate anger. Become intensely angered if they feel abandoned. • **Main defense mechanism is splitting.**	A 30-year-old female presents to the clinic. She reports that she has been to many doctors, she said they were all wonderful until they started ignoring her or cutting her visits short, then she realized what terrible doctors they were. She starts the visit saying that the assistant at the front desk is the "worst she's ever seen" because she didn't smile at her. The other assistant was just wonderful according to her.
Antisocial PD: • Usually characterized by continuous antisocial or criminal acts, inability to conform to social rules, impulsivity, disregard for the rights of others, aggressiveness, lack of remorse, and deceitfulness.	A 26-ear-old male is caught lighting forest fires during a recent spate. He has a history of legal problems since childhood. He reports that his mother is to blame. He denies feeling regret. He has no friends and is found to be hostile to everyone at the police station.
Narcissistic PD: • Usually characterized by a sense of self-importance, grandiosity, and preoccupation with fantasies of success. This person believes he is special, requires excessive admiration, reacts with rage when criticized, lacks empathy, is envious of others, and is interpersonally exploitative.	A patient is in the hospital for chest pain and becomes very agitated because he feels he is not getting enough attention. He reports that he is an important CEO and demands a special VIP room and more consideration and a dedicated nurse to attend his needs.
Cluster C: Anxiety, preoccupation with criticism or rigidity	
Avoidant PD: • Individuals have social inhibition, feelings of inadequacy, and hypersensitivity to criticism. They shy away from starting anything new or attending social gatherings for fear of failure or rejection. They desire affection and acceptance and are open about their isolation and inability to interact with others.	A 45-year-old single male fears an upcoming social party being hosted by his parents. He dreads having to meet other people and doesn't feel comfortable speaking with others. He is planning on staying at home to avoid speaking to others.
Dependent PD: • **Submissive and clinging behavior related to a need to be taken care of.** Individuals are consumed with the need to be taken care of. They are clingy and worry about abandonment. They feel inadequate and helpless and avoid disagreements with others. They usually focus dependency on a family member or spouse.	
Obsessive-Compulsive PD: • Individuals are preoccupied with orderliness, perfectionism, and control. They are often consumed by the details of everything and lose their sense of overall goals. They are strict and perfectionistic, overconscientious, and inflexible. Associated with difficult interpersonal relationships. • **Differentiated from obsessive-compulsive disorder.**	A 38-year-old male presents with his wife for marital counseling. The wife reports that he is inflexible and has unrealistic demands of orderliness and an inflexible schedule. Both partners agree that his demands are causing marital problems.

- When the case describes **hypochondriasis**, think of underlying **dependant, histrionic, or borderline personality disorders.**
- When the case describes **self-aggression** or **self-mutilation**, the diagnosis is often **passive-aggressive personality disorder** (example of acting out).

SUBSTANCE USE DISORDERS

Step 3 will test your ability to recognize substance abuse and know the best management for acute substance use and acute withdrawal.

ALCOHOL DEPENDENCE (ALCOHOLISM)

Alcohol dependence is the frequent use of alcohol resulting in **tolerance and physical and psychological dependence.** **Alcohol abuse** is when episodes of alcohol use result in **failure to fulfill obligations, legal troubles, or exposure to physically dangerous situations.** Tolerance is *not* included in the diagnosis of alcohol abuse.

Diagnosis

- The most accurate diagnosis is made with the **CAGE questionnaire.** Laboratory tests are *never* included in the diagnosis of alcohol abuse.
- When the question describes a patient with alcohol abuse, do the following:

  - **Order toxicology** to look for use of other drugs: breath, blood and urine drug screens.
  - Look for **secondary effects** of alcohol use (but *not* for diagnosis): elevated GGTP, AST, ALT, and LDH.
  - If there's suggestion of IV drug use (e.g., track marks), order HIV, hepatitis B, hepatitis C, and PPD (for tuberculosis).

> CAGE: An answer of yes to any two of the following questions is suggestive of alcohol abuse:
>
> - Have you ever felt that you should Cut down your drinking?
> - Have you ever felt Annoyed by others who have criticized your drinking?
> - Have you ever felt Guilty about your drinking?
> - Have you ever had an Eye-opener to steady your nerves or alleviate a hangover?

Acute Outpatient Management	Acute Inpatient Management Pearls	Chronic Maintenance Management
1) Prevent further ETOH intake 2) Prevent individual from driving a car, operating machinery 3) Sedate patient if she becomes agitated 4) Transfer to inpatient	1) Look for withdrawal symptoms 2) Prevent Wernicke-Korsackoff (ataxia, nystagmus, ophthalmoplegia, amnesia): Give IV or IM thiamine and magnesium ASAP; Also give B12 and folate 3) Benzodiazepine of choice is **chlordiazepoxide** or **diazepam** 4) Choose short-acting benzodiazepam *only* if the question describes patient with severe liver disease (prevent toxic metabolites)—**lorazepam** or **oxazepam** 5) Do *not* give seizure prophylaxis; Repeated seizures should be treated with diazepam 6) Haldol is *never* the answer (reduces seizure threshold)	1) Refer to inpatient rehabilitation or outpatient group therapy (e.g., AA) 2) Never give drug therapy without group psychotherapy 3) Naloxone and acamprosate decrease relapse rate only when given with psychotherapy 4) Disulferam has poor compliance and hasn't been shown to be effective

If the question asks for the most effective management of alcohol abuse or prevention of relapse, the correct answer is Alcoholics Anonymous (AA).

Withdrawal Syndrome	Minor Withdrawal Symptoms	Alcoholic Hallucinosis	Withdrawal Seizure	Delirium Tremens
Onset After Last Drink	6 hours	12–24 hours	48 hours	48–96 hours
Symptoms	Insomnia, tremulousness, mild anxiety, headache, diaphoresis, palpitations	Visual hallucinations There may also be auditory and tactile hallucinations.	Tonic clonic seizures	Hallucinations, disorientation, tachycardia, hypertension, low-grade fever, agitation, and diaphoresis
Exam Tips		If there are hallucinations with generalized cloudy sensorium, alcoholic hallucinosis is *not* the answer.	Get CT scan if repeated seizures to rule out structural or infectious cause.	Time of onset is important. This is the diagnosis if the case describes symptoms 2 days after last drink.

A 38-year-old male presents to the emergency department with acute-onset, right lower quadrant abdominal pain. He undergoes an appendectomy. Two days after surgery, he is found in his room disorientated and agitated, and he is claiming to see snakes in his room. Physical exam reveals tachycardia and temperature of 101.2. Which of the following is the most likely diagnosis?

a. Alcoholic hallucinosis
b. Delirium tremens
c. Korsakoff's psychosis
d. Fentanyl withdrawal
e. Pulmonary embolism

*Answer: The correct answer is **B**. Delirium tremens should always be suspected. The clue is that symptoms occur more than 2 days after the last drink. The question doesn't need to give you a history of alcohol use.*

Substance	Signs and Symptoms of Intoxication	Treatment of Intoxication	Signs and Symptoms of Withdrawal	Treatment of Withdrawal
Alcohol	Talkative, sullen gregarious, moody	Mechanical ventilation if severe	Tremors, hallucinations, seizures, delirium	Long-acting benzo's. No seizure prophylaxis. Disulfiram or naloxone for adjunct to supervised therapy after acute withdrawal
Amphetamines, cocaine	Euphoria, hypervigilance, autonomic hyperactivity, weight loss, pupil dilatation, disturbed perception, stroke, myocardial infarction	Short-term use of antipsychotics,	Anxiety, tremors, headache, increased appetite, depression, risk of suicide	Antidepressants
Cannabis	Impaired motor coordination, impaired time perception, social withdrawal, increased appetite, dry mouth, tachycardia, conjunctival redness	None	None	None

Substance	Signs and Symptoms of Intoxication	Treatment of Intoxication	Signs and Symptoms of Withdrawal	Treatment of Withdrawal
Hallucinogens (e.g., LSD)	Ideas of reference, hallucinations, impaired judgment, dissociative symptoms, pupil dilatation, panic, tremors, incoordination	Supportive counseling (talking down), antipsychotics, benzodiazepines	None	None
Inhalants	Belligerence, apathy, assaultiveness, impaired judgment, blurred vision, stupor, coma	Antipsychotics if delirious or agitated	None	None
Opiates	Apathy, dysphoria, constricted pupils, drowsiness, slurred speech, impaired memory, coma, death	Naloxone	Fever, chills, lacrimation, runny node, abdominal cramps, muscle spasms, insomnia, yawning	Clonidine, methadone
PCP	Panic reactions, assaultiveness, agitation, nystagmus, HTN, seizures, coma, hyperacusis	Talking down, benzodiazepines, antipsychotics, support respiratory function	None	None
Barbiturates and Benzodiazepines	Inappropriate sexual or aggressive behavior, impaired memory or concentration	Flumazenil	Autonomic hyperactivity, tremors, insomnia, seizures, anxiety	Substitute short- with long-acting barbiturates

HUMAN SEXUALITY

HOMOSEXUALITY

Homosexuality is *not* a mental illness but instead is classified as a variant of human sexuality.

GENDER IDENTITY DISORDER AND TRANSEXUALISM

This is the answer when the case describes an individual who **insists that he/she is the opposite gender** and experiences **intense discomfort about his or her sex.** It is *not* the diagnosis when the question describes an individual **who desires to be another gender because of the perceived advantages of the other sex** (e.g., a boy who says he wants to be a girl so that he will receive the same special treatment as his younger sister).

Following are pharmacological agents that cause sexual dysfunction:

- α1-Blockers → Impaired ejaculation
- SSRIs → Inhibited orgasm
- β-Blockers → Erectile dysfunction
- Trazadone → Priapism
- Dopamine agonists ‡ → ↑ erection and libido
- Neuroleptics → Erectile dysfunction

PARAPHILIAS

Paraphilias involves **recurrent, sexually arousing preoccupations,** which are usually focused on humiliation and/or suffering and the use of nonliving objects and nonconsenting partners. Occurs for **more than 6 months** and causes **impairment in patient's level of functioning.** Treatment of choice: **Individual psychotherapy and aversive conditioning.** If severe impairment, give antiandrogens or SSRIs to help reduce patient's sexual drive.

Types of Paraphilias

- **Voyeurism:** Recurrent urges to observe an unsuspecting person who is engaging in sexual activity or disrobing. This is the earliest paraphilia to develop.

- **Pedophilia:** Recurrent urges or arousal toward prepubescent children. Most common paraphilia.

- **Exhibitionism:** Recurrent urge to expose oneself to strangers

- **Fetishism:** Involves the use of nonliving objects usually associated with the human body.

- **Frotteurism:** Recurrent urge or behavior involving touching or rubbing against a nonconsenting partner

- **Masochism:** Recurrent urge or behavior involving the act of humiliation

- **Sadism:** Recurrent urge or behavior involving acts in which physical or psychological suffering of a victim is exciting to the patient.

SECTION 10
EMERGENCY MEDICINE/ TOXICOLOGY

GENERAL MANAGEMENT OF OVERDOSE PATIENT

A 46-year-old woman is brought to the emergency department by her husband after a suicide attempt. She is confused, lethargic, and disoriented. Her respiratory rate is 8 per minute, and her blood pressure is 120/80 mm hg. What is the most important step?

a. Oxygen
b. Bolus of normal saline
c. Naloxone, thiamine, dextrose
d. Endotracheal intubation
e. Gastric emptying
f. Urine toxicology screen

*Answer: The correct answer is **C**. The most important step for an acute change in mental status of unclear etiology is to administer antidotes such as naloxone, dextrose, and thiamine. Oxygen does not make a specific difference. Gastric emptying is not as useful as a specific antidote and should only be used if it is very clear that the overdose occurred during the last hour. When you have an acute change in mental status, **hypoglycemia** is a very common cause, as is an **opiate overdose**. On a CCS case, give naloxone, thiamine, and dextrose and give oxygen and saline while checking the toxicology screen—all at the same time.*

WHEN DO I ANSWER "GASTRIC EMPTYING"?

This response is almost *always* wrong. Gastric emptying is *only* useful in the first hour after an overdose.

- 1 hour: 50 percent of pills can be removed
- 1–2 hours: 15 percent of pills can be removed
- 2 hours: It is useless

You can *never* perform gastric emptying when caustics (acids and alkalis) have been ingested.

Ipecac can *never* be used in a patient with altered mental status, The patient will aspirate (and you will fail). Ipecac is *always* wrong in children.

Intubation and lavage can *rarely* be performed *if* the patient has ingested the substance within the last 1–2 hours and there is *no* response to naloxone, dextrose, and thiamine.

WHEN DO I ANSWER "NALOXONE, THIAMINE, AND DEXTROSE"?

These medications are used for an acute mental status change of unclear etiology.

WHEN DO I ANSWER "CHARCOAL"?

Charcoal will *not* harm anyone. In other words, give it. Charcoal can help in most overdose cases. If you have a toxicology case and do not know what to do—give charcoal.

In overdose cases, do multiple things simultaneously. If there is a change in mental status from an overdose, give naloxone, thiamine and dextrose at the same time as checking a toxicology screen, giving oxygen, and checking routine labs.

Following is the overdose case "menu":

- **Specific antidote** if the etiology is clear
- **Toxicology screen**
- **Charcoal**
- **CBC, chemistry, urinalysis**
- **Psychiatry consultation** if the overdose is the result of a suicide attempt
- **Oxygen** for carbon monoxide poisoning or any dyspneic patient

The following table summarizes specific antidotes for various kinds of poisoning.

Substance	Antidote
Acetaminophen	N-acetyl cysteine
Aspirin	Bicarbonate to alkalinize the urine
Benzodiazepines	Do *not* give flumazenil; it may precipitate a seizure
Carbon monoxide	100 percent oxygen, hyperbaric in some cases
Digoxin	Digoxin-binding antibodies

Substance	Antidote
Ethylene glycol	Fomepizole or ethanol
Methanol	Fomepizole or ethanol
Methemoglobinemia	Methylene blue
Neuroleptic malignant syndrome	Bromocriptine, dantrolene
Opiates	Naloxone
Organophosphates	Atropine, pralidoxime
Tricyclic antidepressants	Bicarbonate protects the heart

ACETAMINOPHEN

CLINICAL COURSE

- **First 24 hours:** Nausea and vomiting, which resolve
- 48–72 hours later: Hepatic failure

TREATMENT

It is safe to give **charcoal and N-acetyl cysteine (NAC).** Know the following about treating an acetaminophen overdose:

- Give **N-acetyl cysteine (NAC)** to *any* patient with a possible overdose of a toxic amount.
- NAC is benign.
- NAC is useful to prevent liver toxicity for up to 24 hours after the ingestion. After 24 hours, there is *no* specific therapy to prevent or reverse the liver toxicity of acetaminophen.
- Vomiting patients can get NAC through the IV route.

If the amount of ingestion is equivocal, then **get an acetaminophen level** to determine if there will be toxicity but do *not* wait for the results to give NAC if the overdose is large.

- 10 grams → toxic
- 15 grams → fatal

The amounts needed for toxicity and fatality are lower if there is **underlying liver disease** or **alcohol abuse.**

Extra NAC never hurt anyone. Untreated acetaminophen overdose will kill the patient.

A man is brought to the emergency department a few hours after ingesting a bottle of extra-strength acetaminophen tablets. What is the next best step in management?

a. Urine toxicology screen

b. N-acetyl cysteine

c. Acetaminophen level

d. Transfer to the ICU

e. Liver function tests

f. Gastric emptying

*Answer: The correct answer is **B**. The specific antidote is more important than waiting for a level with acetaminophen overdose. On a CCS case, do both. Do not transfer patients to the ICU without doing something for them first.*

Aspirin/Salicylate Overdose

Aspirin acts as a direct **stimulant to the brainstem,** causing hyperventilation. A patient with an aspirin overdose will *always* be hyperventilating. In addition, aspirin is a **toxin to the lungs,** causing **acute respiratory distress syndrome (ARDS).**

Other findings in cases of aspirin overdose are the following:

> The easiest way to identify the aspirin overdose patient is **tinnitus.**

- **Metabolic acidosis:** This is from the loss of Kreb's cycle in mitochondria. You end up with lactic acidosis from hypoxic metabolism. The anion gap is elevated.

- **Respiratory alkalosis:** This always precedes the metabolic acidosis.

- **Renal insufficiency:** Salicylates, like other NSAIDS, are directly toxic to the kidney tubule.

- **Elevated prothrombin time:** Aspirin interferes with the production of vitamin K-dependent clotting factors.

- **CNS:** Confusion can occur from aspirin overdose. Severe cases can lead to seizures and coma.

- **Fever**

DIAGNOSTIC TESTING

On CCS, you should order the following:

- **CBC**
- **Chemistry panel**
- **ABG**
- **PT/INR/PTT**
- **Salicylate (ASA) level**

TREATMENT

Treatment is as follows:

- **Alkalinize the urine** to increase excretion.
- Use **charcoal** to block absorption.
- **Dialysis** is used in severe cases.

Alkalinization of the urine is done with D5W with 3 amps of bicarbonate. Alkalinization of the urine facilitates excretion of the following:

- Salicylates (ASA)
- Tricyclic antidepressants (This will show up on the urine tox you ordered.)
- Phenobarbital
- Chlorpropramide

BENZODIAZEPINES

Benzodiazepine overdose (by itself) is *not* fatal. Let the patient sleep! Move the clock forward on CCS, and the overdose will pass.

Do *not* administer flumazenil for benzodiazepine overdoses to patients in the emergency department. You do not know who has chronic dependency, and flumazenil can induce benzodiazepine withdrawal and seizures.

> Remember to order an aspirin, acetaminophen, *and* alcohol (ETOH) levels on *all* overdose patients. There is a very high frequency of coingestion.

CARBON MONOXIDE

The **most common cause of death in fires** is carbon monoxide (CO) poisoning; 60 percent of deaths in the first 24 hours after a fire are due to carbon monoxide poisoning.

Carboxyhemoglobin (COHg) does not release oxygen to tissues. Hence, CO poisoning is the same as anemia and asphyxiation. CO poisoning presents with the following:

- **Shortness of breath**
- **Lightheadedness and headaches**
- **Disorientation**
- Severe disease causes **metabolic acidosis** from tissue hypoxia.

CO poisoning also commonly presents in a family that is "snowed in" and can't leave their house with a wood-burning stove. Everyone is **fatigued and has a headache.** Look for the phrase "He feels better when he is shoveling snow."

TREATMENT

If CO poisoning is suspected, **call an ambulance.** Give **100 percent oxygen** to all survivors from a fire until you have their CO levels.

DIGOXIN

The most common presentation of digoxin overdose is **GI disturbance** (nausea, vomiting, diarrhea, pain). This condition also presents with the following:

- Patient sees yellow "halos" around objects and has blurred vision.
- Arrhythmia: Anything is possible. You may see PR prolongation; there may also be "paroxysmal atrial tachycardia with block."
- Encephalopathy

*Hypo*kalemia may lead to digoxin toxicity, but digoxin toxicity leads to *hyper*-kalemia from poisoning of the sodium/potassium ATPase.

TREATMENT

Administer **digoxin-binding antibodies** (Digibind®) for severe disease. Severe means **central nervous system and cardiac abnormalities.**

ETHYLENE GLYCOL AND METHANOL

Overdoses with both of these substances present with the following:

- **Intoxicated patient**
- **Metabolic acidosis with increased anion gap**

Ethylene glycol presents with the following:

- **Renal insufficiency** from direct toxicity
- **Hypocalcemia** from precipitation of the oxalic acid with the calcium
- **Kidney stones**

Methanol presents with the following:

- **Visual disturbance**
- **Retinal hyperemia** from the toxicity of the formic acid

TREATMENT

Overdoses from both substances are treated with the following:

- **Ethanol** or **fomepizole**
- **Dialysis** to remove them from the body before they are metabolized into the toxic metabolite

METHEMOGLOBINEMIA

This condition involves hemoglobin locked in an oxidized state that will not allow it to pick up oxygen. The patient will present with the following:

- **Cyanosis**
- **Shortness of breath**
- **Dizziness**
- **Headache**
- **Confusion**
- **Seizures**

Look for a **history of use of nitrate, anesthetics, dapsone,** or **other oxidants,** as well as any of the drugs ending in *-caine.* (e.g., lidocaine, benzocaine, bupivicaine). Methemoglobinemia can be from as little as the anesthetic spray put into the throat of a patient who will be intubated. Nitroglycerin can also do cause methemoglobinemia.

DIAGNOSTIC TESTING
- **Normal pO2 on ABG with chocolate-brownish blood** (oxidized blood)
- **Methemoglobin level**

- Cyanotic + Normal pO2 › Should make you think of methemoglobinemia.

TREATMENT
- Administer 100 percent oxygen.
- Methylene blue restores the hemoglobin to its normal state.

NEUROLEPTIC MALIGNANT SYNDROME/ MALIGNANT HYPERTHERMIA

All heat disorders present with **rhabdomyoloysis** and possibly **confusion** or **seizures** when the disorder is severe. Also, a potentially **life-threatening rhythm disturbance** can occur from the hyperkalemia.

NEUROLEPTIC MALIGNANT SYNDROME (NMS)

Look for the ingestion of **neuroleptic medication,** such as **phenothiazines.** NMS has *no* specific diagnostic test. **CPK and potassium levels** can be elevated. **Muscle rigidity** is common.

Treat with the dopamine agonists **cabergoline** or **bromocriptine. Dantrolene** is also effective.

MALIGNANT HYPERTHERMIA

Look for a history of **anesthetic use.** There is *no* clinical distinction between NMS and malignant hyperthermia, just different risks of medications. Treat with **dantrolene.**

HEAT STROKE

This is a heat disorder from **exertion and high outside temperatures.** You can *only* get heat stroke when the outside temperature is high and you are dehydrated or exerting yourself. Although these patients can get the same **confusion, seizures, hyperkalemia, and arrhythmias** that NMS and malignant hyperthermia get, the treatment is entirely different.

Treatment

Treat heat stroke with the **physical removal of heat** from the body by spraying the patient with water and fanning the patient in an air-conditioned room or using ice baths/packs. Do *not* infuse iced saline into the body, since this can stop the heart.

The following table compares heat stroke and heat exhaustion.

	Heat Exhaustion	Heat Stroke
Presenting Symptoms	Excessive sweating Nausea/vomiting	Dry skin Altered mental status
Body Temperature	Elevated	Elevated
Treatment	Normal saline IV (room temp) and removal of patient from hot to cool environment	Spraying patient with water and applying ice baths/packs

The following table compares heat stroke, neuroleptic malignant syndrome, and malignant hyperthermia.

	NMS	Malignant Hyperthermia	Heat Stroke
Risk	Antipsychotic medications	Anesthetics	Exertion on hot days
Presentation	High temperature Confusion Arrhythmia Hyperkalemia	Same	Same
Lab testing	CPK and potassium elevated	Same	Same
Treatment	Bromocriptine Dantrolene	Dantrolene	Hydration and external cooling (ice baths/packs, spraying with water and evaporation)

OPIATE INTOXICATION

Opiate toxicity leads to **death from respiratory depression.** One *cannot* die from opiate withdrawal.

Treat **acute overdoses** with **naloxone.**

ORGANOPHOSPHATES

Organophosphates **inhibit acetylcholinesterase,** blocking the metabolism of acetylcholine and, therefore, enormously increasing the effect of acetylcholine.

Look for either of these in the presentation:

- **Crop duster** exposed to insecticides
- **Nerve-gas attack**

Organophosphate overdose presents with the following symptoms:

- **Salivation**
- **Lacrimation**
- **Urination**
- **Diarrhea**
- **Wheezing from bronchospasm**

TREATMENT

- Best initial therapy: **Atropine**
- Most effective therapy: **Pralidoxime**
- **Remove the clothes and wash the rest off the patient.**

Make *sure* you do not contaminate yourself. When caring for victims of a nerve-gas attack, you must make certain to be protected. The toxin is absorbed through the skin.

TRICYCLIC ANTIDEPRESSANTS

Death over overdose on tricyclic antidepressants occurs from the following.

- **Seizures**
- **Arrhythmia**

A patient with a history of depression comes in with an overdose resulting from a suicide attempt. There was a bottle of amytriptyline nearby. What is the most urgent step?

a. Charcoal

b. Gastric lavage

c. Transfer to ICU

d. EKG

e. EEG

f. Head CT

g. Administer bicarbonate

*Answer: The correct answer is **D**. In tricyclic overdose, the most urgent step is to perform an EKG to see if there is **widening of the QRS**. Those with a wide QRS are most likely to develop **ventricular tachycardia** or **torsades de pointes**. If there is a wide QRS or an arrhythmia, **give bicarbonate and transfer to the ICU**. Gastric lavage is not as important as protecting the heart. Bicarbonate and alkalinizing the patient carries its own risks. Therefore, finding out for sure if the patient really needs the bicarbonate is more important.*

Other effects of tricyclics are related to their anticholinergic effects:

- **Dilated pupils**
- **Dry mouth**
- **Constipation**
- **Urinary retention**

SPIDER BITES

BLACK WIDOW

The bite of a black widow spider presents with **abdominal pain, rigidity, and hypocalcemia.** The patient presents as though there is a perforated abdominal organ, but there is pain *without* tenderness.

Treat with **calcium and antivenin.**

BROWN RECLUSE SPIDER

The bite of this spider presents with local necrosis, bullae, and dark lesions.

Treat by **debriding the wound.** Occasionally, steroids and dapsone are of benefit.

BURNS

The most important step when a patient has been in a fire is to give **100 percent oxygen.** The most common cause of death in fires is carbon monoxide poisoning. After that, the most important thing is to **determine who needs to be intubated and who can be managed just with fluids.**

After giving oxygen, **intubate** the patient if any of the following is present:

- **Hoarseness**
- **Wheezing**
- **Stridor**
- **Burns *inside* the nose or the mouth**

If evidence of respiratory injury is *not* present, then the most important step in management is to **give fluids** as follows:

- 4 ml of lactate ringers or normal saline *for*
  - each percentage with a second- or third-degree burn *for*
  - each kilogram.

The most common cause of death late is **infection.**

HYPOTHERMIA

Look for an **alcoholic falling asleep outside in winter.** Hypothermia kills with **rhythm disturbance.**

The most urgent step is to perform an **EKG: "J-waves of Osborn,"** which look like ST segment elevation, is the most specific finding.

OPHTHALMOLOGY

GLAUCOMA

Acute angle closure glaucoma is an **ophthalmologic emergency** that presents with a **red eye and a fixed midpoint pupil.**

Treatment

The best initial therapy is **pilocarpine drops** to constrict the pupil. **Mannitol** can be used as an osmotic diuretic to help open the angle. Following are other therapies that are used:

- **Acetazolamide:** Decreases production of aqueous humor
- **Prostaglandin analogues:** Latanoprost, travoprost
- **Beta blockers topically:** Timolol
- **Alpha agonists:** Apraclonidine

RETINAL DETACHMENT

This presents with a sudden loss of vision like **"a curtain coming down."** **Consult ophthalmology** and perform a **dilated retinal examination.**

Treatment

Treat by doing the following:

1. Tilt the head back.
2. **Reattach the retina** with surgery, cryotherapy, or by injecting an expansile gas into the eye.
3. If these fail, place a band around the eye to get the retina close to the sclera.

RED EYE

Diagnosing and treating "red eye" requires knowing the basic ophthalmology expected on Step 3. The following table summarizes the various causes of red eye.

	Glaucoma	Conjuctivitis	Uveitis	Abrasion
Presentation	Midpoint fixed pupil Rock-hard, painful eye Corneal haziness	Viral: Bilateral watery discharge, itchy eyes Bacterial: Unilateral purulent discharge, eyelids stuck together	Photophobia	History of trauma, most commonly from contact lenses
Diagnosis	Tonometry	Clinical presentation	Slit lamp examination	Fluorescein stain picks up on the damaged cornea
Treatment	Pilocarpine drops Acetazolamide Mannitol Topical beta blockers	Bacterial form is treated with topical antibiotics	Steroids	*No* specific therapy Do *not* patch abrasions from contact lenses

SECTION 11
ETHICS

AUTONOMY

Autonomy is the most frequently tested subject on Step 3. The following is the most fundamental ethical concept:

- **An adult with the capacity to understand his or her medical problems can refuse any therapy or test.**

It does not matter if the treatment or test is simple, safe, and risk-free. It does not matter if the person will die without the treatment or test. The patient can refuse the treatment or test.

Respecting autonomy is *more important* than trying to do the right thing for a patient. Trying to do the right thing for a patient is called **beneficence.**

A 35-year-old mentally intact patient is refusing radiation for a stage I lymphoma. The treatment has a 95 percent chance of cure and virtually no adverse effects. What do you do?

a. Try to discuss it with him.

b. Honor his wishes.

c. Order a psychiatric consultation.

d. Arrange an ethics committee consultation.

e. Get a court order.

Answer: The correct answer is A. Even though an adult patient with capacity can refuse anything, USMLE wants you to discuss things first. Even though you may eventually honor his wishes, if an answer says "meet," "confer," or "discuss," then do that first.

CAPACITY

Capacity is determined by physicians. *Competence* is a legal term and is determined by courts and judges. An adult who is alert and not mentally handicapped is deemed to have *capacity* to understand her own medical procedures and treatments.

PSYCHIATRY CONSULTATION

"Psychiatry consultation" is the answer when **a patient's capacity to understand is not clear.** A psychiatry consultation is *not* necessary in the following situations:

- The patient is clearly competent.
- The patient is in a coma and clearly does not have the capacity to understand.

MINORS

Minors, by definition, **are not determined to have the capacity** to understand their medical problems until the age of 18.

However, Step 3 does like to test your understanding of the **emancipated minor.** Emancipation means that although the patient is under 18, he can make his own decisions. Emancipated minors are **living independently** and **self-supporting, married,** or **in the military.**

Partial emancipation is considered to be present for the following issues:

- **Sex**
- **Reproductive health**
- **Substance abuse**

If the patient is a minor and seeks treatment for contraception, sexually transmitted diseases, HIV, or prenatal care, she is partially emancipated. In other words, she can make these decisions on her own, and her privacy is to be respected like that of an adult. **An exception is abortion:** 32 states have parental notification laws for abortion.

How does USMLE get around issues that are not universal across the United States? For such questions, the answer is a safe, universally correct answer, such as "Recommend that the patient inform the parents."

LIMITATIONS ON THE ABILITY OF PARENTS TO REFUSE TREATMENT FOR A MINOR

Parents cannot refuse lifesaving therapy for minors. For example, if a blood transfusion would be lifesaving, the parents cannot refuse. Doing so would be considered child abuse. Jehovah's Witnesses may refuse therapy for themselves but not for a child.

INFORMED CONSENT

Informed consent is based on **autonomy.** Only a fully informed patient with the capacity to understand the issues can grant "informed consent." For the consent to be informed, the patient must be informed as follows:

- The patient is informed of the **benefits** of the procedure (how will it help).
- The patient is informed of the **risks** of the procedure.
- **Alternatives** to the procedure are given.
- The information is in a **language the patient can understand.**
- The informed consent **must be given for each procedure (specificity).**

EMERGENCY PROCEDURES

Consent is implied in an emergency when there is not sufficient time to determine capacity or prior wishes. If prior wishes are fully known, then this information takes precedence. Consent obtained via telephone is considered valid. If the patient's proxy is not present at the time of the procedure, consent obtained via the telephone counts.

PREGNANT WOMEN

Pregnant women can refuse therapy, even if the life of the fetus is at risk. Until the fetus comes out of the body, it is considered part of the woman's body. For example, a woman can refuse a blood transfusion while pregnant. She can also refuse antiretroviral therapy during pregnancy, even if the life of the fetus is at risk. Once the baby comes out, however, she cannot refuse treatment for the baby.

CONFIDENTIALITY

The patient has an absolute right to privacy concerning his own medical information. The following persons do *not* have a right to any of the medical information of the patient:

- Relatives, employers, friends, and spouses
- Other physicians: If a physician seeks medical information about a patient, you cannot release it without the express consent of the patient.

- Members of law enforcement: You cannot release medical information to courts or police without a court order or subpoena.

Hence, *only* a patient can obtain or ask for his medical information to be released. A current physician cannot obtain a patient's previous medical records without her direct consent.

BREAKING CONFIDENTIALITY TO PREVENT HARM TO OTHERS

An *exception* to the privacy rule is in the circumstance of **protecting other people.**

- If a patient has a **transmissible disease,** such as tuberculosis or HIV, the physician can violate the patient's confidentiality to protect innocent third parties. If you have tuberculosis, for example, your doctor can contact your close associates without your consent if they are at risk. If you have syphilis, HIV, or gonorrhea, your doctor can safely inform others that they may be at risk without your consent.
- The classic example is of a patient with a **psychiatric illness who may be planning to harm others.** They physician has the right to break your confidentiality to alert the person at risk to prevent harm.

This issue comes down entirely to whether another person may be harmed by the patient's illness or actions. If you have a dangerous disease and your doctor does *not* inform the innocent third party at risk, then that physician is liable for harm that befalls the innocent person.

END-OF-LIFE ISSUES

Autonomy as applied to end-of-life issues is the most important subject for the test and for patient autonomy.

WITHHOLDING AND WITHDRAWING OF CARE

Withholding of care and withdrawing of care are considered **indistinguishable** from the point of view of the test and of proper ethical behavior. **An adult with capacity can withhold or withdraw any form of therapy.** If the patient begins therapy, she has the right to withdraw that care. The reasons for the withdrawal or withholding of care are *not* important.

ADVANCE DIRECTIVES

An advance directive is when **an adult patient with capacity directs the care of himself prior to losing capacity.**

Health Care Proxy

The strongest advance directive is a **health care proxy.** The proxy is both a document describing the care the person desires as well as the **appointment of an agent** to be the decision maker. The agent as a decision maker does not take hold until the patient loses the capacity to make a decision. If I appoint a proxy but I am still here, alert, and communicative, you *cannot* ask the agent for consent for my procedures.

Living Will

A living will is a written document **outlining the care** desired by the patient. If a patient does not have a health care proxy, the living will can be very useful to outline the care she wants. If the patient writes out, "I never want to be intubated," this is valid. If she writes, "No heroic measures," this is not valid. To be useful, a living will must be **clear and precise.**

Do Not Resuscitate (DNR) Orders

The DNR order means the **refusal of endotracheal intubation and cardio-pulmonary resuscitation** in the event of the loss of the ability to breath or the heart stopping. A DNR order does *not* mean the elimination of testing or medical therapy.

PATIENT WITH NO CAPACITY AND NO ADVANCE DIRECTIVE (PROXY OR LIVING WILL)

This is the most complex and the most common circumstance. In this case, the care is based on the best understanding of the patient's wishes for herself. Family and friends attempt to outline what they heard the patient say she wanted. This is *not* the same as saying, "This is what is best for the patient." Decisions are based on the best possible understanding of clearly expressed wishes. If there is no clear expression of wishes, then the weakest basis on which to act is the "best interests of the patient."

Ethics Committee

The ethics committee is used for cases in which the following are true:

- **The patient is not an adult with capacity.**
- **There are no clearly stated wishes on the part of the patient.**

Also, the ethics committee is the answer if

- **the caregivers, such as the family, are split or in disagreement about the nature of the care.** If some family say, "He never wanted to be on a ventilator, ever," and some family say, "He might have wanted a ventilator sometime," then this is a case for an ethics committee.

Court Order

This option comes into play only when **all the other options have not given clarity.** If there is disagreement after all the other steps, including an ethics committee, which cannot reach a clear determination of care, then a court order is the answer. You do *not* need a court order if the proxy clearly states wishes or the family is in agreement.

FLUID AND NUTRITION ISSUES

An adult patient with capacity may refuse all forms of nutrition. There is *no* ethical basis for forcing fluids or nutrition upon a patient. If the patient is not an adult with the capacity to understand, the proxy or living will can direct the removal of fluid and nutrition, provided the patient's clearly expressed wishes while competent stated that no artificial nutrition be started. In the absence of clearly stated wishes on the issue of fluids and nutrition, they should be given.

PHYSICIAN-ASSISTED SUICIDE AND EUTHANASIA

- **Physician-assisted suicide** means providing the patient with the means to end her own life. **This is always wrong.**
- **Euthanasia** means the physician directly administers the means of ending the patient's life. **This is always wrong.**

These are *not* the same as providing pain medications that may end the patient's life. It is ethical to give pain medication, even if the only way to relieve pain may result in the inadvertent shortening of life. The primary difference is **intent:**

- In physician-assisted suicide, the primary intent is to end life.
- With a life shortened by pain medication, the primary intent is to relieve suffering.

FUTILE CARE

There is *no* obligation on the part of the physician to provide care that will not work. There is no obligation to provide treatments without possible benefit.

A patient with widely metastatic cervical cancer develops renal failure. The family insists that dialysis be started. What do you tell them?

Answer: You do not *have to provide dialysis to a person who will certainly die and not benefit from the treatment.*

BRAIN DEATH

You are *not* obliged to provide care for a brain-dead patient. Brain death = dead.

REPRODUCTIVE ISSUES

ABORTION

A woman's right to an abortion varies by trimester of pregnancy:

- **First trimester:** A woman has an **unrestricted** right to an abortion.
- **Second trimester:** A woman has access, but her rights are **less clear.**
- **Third trimester:** There is **no clear access** to abortion in the third trimester. In the third trimester, the fetus is potentially viable.

You do not need the consent of the father for the abortion.

DONATION OF GAMETES

Patients have an **unrestricted right** to donate sperm and eggs. There is *no* ethical problem with being a **paid donor** for sperm and eggs. Note that one cannot be a paid donor for organs, such as the kidney or corneas.

HIV ISSUES

A **patient has a right to confidentiality** of his HIV status. However, this confidentiality can be broken to protect the uninfected, such as sexual and needle-sharing partners.

There is **no obligation for HIV-positive health care workers to disclose their HIV status.** This includes surgeons. A surgeon does *not* have to disclose her HIV status to patient.

Physicians have the legal right to refuse to treat any patient. It is *not* illegal to refuse to take care of HIV-positive persons—it is **unethical** to refuse care to HIV-positive patients simply because they are HIV-positive, but it is **legal** to do so.

DOCTOR-PATIENT RELATIONSHIP

ACCEPTING A PATIENT

A physician does not have an obligation to accept a patient. The need of a person does not compel the physician to accept that person as a patient. For example, if there is only one neurosurgeon at a hospital and a patient needs neurosurgery, this situation does not compel the physician to accept the patient.

Once having accepted a patient, however, **the physician cannot simply abandon the patient.** The physician has an obligation to inform the patient that he must find another physician, and the physician must render care until a substitute caregiver can be identified.